T LYMPHOCYTES IN THE LIVER

T LYMPHOCYTES IN THE LIVER

Immunobiology, Pathology, and Host Defense

Edited by

I. NICHOLAS CRISPE
Yale University School of Medicine
New Haven, Connecticut

WILEY-LISS

A John Wiley & Sons, Inc., Publication

New York • Chichester • Weinheim • Brisbane • Singapore • Toronto

This book is printed on acid-free paper. ♾

Published simultaneously in Canada.

Library of Congress Cataloging-in-Publication Data:

T lymphocytes in the liver : immunobiology, pathology, and host
defense / edited by I. Nicholas Crispe.
p. cm.
Includes index.
ISBN 0-471-19218-X (alk. paper)
1. Liver—Diseases—Immunological aspects. 2. T cells.
3. Autoimmune diseases. 4. Liver—Immunology. I. Crispe, I. N.
[DNLM: 1. Liver—immunology. 2. Liver Diseases—immunology. 3. T-Lymphocytes—immunology. 4. Autoimmunity. WI 700 T1105 1999]
RC846.9.T2 1999
616.3′62079—dc21
DNLM/DLC
for Library of Congress 98-7962

Printed in the United States of America.

10 9 8 7 6 5 4 3 2 1

CONTENTS

FOREWORD

Since antiquity, the liver has been viewed as an organ of extraordinary complexity. This reputation is well deserved, not just because of the many vital functions that it sustains, but also because it is often difficult to understand its mechanisms. The role that immunologic processes play both in normal function and disease states is no exception. Early descriptions of "autoimmune" diseases included chronic autoimmune hepatitis, primary biliary cirrhosis, and sclerosing cholangitis. Even the common virus-mediated inflammations, hepatitis C and B, are now viewed as having autoimmune components, despite knowledge of their inciting agents. Yet, despite rapid growth in knowledge of basic immunobiology, there continues to be a gap in the ability to translate that information into practice for the benefit of patients with chronic liver disease.

It is with that background that this extremely intriguing and perhaps paradigm-breaking anthology, "T Cells in the Liver" is presented. Crispe and his contributing authors have assembled a compelling collection that highlight a number of new concepts concerning the liver's role in regulation of the immune system. The large and distinctive population of lymphocytes that resides within the liver is now being characterized in detail. And in some instances unique populations not found elsewhere in the body have been described. The liver is situated strategically between the external and systemic environment, where it is continually receiving foreign antigens that have passed the intestinal barrier. It filters and processes these invaders in novel ways. New concepts are developing on mechanisms of oral tolerance, and why the liver is so privileged that it is able to suppress immune rejection when it is transplanted. Even systemic tolerance can result when dendritic cells migrate and take residence in distant regions. The important role of the Kupffer cell in antigen presentation and cytokine production is being clarified, as well as the role of adhesion molecules within the liver sinusoids, so critical in attracting immunocytes and in regulating immune responses. How hepatocytes can express Fas ligand on their surface yet in many circumstances be protected from overt T-cell-mediated destruction and cell suicide is an important new concept. At the same time the liver may be the final "graveyard" of T cells. Yet under different circumstances other lymphocytes may differentiate in the relatively protected environment of the liver and then migrate to external sites to complete their life story. How these dichotomies exist is a major subject of this text.

This book may raise as many questions as it answers. But it gives promise of future insights that seem likely to change our fundamental understanding of both the liver's role in modulating our immune system and the pathogenesis and ultimate treatment of many forms of chronic liver disease. Immunologists (who now must accept the liver as an organ of primary immunologic importance) should find it a helpful reference point for focusing future research strategies. Hepatologists will discover that they may need to reorder their concepts of the role of the liver in oral tolerance, immune privilege, and "autoimmune liver disease." For all these reasons, this volume should be a landmark contribution to the field.

James L. Boyer
Director, Yale Liver Center
Ensign Professor of Medicine

PREFACE

The liver is a large, highly metabolically active organ which is essential for life. It is also subject to a number of human diseases of great epidemiological importance, many of which clearly have an immune component. The sophisticated and multifarious metabolic activities of the liver render a synthetic alternative implausible, and this has led to great interest in liver transplantation. Surprisingly, liver transplants, while technically difficult, are immunologically straightforward; exact tissue matching is not essential and rejection crises are relatively few. The reason for this is not completely understood.

In this volume we survey the immunology of the liver with particular reference to T lymphocytes. These cells are the prime movers in transplant rejection, but also in the defensive immune response against many viruses, including those of hepatitis B and C. In addition, T cells are believed to be instigators of damage in autoimmune diseases, including autoimmune liver disease. Our underlying assumption is that T cell immunity in the liver is distinctive enough to warrant a specialized discussion. Neither the populations of T cells present in the liver, nor their biological activities, seem to be exactly the same as in other organs.

This book has its origins in a search we embarked on around 1993 to find extrathymic sites of T cell development. The dominant paradigm in T cell biology was that T cells arise from uncommitted, circulating precursor cells by differentiation in the thymus. This organ alone seemed capable of inducing the expression of the T cell receptor gene recombination machinery essential for the somatic gene rearrangement that creates T cell receptors, and then of selecting the immature T cells on the basis of receptor specificity to generate a functionally competent, self-tolerant mature T cell repertoire. A few years ago this paradigm began to fray around the edges, and we and others became interested in the possibility that some T cells, particularly "non-standard" types of T cells such as gamma-delta cells and NK-T cells, might differentiate in other tissues. A variety of candidate sites have been investigated, including the bone marrow, intestinal epithelium, skin, and liver. We investigated the liver, using intrathymic adoptive transfer experiments to try to detect progenitor cells with the differentiation potential of thymocytes, an experiment that was ultimately unsuccessful. But while following this line of investigation, Dr. Lin Huang in my laboratory identified an interesting subset of T cells that seemed unique to the liver. These were CD4-

and CD8-negative T cells with a low surface density of alpha-beta T cell receptor, but a high density of the marker B220. This phenotype is unknown elsewhere in the normal mouse, but was familiar to us as the end-stage phenotype assumed by the T cells that accumulate in mice genetically deficient in the CD95 (Fas) death receptor, or its sole ligand CD95L (FasL). These cells accumulate because the mutant mice are defective in their ability to remove T cells at the end of an immune response, so that our finding of similar cells in the normal mouse liver immediately suggested that these cells might be dying, and that the liver might be their final resting place. We have conducted a series of experiments that tend to support this view.

At first, we thought of the liver simply as a collecting site for dying T cells, and imagined that it must extract them from the circulation, much as effete plasma glycoprotein molecules are extracted after sialic acids are lost from their carbohydrate side-chains. However, on exploring the literature it became clear that the liver displays many unusual immunologic properties. It is strongly tolerogenic in an allograft situation; it is essential for oral tolerance, and it is the site of several important chronic infections in which immunity seems to be disabled. Could all of these phenomena share an underlying mechanism?

This volume is an attempt to concentrate the information bearing on this question. A panel of authors with diverse expertise have contributed chapters covering the fundamental immunobiology of liver T cells, their defensive immune responses against pathogens, and their role in putatively autoimmune tissue damage. The sum of these contributions suggests that the liver is indeed a unique immunological environment with distinctive properties. The underlying theme is that the liver is strongly tolerogenic for certain immune responses, particularly those mounted by CD8+ cytotoxic and CD4+ inflammatory cells, but that this tolerance may be overcome to mount a defensive immune response resulting in the clearance of pathogens. This concept allows for a more subtle view of the chronicity of many liver pathogens, but also suggests that the liver may play an important role in systemic diseases with an immune component.

This line of thinking has attracted interest among our clinical colleagues, and it is possible that if there evolves a new paradigm for the nature of liver immune responses we may be able to offer some insights into human disease.

The book is dedicated to my friend Dr. Clare Openshaw, whose liver finally let her down, but not her warmth, intellect, and humor.

I. Nicholas Crispe
Yale University School of Medicine

CONTRIBUTORS

Toru Abo, Niigata University, School of Medicine, Niigata, Japan

Roy Calne, Addenbrooke's Hospital, Cambridge, United Kingdom

Francis V. Chisari, The Scripps Research Institute, La Jolla, CA

I. Nicholas Crispe, Yale University School of Medicine, New Haven, CT

Kenneth A. Fleming, Nuffield Department of Pathology, University of Oxford, Oxford, United Kingdom

M. Eric Gershwin, University of California, Davis School of Medicine, Davis, CA

Mimi Guebre-Xabier, Walter Reed Army Institute of Research, Washington, DC

John T. Harty, University of Iowa, Iowa City, IA

A. C. Hayday, Yale University, New Haven, CT

Lin Huang, Brigham and Women's Hospital, Boston, MA

Urszula Krzych, Walter Reed Army Institute of Research, Washington, DC

Y. Ma, King's College Medical School, London, United Kingdom

Allan McI Mowat, University of Glasgow, Glasgow, Scotland

Wajahat Z. Mehal, Yale University School of Medicine, New Haven, CT

Robert Schwenk, Walter Reed Army Institute of Research, Washington, DC

Judy Van de Water, University of California, Davis School of Medicine, Davis, CA

D. Vergani, King's College Medical School, London, United Kingdom

Hisame Watanabe, Niigata University, School of Medicine, Niigata, Japan

Anura Weerasinghe, Niigata University, School of Medicine, Niigata, Japan

L. Wen, Yale University School of Medicine, New Haven, CT

CHAPTER 1

THE ANATOMY OF THE NORMAL LIVER AND THE HEPATIC LYMPHOCYTE

KENNETH A. FLEMING
Nuffield Department of Pathology, University of Oxford, Oxford, United Kingdom

INTRODUCTION

In the 1960s, the first realization that lymphocytes were not simply passive passengers in the blood and lymph arose out of the work of Gowans and coworkers, who demonstrated that lymphocytes show specific trafficking throughout the body (1). This work concentrated on the passage of lymphocytes to and from the lymphoid system (specifically the thymus, lymph nodes, and spleen) and demonstrated a highly organized system. Extension of this work demonstrated that other organs are involved in this trafficking, including the lungs and the liver (2). Throughout the 1980s further refinements established that liver-committed lymphocytes are largely an intravascular marginal pool (3,4). In parallel with this work, the 1970s and 1980s saw the identification of different subsets of lymphocytes, and extensive work on migration and function of these subsets has been reported (5). However, there is little information available on the microanatomic trafficking and distribution of intrahepatic lymphocytes, their subset characterization and their function within and outside of the normal liver.

Despite this relative ignorance, some interesting areas have been explored, and it is becoming increasingly evident that the liver has a specific and important role in immunobiology. In particular, early work has shown that tolerance to antigens can be induced by administering the antigen orally, so that there is subsequent passage to the liver via the portal vein; in contrast, tolerance is not induced by parenterally administered antigen (6). These investigations have suggested that some specific processing occurs in the periphery, probably the liver, resulting in T-cell inactivation and deletion. Further evidence of the unique nature of the liver as a lymphoid organ comes from the results of liver transplantation. This requires relatively little systemic immunosuppres-

T Lymphocytes in the Liver: Immunobiology, Pathology, and Host Defense, Edited by I. Nicholas Crispe
ISBN 0-471-19218-X

sion, unlike skin or kidney transplantation, and induces specific tolerance to transplantation of other organs (7). This effect is dependent on intrahepatic lymphocytes and may be accompanied by systemic chimerism, suggesting a role for donor intrahepatic lymphocytes in the induction of tolerance (8). Furthermore, over the last 30 years, it has been demonstrated that several important hepatic and biliary diseases are probably autoimmune in nature (particularly autoimmune hepatitis and primary biliary cirrhosis) or are immune-mediated (hepatitis B virus infection, which infects around 300 million people worldwide). The role of the natural immunobiology of the liver in these diseases is completely obscure and undoubtedly warrants active investigation.

This book details current knowledge of the role and function of intrahepatic lymphocytes. This chapter will describe the gross and microscopic anatomy of the liver, within which the intrahepatic lymphocytes carry out their functions. It will also describe the little that is known of the distribution of lymphocytes within this microanatomy and the interactions with constituent liver cells.

GROSS ANATOMY OF THE LIVER

The liver is the largest single organ in the body. In man, it weight around 1.5 Kg and is situated in the upper right side of the peritoneal cavity under the diaphragm. It is covered by a fibrous tissue capsule and the peritoneum, apart from the "bare area," which is the region at the upper posterior part of the liver in contact with the diaphragm. The liver is the major biochemical factory in the body, carrying out a large range of synthetic and degradative functions and playing a major role in metabolism of fats, carbohydrates, and proteins. Reflecting these metabolic functions, it has two blood supplies. It also has a major role in detoxification of substances, including many drugs. The liver is responsible for the normal breakdown of hemoglobin, with resultant synthesis and secretion of bilirubin into the bile. The bile is secreted via the biliary ducts into the gut (duodenum). The blood supply and the biliary ducts enter and leave the liver at the porta hepatitis, which is where the free edge of the lesser omentum joins the liver.

On anatomical grounds, the liver can be divided into right, left, caudate, and quadrate lobes. However, a much more important division is into segments. These have functional and therapeutic significance, reflecting separate vascular and biliary supplies and drainages. Internal to the porta hepatitis, the first division of the blood supply divides the liver into a left and right lobe. Further subdivisions result in eight segments, four on the right, three on the left, plus the caudate lobe. It is possible that these segments have somewhat different functionality, as well as separate vascular supplies and drainages, and that diseases may preferentially manifest in certain lobes or segments. However, this has not been demonstrated. Surgically, segmental anatomy is very important, as resection can be performed by following the segmental boundaries.

Bile synthesized in the liver is transported to the duodenum via the common bile duct. This latter structure is formed by the merging of the cystic duct (from the gall bladder) and the common hepatic duct, which in turn has been formed by the merging of the right and left hepatic ducts. These latter are the extrahepatic ducts that are formed by the coalescence of intrahepatic ducts, which collect bile from the right and left lobes of the liver.

MICROANATOMY OF THE LIVER

There are two major components of the liver—the liver lobule or acinus and the portal tracts (Figs. 1.1., 1.2., and 1.3). The liver lobule contains several cellular components, but the most important and numerous is the hepatocyte. It is estimated that there are 2×10^9 to 9×10^9 hepatocytes in the human liver (9). The great majority of the metabolic functions of the liver are carried out by the hepatocyte. The portal tract partly functions as the supporting structure for the liver, but primarily contains the biliary system and blood supply, as the hepatic artery and portal vein (Fig. 1.3). The portal tract also contains the lymphatics.

Blood Supply

The liver has two systems of blood supply and receives about 25% of its blood as arterial blood via the hepatic artery, a branch of the celiac axis. This enters the liver at the porta hepatitis in the free margin of the lesser omentum. Adjacent to the hepatic artery is the portal vein that carries venous blood from the gut into the liver (75% of the blood flow), and the common bile duct, which carries bile synthesized

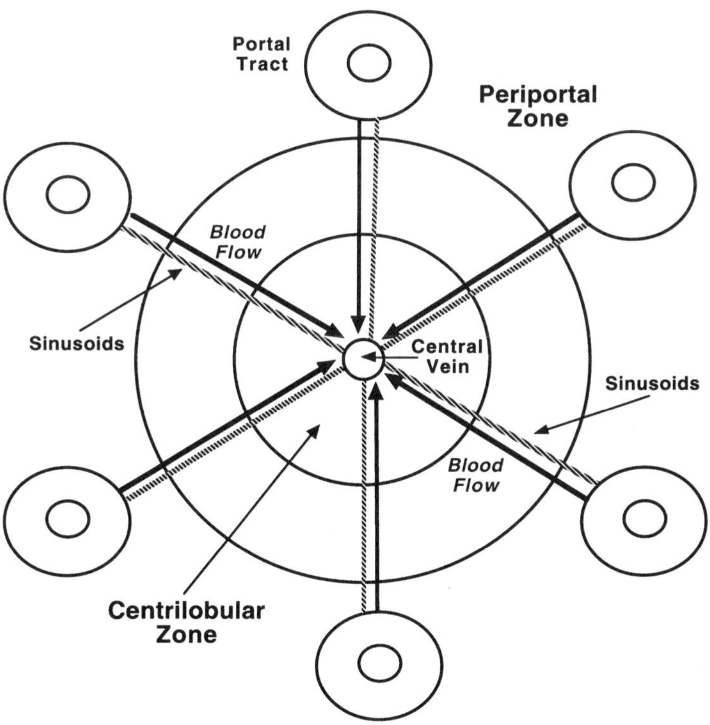

Figure 1.1. Diagram of the hexagonal liver lobule. The portal tracts are around the periphery and the blood drains from them to the central vein, via the sinusoids. The periportal, mid- and central zones are indicated.

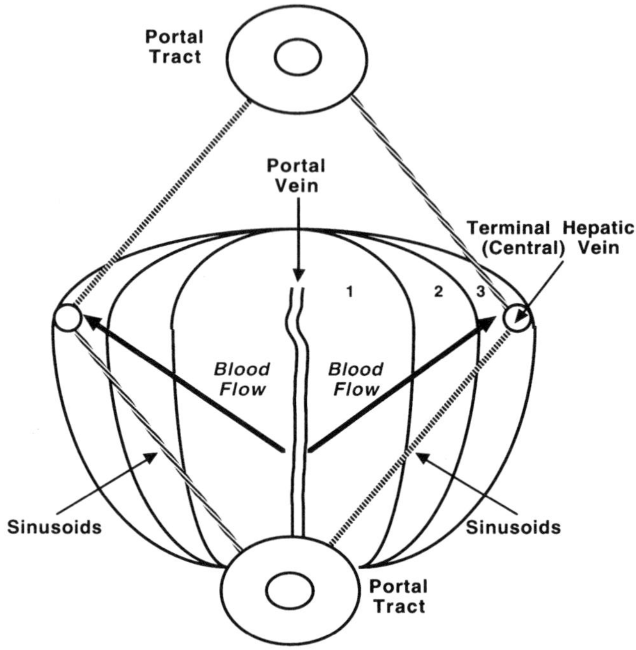

Figure 1.2. The acinus model of the liver. The blood flows from the portal vein in the portal tract and its final branch in the acinus via the sinusoids, into adjacent terminal hepatic veins. Zones 1, 2 and 3 are indicted.

by the liver into the duodenum. On entering the liver, these structures form the portal tracts, which divide repeatedly into smaller and smaller branches. Infarction of the liver is relatively uncommon because of its dual blood supply. The hepatic artery ends as a capillary plexus around the smallest branches of the portal vein and a plexus around the bile ducts, both of which then drain into the portal veins and sinusoids (Figs. 1.1, 1.2, and 1.3). Some hepatic arterioles drain directly into the sinusoids.

The portal vein also enters the liver at the porta hepatis and repeatedly divides as part of the portal tracts. The portal veins drain into the liver sinusoids, which then drain into the central or terminal hepatic vein (Figs. 1.2 and 1.3). The terminal hepatic veins repeatedly merge, eventually forming the segmental hepatic veins and common hepatic veins, which drain from the upper posterior region of the liver into the inferior vena cara.

The Lobule or Acinus

There are two models proposed for the vascular microanatomy of the liver—the hexagonal lobular and the acinar models. The lobular model was first described in 1833 (10) while the acinar model was proposed in 1954 (11). The lobular model is

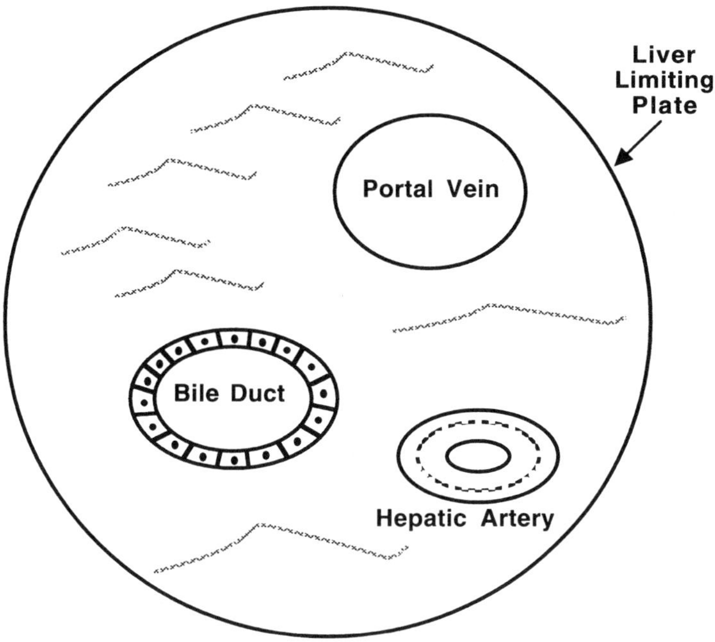

Figure 1.3. The portal tract consists of fibrous tissue containing the bile duct, hepatic artery and portal vein. The interlobular bile duct (diameter less than 100μM) is central and has an associated branch of the hepatic artery.

more easily understood (Fig. 1.1). This model is based on a single hepatic central vein that is draining blood from six adjacent portal tracts. This blood is a mixture of arterial blood (hepatic artery) and venous blood from the gut (portal vein) and it drains via sinusoids into the central vein. The lobular hepatocytes are split into three imprecise but roughly equal regions based on their position relative to the draining central vein; the periportal, the centrilobular and midlobular hepatocytes. In contrast, the acinar model is centered on the portal vein exiting from a single portal tract (Fig. 1.2). The blood from this portal vein drains into several adjacent terminal hepatic veins. The surrounding hepatocytes are called acinar zone 1 hepatocytes. The hepatocytes of acinar zone 3 surround the draining terminal hepatic vein and zone 2 hepatocytes are in the intervening zone.

In practice, there is considerable overlap in usage of the different terminologies, with periportal signifying zone 1, centrilobular signifying zone 3 and midlobular signifying zone 2. The major distinction is in understanding actual blood flow and thus in explaining and understanding the pattern of cell injury and death that occurs in a variety of diseases. The acinar model correlates better with the observed reality.

It is of interest that the hepatocytes in different parts of the lobule/acinus are functionally diverse and are able to change depending on circumstances (12).

Sinusoid

The structure of the sinusoid (10 μm in diameter) is unusual (Fig. 1.4). Much of the surface is bare, with direct continuity between the sinusoidal lumen and the underlying hepatocyte. Five cells are found lining the sinusoid: the endothelial cell, the Kupffer cell, the hepatocyte, the stellate cell, and the Pit cell.

Endothelial Cell Endothelial cells, which are the majority of the lining cells of the sinusoid, do not have a basement membrane. Furthermore, the cells are discontinuous, and even the covered areas have fenestrae (windows) (Fig. 1.4). There are two types of fenestrae: clusters of small fenestrae 0.1–2 μm in diameter forming "sieve plates," and large solitary fenestrae 2 μm in diameter. The normal endothelial cells expresses ICAM-1 (intracellular adhesion molecule 1) and 2 and LFA-3 (leukocyte function-associated antigen 3) and can be induced to express VCAM-1 (vascular cell adhesion molecule 1) in inflammation (13). These molecules are presumably involved in leukocyte trafficking in the normal and inflamed liver.

Kupffer Cell The second most frequent lining cell is the Kupffer cell (a macrophage and part of the mononuclear phagocytic system). It forms about 15% of the cells in the liver, but about 80% of the tissue macrophages of the body (14). Kupffer cells are distributed in an apparently random fashion along sinusoids, resting on endothelial cytoplasm or between endothlial cells. It is tempting to speculate that the distribution is not random, as the density is greater in the periportal region. Like all macrophages they are capable of movement as part of their scavenging role in their particular territory. There is clear evidence that Kupffer cells can both hypertrophy and mitose, but they also increase in number by recruitment of monocytic cells from the peripheral blood (15). Kupffer cells, like all macrophages, express human leukocyte antigens (HLA)

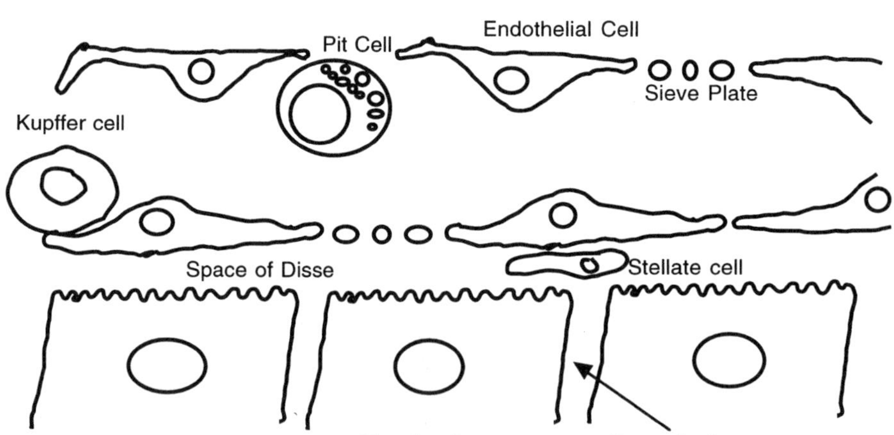

Figure 1.4. The micro-anatomy of the liver sinusoid. The lining endothelial cells are discontinuous. The lumen contains the Kuppfer cells (macrophages) and the Pit cells (NK-Tcells). The stellate cells are the principle site of connective tissue synthesis in liver damage.

class I and II, Fc receptors, CD80, VCAM-1, ICAM-1, LFA-3, etc. (13). Accordingly, they presumably have a key role in the immunobiology of the liver.

Stellate Cell (Space of Disse) The space of Disse is the region between the endothelium of the sinusoid and the underlying hepatocyte (Fig. 1.4). It contains the stellate cells (cells of Ito, fat-containing cells, lipocytes, perisinusoidal cells). These are recognized on ultrastructural examination by their stellate shape, their content of fat vacuoles, of vitamin A (retinoic acid, which is visible as fluorescence on light microscopy), and of smooth muscle alpha actin and desmin on immunohistochemistry. They appear to be capable of transformation or activation by injurious stimuli into myofibroblasts, capable of contractile movement and synthesis of collagen. They are thought to be the principle source of collagen in the liver (16), migrating to where they are required. They lay down collagen in the space of Disse causing "capillarization" of the sinusoids, which presumably decreases exchange between the blood and hepatocytes.

The blood flow through the sinusoids is not continuous. There is good evidence of variable closure and opening of sinusoids, which is probably regulated by the lining cells, including contraction of stellate cells, hypertrophy of Kupffer cells, and endothelial cell edema and injury (17). It is possible that these periods of stasis allow particular molecular and cell interaction between the sinusoidal blood and the lining cells, facilitating, for example, immunological surveillance.

Hepatocyte The hepatocyte is the powerhouse of the liver. It is a large polyhedral cell and measures about 30 μm in diameter. It has a microvillous surface on the sinusoidal border (Fig. 1.4). The canalicular surface abuts onto the adjacent hepatocyte and contains an intracellular space into which bile is secreted (the canaliculus). The hepatocyte nucleus is central. With ageing, it increasingly becomes binucleate and tetraploid; 25% of cells are binucleate at adulthood and 15% are tetraploid at 15 years of age in man (18). There is no basement membrane. Unlike most other nucleated cells, normal hepatocytes have very low amounts of HLA class I molecules on their surface (19). These molecules are upregulated in some diseases (20), but it is an intriguing possibility that some of the immunological peculiarities of liver may reflect this minimal expression of HLA, e.g., diminished ability to present foreign antigen. HLA class II is not expressed in normal hepatocytes, but can be expressed in diseased liver (21). Similarly, cell adhesion molecules ICAM-1, LFA-3 (13) and Fas (22) are upregulated in disease states allowing hepatocyte interactions with appropriate T cells. It is postulated that the mechanism involving Fas/Fas ligand (on T cells) may be responsible for liver cell death in certain situations, including transplant rejection. Indeed, in alcoholic liver, hepatocytes also express Fas-ligand mRNA, raising the possibility of autocrine/paracrine induction of apoptosis (22).

Biliary System

The biliary system starts as the hepatocytes synthesize and secrete bile into the bile cannaliculus, which is located between adjacent hepatocytes (Fig. 1.4). The bile travels along the cannaliculi (possibly propelled by contractile motions of cannalicular walls) towards the portal tracts. The cannaliculi join to form bile ductules at the edge of the portal tract. These canals of Hering, first described in Hering's textbook in 1872 (23), then merge to form the interlobular bile duct (<100 μm in diameter). Subsequent merging of the canals forms septal ducts (>100 μm in diameter) which merge to form the segmental ducts, right and left hepatic ducts, and the common hepatic duct. There are an estimated 10 divisions between the smallest interlobular duct and the porta hepatis (24). The common hepatic duct joins with the cystic duct coming from the gall bladder (situated under the right anterior margin of the liver and acting as a reservoir for bile) to form the common bile duct, which delivers bile into the duodenum. The biliary epithelial cells normally express HLA class 1 molecules but not class II molecules (19,21). The latter are induced in a variety of biliary diseases, suggesting a role for endogenous antigen presentation (21). Other cell surface molecules involved in inflammatory reactions (ICAM-1, LFA-3) are also induced in inflamed biliary epithelium (13).

Lymphatic System

The lymphatics of the liver arise as the space of Disse (Fig. 1.4). This space enters the portal tracts as openings in the connective tissue at the liver limiting plate (Fig. 1.3). These spaces form lymphatics by acquiring a lining of endothelial cells and becoming valved. They coalesce to form a lymphatic plexus around the hepatic artery and subsequently around biliary ducts and portal vein branches. By subsequent merging, lymphatic channels exit the liver via the porta hepatis to drain into lymph nodes around the hepatic artery. There is also a small plexus of lymphatics around the central hepatic veins, which exit around the hepatic veins. Lastly, an intracapsular plexus connects with the intrahepatic lymphatics. The lympatic flow in the liver is the largest in the body constituting about 15% to 20% of the total. It contains an unusually high protein content (about 90% of plasma) and has a large number of cells, of which most (80%) are lymphocytes. With a flow of 2×10^8 cells per 24 hours, the liver has more lymphocytes migrating through it than any other nonlymphoid organ (25).

Hemopoiesis in the Liver

The liver first begins to develop around the third week after conception and the parenchymal component arises as an endodermal outgrowth of the future duodenum, the hepatic diverticulum. The connective tissue component is of mesenchymal origin. This latter has two components: the septum transversum (ST) and mesenchymal celomic cells which invade the septum transversum. The ST is a transverse sheet of cells separating the pericardial and peritoneal cavities.

By the fourth week after conception, the hepatic diverticulum has extensively proliferated and extended into the ST and the vascular sinusoidal structure is beginning to appear. Blood-forming cells start to appear extravascularly around 6 weeks and by 12 weeks the liver is the main source of hemopoiesis. The hemopoietic stem cells in the mouse develop in the yolk sac and migrate into the developing liver. After birth, the hemopoietic function of the liver decreases and by 6 months of age has ceased. However, extramedullary hemopoiesis can be initiated in the liver at any time when bone marrow hemopoiesis is reduced, although the signals for this are unknown. The importance of this aspect of hepatic function is neither well understood nor investigated.

THE HEPATIC LYMPHOCYTE

A variety of techniques have been used to examine the lymphocytes found in the liver. These range from enzymatic disruption of the liver followed by density gradient separation of mononuclear cells, recovery of nonadherent cells and subsequent analyses of fluorescence-activated cell sorter (FACS), to washing out the liver to release sinusoidal cells, which are then subsequently analyzed for cell number and type (26,27). Both approaches can be criticized, since they might result in selection bias, but the number by lymphocytes isolated by different techniques has been reasonably concordant. Thus, Hata et al. (27) examined "normal" human liver and showed a mean of $1 \times 10^6 \pm 0.6 \times 10^6$ lymphocytes per gram of wet weight. If the normal liver weighs around 1.5 kg, then this suggests the liver contains about 1.5×10^9 lymphocytes in total. Other estimates have suggested that the liver contains up to 9×10^9 lymphocytes (9).

Lymphocyte Subsets in Liver

B Cells A number of publications have analyzed the different subsets of lymphocytes in the liver (26–31). These studies have shown that B cells are few, and comprise less than 5% of all lymphocytes. The number increases with age and varies depending on whether the animal has been exposed to foreign antigens. Thus animals brought up in a pathogen-free environment have essentially no B cells in the liver, while B cells comprise up to 5% of the total lymphocytes for those reared in normal conditions. Most of these B cells have IgA surface immunoglobulin and it is postulated that these are responding to the antigen load from the gut (32). This process presumably explains the increase of B cells in the liver from birth. The little work that has been published on the distribution of B cells in normal liver shows a preponderance in the lobule compared to the portal tract (29,30). However, further anatomical localization, especially the identification of any B cell interaction with other hepatic cells, is not available.

T Cells The normal liver contains two types of T cell (33,34). The conventional T cell, which is either CD4 or CD8 positive or double negative, has high-intensity T cell antigen receptor (TCR) on FACS analysis and corresponds to the equivalent T cell in the peripheral blood. It accounts for about 25% of the hepatic lymphocytes and has predominantly α/β TCR. The ratio of CD4/CD8 lymphocytes of the hepatic T cells is different from that in peripheral blood, in that whereas the CD4/CD8 ratio in peripheral blood is approximately 2:1, in the liver it is about 0.5:1. Investigation of the distribution of these lymphocytes in the normal liver shows that CD4 and CD8 cells are found in both portal tracts and the liver lobule, but both types are predominantly located in the portal tract (29,30). As with the B cell, further refinement of the relationship of these T cells to other hepatic cells is not described.

The hepatic lymphocytes also consist of an unusual T cell type (or subtype) that has many features in common with natural killer (NK) cells. This cell has been identified by a variety of workers and given several names including NK-T cell, lymphokine-activated killer cell (LAK), and large granular lymphocyte (LGL) (26,35,36). The essential feature is that the cells have an intermediate intensity TCR on FACS analysis and have interleukin-2 receptor β (IL-2Rβ) present. There are at least two subtypes, namely a $NK1.1^+$ and $NK1.1^-$ cell (33). The current state of knowledge on the function of these cells is described later in this book (Chapters 2 and 4). The NK-T cells constitute about 40% of the lymphocytes in the liver, whereas in the peripheral blood this cell constitutes about 5% of the lymphocytes.

Pit Cells The NK-T cells, or at least a subset of them, appear to be identical to the pit cells first described in 1976 in mouse (37). An analogous cell was identified in humans in 1984 (38). It is a T cell with NK properties as described above. Part of the initial recognition of this cell was based on its ultrastructural features. It has abundant cytoplasm which contains membrane-bound granules of electron-dense material, fancifully resembling the "pits" of a salt cellar. Similar cells are found as a large proportion of T cells in the bone marrow, but they are rare elsewhere, particularly being less than 1% of thymic T cells. Unlike the B cell and the conventional T cell (see previous section), some detail is known about the interaction of this cell with other hepatic cells. Thus, in the normal liver, these cells adhere to Kupffer and endothelial cells and, under IL-2 treatment and in autoimmune hepatitis, are additionally found in the space of Disse, in contact with hepatocytes (38,39).

CONCLUSION

The above brief survey of the anatomy of the liver identifies three unusual properties. First, the liver has two blood supplies, the majority coming from the gut. Both supplies drain into the sinusoids and from the sinusoids into the hepatic veins, thus exiting the liver. Second, the capillary (or sinusoidal) microvascular lining is attenuated and absent in places, a feature that allows particularly close apposition of the blood cells and the underlying tissues. Third, the liver contains probably the largest number of trafficking lymphocytes in the body, with large amounts of an unusual cell, the NK-T cell. While these three properties are most obviously related to the metabolic role of the liver, additionally they may reflect the unusual immunobiology of the liver.

In this regard, the role of the liver in removal of activated CD8 T cells from the circulation, is of interest. It has been shown that such cells appear to accumulate in the liver, undergo apoptosis, and then disappear. It is possible that this is the result of the liver recognizing that a T cell as already primed for apoptosis, and that by simply arresting it, the liver becomes the site of apoptosis. This arrest would result from either endothelial cells, hepatocytes, stellate or Kupffer cells (or a combination of these) recognizing changes in the surface membrane of the apoptotic lymphocyte. This has been called the "elephant's graveyard" hypothesis (40).

Alternatively, the liver may have a more active role, in which it specifically recognizes activated, Fas-expressing, but non-apoptotic T cells and, in response, traps them and administers an apoptotic hit (the "responder trap" hypothesis) (40). It has been suggested that this hit might be mediated by other lymphocytes (expressing Fas ligand) in the liver or by galectin-1 expressed on sinusoidal endothelial cells, or by the expression of Fas-ligand on hepatocytes.

This responder trap hypothesis could explain some of the unique immunological properties of the liver, particularly in relation to induction of tolerance. Thus an activated CD8 cell, which is capable of recognizing and responding to a specific antigen, is deleted from the circulation before interaction with its target, effectively confirming tolerance. It is noteworthy that this role is probably at least partly dependent on the unique microanatomy and cellular composition of the liver.

REFERENCES

1. Gowans, J.L. 1966. Life span, recirculation and transformation of lymphocytes. *Int. Rev. Exp. Pathol.* 5:1–24.
2. Smith, M.E., and Ford, W.L. 1983. The recirculating lymphocyte pool of the rat: a systematic description of the migratory behaviour of recirculating lymphocytes. *Immunology* 49:83.
3. Binns, R.M., and Licence, S.T. 1985. Patterns of migration of labelled blood lymphocyte sub-populations: evidence for two types of Peyer's patch in the young pig. *Adv. Exp. Med. Biol.* 186:661.
4. Pabst, R., and Binns, R.M. 1989. Heterogeneity of lymphocyte homing physiology: several mechanisms operate in the control of migration to lymphoid and non-lymphoid organs in vivo. *Immunol. Rev.* 108:83–109.
5. Stevens, S.K., Weissman, I.L., and Butcher, E.C. 1982. Differences in the migration of B and T lymphocytes: organ-selective localisation in vivo and the role of the lymphocyte-endothelial cell recognition. *J. Immunol.* 128:844–851.
6. Kagnoff, M.F. 1988. Oral tolerance. *Monogr. Allergy* 24:222–226.
7. Calne, R.Y., Sells, R.A., Pena, J.R., et al. 1969. Induction of immunological tolerance by porcine liver allografts. *Nature* 223:472–476.
8. Jonsson, J.R. et al. 1997. Peripheral blood chimaerism following human liver transplantation. *Hepatology* 25:1233–1236.
9. Schlitt, H.J., Kanehiro, H., Raddatz, G., et al. 1993. Persistence of donor lymphocytes in liver allograft recipients. *Transplantation* 56:1001–1007.
10. Kiernan, F. 1933. The anatomy and physiology of the liver. *Phil. Trans. R. Soc. Lond. B. Biol. Sci.* 123:711–770.
11. Rappaport, A.M., Borowy, Z.J., Lougheed, W.M., and Lotto, W.N. 1954. Sub-division of hexagonal liver lobules into a structural and functional unit: role in hepatic physiology and pathology. *Anat. Rec.* 119:11–70.
12. Jungermann, K., and Katz, N. 1989. Functional specialisation of different hepatocyte populations. *Physiol. Rev.* 69:708–764.

13. Steinhoff, G., Behrend, M., Schrader, B., Duijvestijn, A., and Wonigeit, K. 1993. Expression patterns of leukocyte adhesion ligand molecules on human liver endothlia. *Am. J. Pathol.* 142:481–488.
14. Cope, E.M., and Dilby, S.A. 1990. Kuppfer cell numbers during human development. *Clin. Exp. Immunol.* 81:485.
15. Crofton, R.W., Diesselhopf den Dulk, M.M.C., and van Furth, R. 1978. The organ kinetics and characteristics of the Kuppfer cell in the normal steady state. *J. Exp. Med.* 148:1–17.
16. Gressner, A.M., and Bachem, M.G. 1995. Molecular mechanisms of liver fibrogenesis: a homage to the role of activated fat-storing cells. *Digestion* 56:335–346.
17. Koeffel, T.A., Trauner, M., Bss, J.C., et al. 1997. Extrahepatic biliary obstruction impairs microvascular perfusion and increases leukocyte adhesion in rat liver. *Hepatology* 26:1085–1091.
18. Alder, C.P., Ringlage, W.P., and Bohm, N. 1981. DNA content and cell number in heart and liver of children. *Pathol. Res. Pract.* 172:25–41.
19. Fleming, K.A., McMichael, A., Morton, J.A., Woods, J., and McGee, J.O. 1981. Distribution of HLA class 1 antigen in normal human tissue and in mammary cancer. *J. Clin. Pathol.* 34:779–784.
20. Barbatis, C., Woods, J., Morton, J.A., Fleming, K.A., McMichael, A., and McGee, J.O. 1981. Immunological analysis of HLA (ABC) antigens in liver disease using a monoclonal antibody. *Gut* 22:985–991.
21. Chapman, R.W., Kelly, P.M., Heryet, A., Jewell, D.P., and Fleming, K.A. 1988. Expression of HLA-DR antigens on bile duct epithelium in primary sclerosing cholangitis. *Gut* 29:422–427.
22. Galle, P.R., et al. 1995. Involvement of the CD95 (APO-1/Fas) receptor and ligand in liver damage. *J. Exp. Med.* 182:1223–1230.
23. Hering, E. 1872. *Manual of Human and Comparative Histology*, Vol 2. Berlin: Striter.
24. Ludwig, J. 1996. Qualitative Anatomy of the Biliary Tract: The Future is Now. Post-Graduate Course. American Association for the Study of Liver, Thorofare, NJ 08086-9447. Chicago.
25. Smith, J.B., McIntosh, G.H., and Morris, B. 1970. The traffic of cells through the tissues: a study of peripheral lymph in sheep. *J. Anatomy* 107:87–100.
26. Bouwens, L., Remels, L., Backeland, M., van Bossuyt, H., and Wisse, E. 1987. Large granular lymphocytes or "Pit Cells" from rat liver: isolation, ultra-structural characterisation and natural killer activity. *Eur. J. Immunol.* 17:37–42.
27. Hata, K., Zhang, X.R., Iwatsuki, S., Van, T.D., Herberman, R.B., and Whiteside, T.L. 1990. Isolation, phenotyping, and functional analysis of lymphocytes from human liver. *Clin. Immunol. Immunopathol.* 56:401–419.
28. Bouwens, L., and Wisse, E. 1987. Immuno-electron microscopic characterisation of large granular lymphocytes (natural killer cells) from rat liver. *Eur. J. Immunol.* 17:1423–1428.
29. Si, L., Whiteside, T.L., Schade, R.R., and van Thiel, D.H. 1983. Studies of lymphocyte sub-populations in the liver tissue and blood of patients with chronic active hepatitis. *J. Clin. Immunol.* 3:408–419.
30. Meeusan, E., Gorrell, M.D., and Brandon, M.R. 1988. Presence of a distinct CD8+ and CD5-leukocyte sub-population in the sheep liver. *Immunology* 64:615.
31. Whiteside, T.L., Lasky, S., Si, L., and van Thiel, D.H. 1985. Immunologic analysis of mononuclear cells in liver tissues and blood of patients with primary sclerosing cholangitis. *Hepatology* 5:468–474.

32. Hall, J.G. 1984. Factors affecting the release and localization of lymph-bourne immunoblasts from the GALT. In *Immunology of the Sheep*, Morris, B, Masayuki, M., eds. Basel: Editions Roches, pp 278–305.
33. Tsukahara, A., Shuhji, S., Tsuneo, I., et al. 1997. Mouse liver T-cells: their change with ageing and in comparison with peripheral T-cells. *Hepatology* 26:301–309.
34. Abo, T., et al. 1995. Extrathymic T-cells start at an intermediate phylogenetic position between natural killer cells and thymus-derived T-cells. *Nat. Immunol.* 14:173–187.
35. Vujanovic, N.L., Herberman, R.B., and Hiserodt, J.C. 1988. Lymphokine-activated killer cells in rats: analysis of tissue and strain distribution, ontogeny and target specificity. *Cancer Res.* 48:878–883.
36. Rolslad, B., Herberman, R.B., and Reynolds, C.W. 1986. Natural killer cell activity in the rat, V. The circulation patterns and tissue localisation of peripheral blood large granular lymphocytes (LGL). *J. Immunol.* 136:2800–2808.
37. Wisse, E., Van't Noordende, J., van der Meulen, J., and Daems, W.T. 1976. The pit cell: description of a new type of cell occurring in rat sinuoids and peripheral blood. *Cell Tissue Res.* 173:423–435.
38. Kaneda, K., Kurioka, N., Seki, S., Wake, K., and Yamanoto, S. 1984. Pit cell-hepatocyte contact in auto-immune hepatitis. *Hepatology* 4:955–958.
39. Bouwens, L., Marinelli, A., Kuppen, P.J.K., Eggermont, A.M.M., van de Velde, C.J.H., and Wisse, E. 1990. Electron microscopic observations on the accumulation of large granular lymphocytes (Pit Cells) and Kupffer cells in the liver of rats treated with continuous infusion of interleukin-2. *Hepatology* 12:1365–1370.
40. Crispe, I.N., and Mehal, W.Z. 1996. Strange brew: T-cells in the liver. *Immunol. Today* 17:522–525.

CHAPTER 2

T CELLS EXPRESSING αβ ANTIGEN RECEPTORS IN THE LIVER

LIN HUANG
Brigham and Women's Hospital, Boston, MA

INTRODUCTION

The liver is the largest solid organ in the body, receiving large amounts of circulating blood through its dual blood supply, the hepatic artery and the portal vein. The latter drains blood from the gastrointestinal tract and the spleen, two of the largest immune organs in the body. Circulating lymphocytes carried in the blood percolate through the hepatic sinusoids, a unique form of capillary with widely fenestrated endothelium, and numerous macrophages (Kupffer cells) anchored inside the luminal wall. There is no genuine basement membrane separating the capillary from the liver parenchyma. This unique circulation pattern and capillary ultrastructure provide ample opportunities for the circulating lymphocytes to directly interact with hepatocytes, Kupffer cells, and sinusoidal endothelial cells.

Most of the large numbers of lymphocytes present in the hepatic sinusoids are T cells expressing the αβ T cell antigen receptor (TCRαβ). While a small fraction of these αβ liver T cells phenotypically resembles the conventional mature αβ T cells found elsewhere in the periphery, the majority expresses a reduced level of TCRαβ with little or no expression of the CD4 or CD8 coreceptor molecules. The latter also distinguish themselves from conventional αβ T cells by a surface phenotype indicative of prior activation. The origin of these unusual liver T cells and their relationship to conventional αβ T cells have been the subject of intensive research and debate. This chapter reviews data to suggest that the majority of αβ T cells in the liver are derived from previously activated T cells through receptor and coreceptor downregulation, and that they are undergoing apoptosis in the liver. It is proposed that, in addition to many vital metabolic functions, the liver plays an important role in regu-

T Lymphocytes in the Liver: Immunobiology, Pathology, and Host Defense, Edited by I. Nicholas Crispe
ISBN 0-471-19218-X

lating T cell response and homeostasis. By eliminating T cells that are potentially self-reactive, the liver may also be involved in the induction and maintenance of peripheral tolerance of T cells.

CONVENTIONAL TCRαβ CELLS

In humans and most laboratory animals, the vast majority of T cells in the peripheral lymphoid tissues express a TCR composed of a disulfide-linked heterodimer of an α chain and a β chain (TCRαβ) (1). The TCRαβ heterodimer is noncovalently associated with the CD3 complex, a multimolecular transmembrane structure consisting of γ, δ, ϵ, ζ, and η chains (1). The TCRαβ heterodimer is responsible for antigen recognition, whereas the CD3 complex is believed to play an important role in transmembrane signaling (1). It is now clear that TCRαβ recognizes antigen in the form of small peptide fragments presented by the major histocompatibility complex (MHC) molecules expressed on antigen-presenting cells (APC). The antigen specificity of an individual T cell receptor is determined by the particular variable regions of both the α and β chains, which differ from T cell to T cell. This variability arises from random recombination of the gene segments encoding the TCR α and β chain during T cell development in the thymus (2,3).

The recognition of antigen peptide presented by MHC molecules is assisted by CD4 and CD8, the so-called coreceptor molecules expressed on the surface of T cells (4,5). In a normal host, the vast majority (>98%) of mature αβ T cells found in the periphery express either the CD4 or the CD8 coreceptors. CD4 exists as a single-chain glycoprotein, whereas CD8 exists as either a heterodimer consisting of one α and one β chain (CD8αβ) or a homodimer of two α chains (CD8αα) (4). In peripheral T cells, CD8 exists almost exclusively as a CD8αβ heterodimer. T cells expressing CD8αα homodimer are primarily found in the gastrointestinal epithelium (6,7). Mutagenesis experiments and the crystal structure of CD4, CD8, and MHC molecules have provided precise information about the interaction between the coreceptors and MHC molecules (5). The CD4 coreceptor binds to the invariant β2 domain of class II molecules, whereas CD8 binds to the nonpolymorphic α3 domain of class I MHC molecules (5,8–10). Through such an interaction, the coreceptors direct antigen recognition to the appropriate class of MHC molecules, and enhance the binding between TCR and the antigen peptide–MHC complex (4,11). It is now clear that class II MHC molecule is responsible for presentation of endosomally derived antigen peptides to $CD4^+$ TCRαβ T cells, whereas antigen peptides from cytosolic pathogens are processed and presented by class I MHC molecules to $CD8^+$ TCRαβ cells (12).

ACTIVATION AND INACTIVATION OF TCRαβ CELLS

T cell recognition of antigenic peptide presented by MHC molecules expressed on APCs usually leads to T cell activation, which is characterized by proliferation of antigen-specific T cells, production of interleukin-2 (IL-2) and other cytokines, and delivery of effector functions. The molecular events leading to T cell activation after antigen recognition are not completely understood. But it is clear that signaling through the TCR-CD3 complex and the coreceptors are both important for T cell activation (13). The tyrosine kinases ZAP-70, a *syk*-family tyrosine kinase associated with the ζ chain of the CD3 complex in *ex vivo* murine T cells, and $p56^{lck}$, a *src* family tyrosine kinase linked to the cytoplasmic tails of CD4 and CD8, are critically involved in TCR-mediated signal transduction (13,14). Mutation in either $p56^{lck}$ or ZAP-70 blocks TCR mediated T cell activation (15–17). Stimulation through TCR leads to phosphorylation and activation of ZAP-70 (13). Cross-linking of CD4 or CD8 to TCR causes an increase in tyrosine phosphorylation of several substrates, including the CD3 ζ chain (18,19). It has been suggested that simultaneous recognition of a single antigenic peptide-MHC complex by a TCR and a CD4 or CD8 molecule help to bring $p56^{lck}$ into the proximity of the TCR-CD3 complex, and allow $p56^{lck}$ to phosphorylate the tyrosine residues in the ζ chain and other substrates, leading to a complex cascade of downstream events (5).

It has been recognized for a long time that signaling generated via the TCR-CD3 complex and the coreceptors is not sufficient for activation of T cells, and that a second or costimulatory signal is required (20). Accumulating data have shown the interaction between CD28 expressed on T cells and B7-1 (CD80) or B7-2 (CD86, also called B70 in human) expressed by professional APCs provides the critical costimulation for T cell activation (21–23). Mice with disrupted genes encoding CD28 have profound impairment in T cell responsiveness to antigens (24,25). APCs lacking B7 are unable to activate T cells *in vitro*, and blocking CD28–B7 interaction with monocloncal antibodies inhibits T cell activation both *in vitro* and *in vivo* (26–28).

Inactivation of T cells is important for two obvious reasons: (i) Immune responses need to be terminated, and the majority of antigen-activated T cells have to be inactivated and destroyed after antigen has been cleared. This is crucial for maintaining the homeostasis of the immune system. (ii) Potentially self-reactive T cells may somehow evade intrathymic clonal deletion, and may enter peripheral tissues. These cells need to be inactivated upon recognition of self-antigens to avoid autoimmunity.

T cell inactivation may be achieved without cell death. This form of T cell inactivation is often called "anergy" in the literature, and has been described in several experimental systems (29). *In vitro*, stimulation of TCR in the absence of costimulation classically leads to T cell inactivation (30,31). This appears to be related to a block in IL-2 production at the transcription level (32), and can be prevented by costimulation via the CD28-B7 interaction (33). Antigen stimulation of TCR in the presence of IL-10, or occupancy of TCR by altered antigenic peptide with single amino acid substitution, can lead to T cell inactivation *in vitro*, even in the presence of costimulation delivered by B7 expressed on APCs (34,35). The *in vivo* physiological relevance of these *in vitro* models is not well established.

Inactivation of mature T cells by antigen can also be achieved through apoptosis of antigen-stimulated T cells, also known as activation-induced cell death (AICD). This form of T cell inactivation can be observed *in vitro*, in T cell lines, or *ex vivo*, in T cells upon antigen or superantigen stimulation (36,37), but the clearest evidence for its occurrence *in vivo* comes from studies with superantigens (38–40), and in TCR transgenic mice responding to nominal antigens (41–43). Injection of mice with superantigens leads to three distinct phases of T cell response: (i) An initial phase of T cell activation characterized by massive cell proliferation and cytokine production, including IL-2, tumor necrosis factor (TNF), IL-6, and IFNγ; (ii) A phase of unresponsiveness when T cells are unable to proliferate or secrete cytokines upon TCR stimulation *in vitro;* followed by (iii) T cell apoptosis resulting in eventual elimination (peripheral deletion) of superantigen-reactive T cells expressing particular T cell receptor variable region beta chains (Vβs) (38–40,44). Such a T cell inactivation and deletion process has also been described in several TCR transgenic mice after injection of antigens (41,42,45). In some instances, a proliferative phase was not observed, although there was often evidence of T cell activation, such as blastogenesis and expression of surface markers associated with activation, before T cells underwent inactivation and deletion (46). It has been suggested that this form of *in vivo* T cell inactivation by AICD occurs in the majority of activated T cells during normal immune responses.

The molecular mechanism underlying antigen-induced T cell inactivation and the eventual elimination of T cells by AICD is not completely understood. But it is now clear that in the majority of cases, the Fas/Fas-ligand interaction and a TNF-mediated pathway are involved in AICD of mature T cells (47,48). Fas (Apo-1 or CD95) is a member of the TNF receptor/nerve growth factor (NGF) receptor family, while Fas ligand (FasL) is a member of the TNF family (49). T cell activation by anti-TCR, superantigen, or antigenic peptide results in rapid upregulation of Fas expression on T cells both *in vitro* and *in vivo* (50,51). This upregulation is paralleled by the kinetics of AICD of T cells. Cell death, but not activation, can be selectively inhibited by a soluble Fas-Fc fusion protein (50,51). Mutations in the genes for Fas and FasL cause disorders characterized by massive accumulation of activated T cells in mice homozygous for the *lpr* and *gld* mutations, respectively (52,53). Furthermore, mature T cells from *lpr* mice are resistant to superantigen B (SEB)-induced AICD *in vivo* (54). In a line of *lpr* mice transgenic for a class II restricted TCR, AICD of $CD4^+$ transgenic T cells is inhibited (47). However, in another line of *lpr* mice carrying a different class II restricted transgenic TCR, AICD of $CD4^+$ T cells occurs, but can be abrogated by additional blocking of TNF, indicating the existence of an alternative, TNF-dependent pathway for AICD (48).

In many experimental systems, the inactivation phase of T cell response to antigen or superantigen stimulation involves TCR downregulation, coreceptor downregulation, or both (40,41,55,56). *In vivo*, TCR and/or coreceptor downregulation accompanies the inactivation phase of the T cell response following injection of superantigens such as SEB or cells expressing viral superantigen-7 (vSAG-7) (40,56). Such TCR/coreceptor downregulation has also been described in several TCR transgenic mice following injection of antigens or antigenic peptides (41,55,57). Furthermore, the degree of TCR and coreceptor downregulation can occur in a dose-dependent fashion in a line of double transgenic mice where the transgenic TCR recognizes K^b molecules expressed on hepatocytes under the control of the complement-reactive protein promoter (58). In some cases, cells that have downregulated TCR and/or coreceptor revert to a functional state when removed to an antigen-free environment (55,56,58), whereas in other instances, TCR and/or coreceptor downregulation is associated with AICD (40,56). The ultimate fate of T cell undergoing AICD *in vivo* is not clear. The following discussion presents evidence that inactivated T cells accumulate in the liver, where they undergo apoptosis, and are eventually eliminated.

LIVER TCRαβ T CELLS: TCR AND CORECEPTOR EXPRESSION

While the presence of T cells in the liver has been recognized for a long time on the basis of immunohistologic staining, a detailed phenotypic characterization was not possible until the cells were isolated, and analyzed by flow cytometry. Slightly different methods have been described for isolation of intrahepatic lymphocytes from murine and human livers (59–62). Most of these methods involve enzymatic digestion of liver tissue and gradient centrifugation. In order to isolate resident lymphocytes from mouse liver, it is necessary to gently perfuse the liver *in situ* via the portal vein to remove passenger lymphocytes circulating in the blood. The liver is then resected and mechanically disrupted by forcing through a fine metal mesh. Liver tissue samples are then digested with collagenase to disrupt parenchymal hepatocytes to release lymphocytes. Finally, mononuclear cells (MNC) are isolated by gradient centrifugation over Ficoll solution (59), Percoll gradient (62), 100% fetal calf serum (63) or 30% metrizamide (53). In humans, it is estimated that from 0.8×10^6 to 6×10^6 MNCs can be isolated from each gram of liver tissue (64). In mice, the total number of MNCs that can be isolated from each liver ranges from 0.5×10^6 to 10×10^6 (60). An alternative method called sinusoidal lavage has been described in the literature for isolation of liver lymphocytes (65,66). This method is based on the idea that intrahepatic lymphocytes will de-attach from their adhesion to the sinusoids if a high enough perfusion pressure is applied. Sinusoidal lavage can be achieved either via the portal vein in mice or transparenchymally through the Glisson's capsule on surgical liver biopsies from humans (65,66).

Flow cytometric analysis of small lymphocytes showed that TCRαβ T cells are the major lymphocyte population in the liver. In contrast to conventional αβ T cells found in the periphery, which express a uniformly high level of TCRαβ, the liver contains two distinct populations of TCRαβ T cells based on the level of TCRαβ expression (60,67). One population expresses TCRαβ at a level comparable to the conventional peripheral of αβ T cells ($TCR\alpha\beta^{hi}$), while the other expresses a reduced level of TCRαβ ($TCR\alpha\beta^{lo}$) (60,67). The latter population is sometimes referred to as $TCR\text{-}\alpha\beta^{intermediate}$ in the literature, as the level of TCR expression on these cells is lower than that on mature peripheral T cells, but higher than that on immature T cells in the thymus (60,67). Further flow cytometric analysis revealed phenotypic heterogeneity of liver αβ T cells based on the expression of CD4 and CD8 coreceptors (60). As shown in Figure 2.1, while most of the $TCR\alpha\beta^{hi}$ cells are either $CD4^+$ or $CD8^+$ single positive T cells, the $TCR\alpha\beta^{lo}$ cells consist mainly of $CD4^-CD8^-$ (double negative, DN) T cells. There were also some $CD4^+$ cells and $CD8^+$ cells expressing a low level of TCRαβ, and $CD4^-CD8^-$ cells expressing a high level of TCR. Of note is that the level

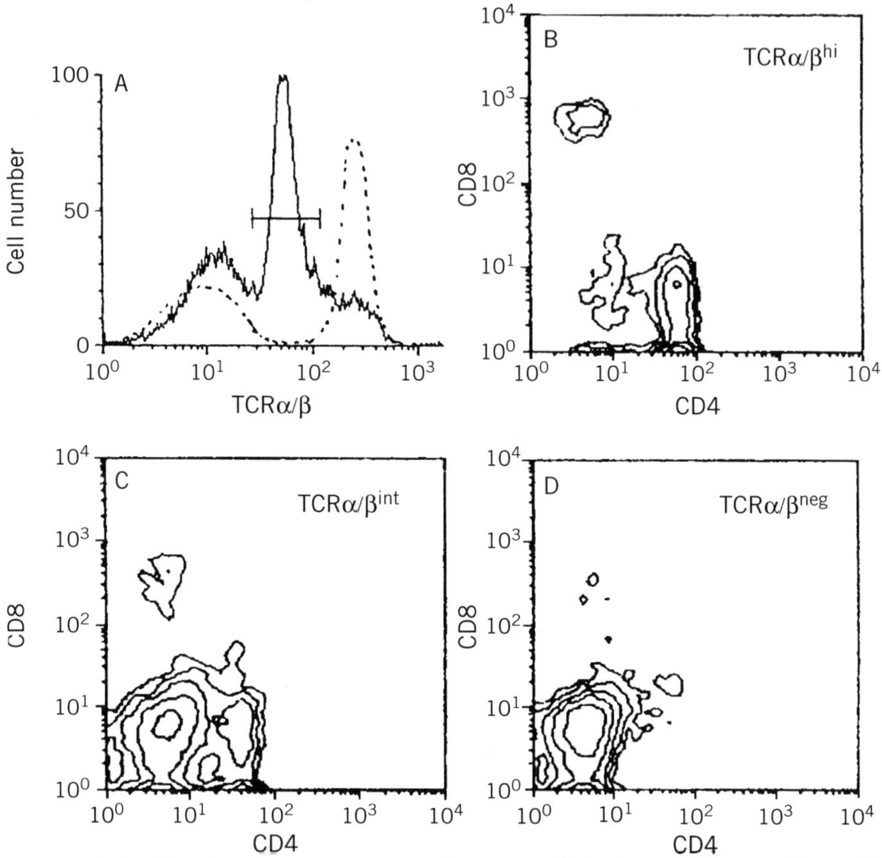

Figure 2.1. TCRαβ and coreceptor expression on T cells in the normal mouse liver. This is a three-color flow cytometric analysis of liver lymphocytes after staining with monoclonal antibodies against TCR-Cβ, CD4, and CD8. (**A**): TCR-Cβ expression on liver lymphocytes (solid line), in comparison with lymph node cells (broken line). (**B–D**): CD4 and CD8 expression on $TCR\alpha\beta^{hi}$, $TCR\alpha\beta^{lo}$ and $TCR\alpha\beta^{neg}$ cells. Note the expression of CD4 and CD8 on $TCR\alpha\beta^{lo}$ cells is lower than that on $TCR\alpha\beta^{hi}$ cells (compare B with C).

of CD4 and CD8 coreceptor expression on $TCR\alpha\beta^{lo}$ cells is also reduced compared with that on $TCR\alpha\beta^{hi}$ T cells (compare Fig. 2.1B with Fig. 2.1C). The existence of such cellular intermediates, namely the $CD4^{hi}TCR\alpha\beta^{lo}$, $CD4^{lo}TCR\alpha\beta^{lo}$, $CD8^{hi}$-$TCR\alpha\beta^{lo}$ and $CD8^{lo}TCR\alpha\beta^{lo}$ cells, have also been noted by other investigators (62), and are compatible with the idea that liver $CD4^{-}CD8^{-}TCR\alpha\beta^{lo}$ cells are generated from single positive cells that have downregulated the expression of TCR and coreceptor molecules.

In addition to TCRαβ T cells, the murine liver also contains some TCRγδ T cells (60), conventional NK cells (59), and a recently identified subset of lymphocytes called NK-T cells, which express both the TCRαβ and NK-1.1 (a marker of natural killer cells) (68). In young adult mice, TCRγδ T cells are a minor population, never exceeding 5% (60).

B220 EXPRESSION ON TCRαβ^{LO} LIVER T CELLS

The B220 epitope of the CD45R molecule is generally appreciated as a B cell–specific surface marker (69). However, an increasing body of evidence has indicated that its expression is not restricted to the B cell lineage. It is also expressed on T cells, but only in association with T cell activation (70–73). Resting T cells do not express B220. *In vitro*, B220 expression can be induced on both $CD4^+$ and $CD8^+$ αβ T cells upon activation with concanavalin A (Con A), anti-CD3 antibody, or staphylococcal enterotoxin B (70). *In vivo* injection of staphylococcal enterotoxin B induced B220 expression on $CD8^+$ but not $CD4^+V\beta8^+$ T cells in normal mice (70,73). In addition, B220 expression has also been reported on lymphokine-activated killer (LAK) cells expressing TCRαβ upon activation by IL-2 or IL-4 *in vitro* (74), and TCRγδ T cells upon activation with anti-CD3 antibody and IL-2 *in vitro* or after antigen exposure *in vivo* in TCR transgenic mice (71,75). Therefore, when expressed on T cells, B220 appears to be a marker of T cell activation.

Interestingly, in *lpr* and *gld* mice, there is abnormal accumulation of TCRαβ T cells expressing B220 (76–78). Most of these cells are $CD4^-CD8^-$ cells expressing a reduced level of TCRαβ (76–78). Although the exact origin of these abnormal cells is not clear and continues to be a subject of debate and research, evidence has been mounting that they represent previously activated, end-stage T cells that fail to be eliminated by AICD (47,54,79). This is due to the mutation in genes encoding Fas and FasL in *lpr* and *gd* mice, respectively (49). Thus the expression of B220 on the abnormal T cells in these mice is in line with their activation status.

As is shown in Figure 2.2A, most liver TCRαβ T cells express B220. The $B220^+TCR\alpha\beta$ T cells consist exclusively of $TCR\alpha\beta^{lo}$ cells, while the $B220^-$ liver T cell population includes both $TCR\alpha\beta^{hi}$ and $TCR\alpha\beta^{lo}$ cells. It is of note that prior antigen exposure and T cell activation can be associated with downregulation of TCRαβ, coreceptor, or both under certain conditions (40,41,55,56,80–82). Therefore, the reduced level of TCRαβ and coreceptor expression, and the expression of B220 on the majority of liver T cells suggest that they represent antigen-experienced T cells.

OTHER ACTIVATION MARKERS ON LIVER αβ T CELLS

In addition to B220, the liver $TCR\alpha\beta^{lo}$ T cells express a variety of other surface markers that are associated with prior activation (Table 2.1). It is of note that the phenotype of $B220^-$ liver TCRαβ T cells resembles that of mature resting T cells found elsewhere in the peripheral lymphoid tissues such as the lymph nodes and spleen. Both $B220^-$ and $B220^+$ TCRαβ T cells express a similar level of Fas on the membrane and abundant Fas mRNA was detected by RNAse protection assay (83). However, the expression of Fas β, a soluble isoform of Fas that is believed to inhibit FasL-induced apoptosis, is markedly different between the two subsets (83). The $B220^+TCR\alpha\beta^{lo}$ T cells express a much lower level of Fas β mRNA than the $B220^-TCR\alpha\beta$ cells (83). Such a difference in Fas β expression may account for their difference in apoptosis.

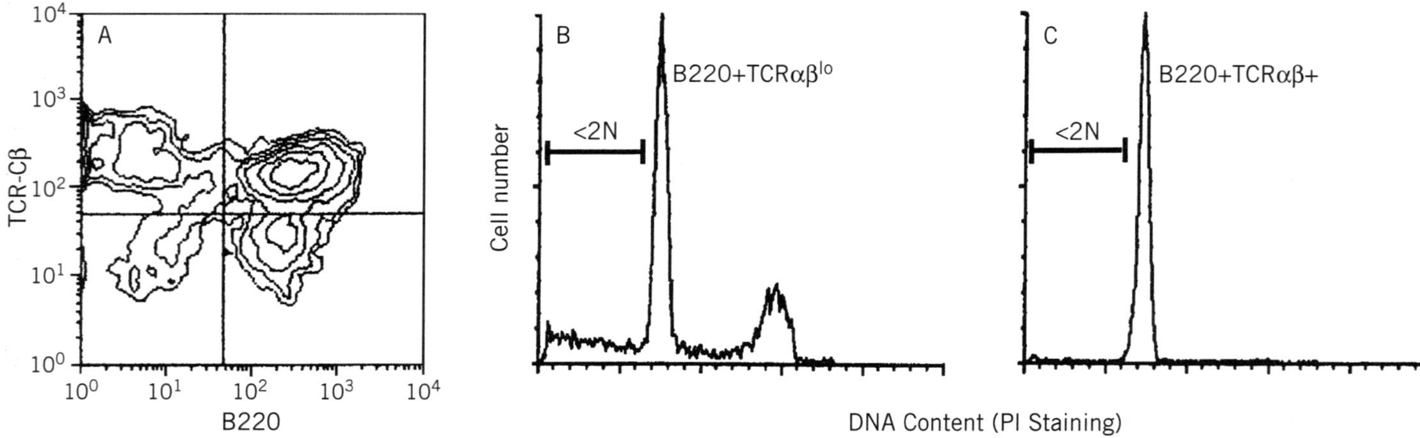

Figure 2.2. Proliferation and apoptosis of B220$^+$TCR$\alpha\beta^{lo}$ cells in normal mouse liver. (**A**): Most TCR$\alpha\beta^+$ cells in the liver express B220. This is a two-color flow cytometric analysis of liver lymphocytes after staining with monoclonal antibodies against TCR-Cβ and B220. (**B**): PI staining of purified B220$^+$TCR$\alpha\beta^{lo}$ liver T cells. (**C**): PI staining of purified B220$^-$TCR$\alpha\beta^+$ liver T cells. The B220$^+$TCR$\alpha\beta^{lo}$ cells contain a large fraction of cells with subdiploid nuclei (<2N), as well as cells in the S and M + G2 phases of the cell cycle.

TABLE 2.1 Phenotype of TCRαβ T Cells in the Liver, Compared with Normal Mature T Cells and *lpr* T Cells

	Liver T Cells			
	B220$^+$	B220$^-$	Peripheral T cells	*lpr* T cells
TCRαβ	Low	High	High	Low
CD4/8	CD4-CD8-, CD4/8^{lo}	CD4^{hi}, CD8^{hi}	CD4^{hi}, CD8^{hi}	CD4$^-$CD8$^-$
B220	+	–	–	+
CD44	High	Low	Low	High
CD25	+	–	–	–
Thy-1	Low	High	High	Low
Ly6C	+	–	–	+/–
Fas	High	High	Low	–
Fasβ	Low	High	Low	?
Apoptosis	+	–	–	–

PROLIFERATION AND APOPTOSIS OF B220$^+$ LIVER αβ T CELLS

Superantigen-induced or antigen-induced TCR and/or coreceptor downregulation that accompanies T cell inactivation is sometimes associated with apoptosis. To investigate whether the B220$^+$CD4$^-$CD8$^-$TCRαβ^{lo} liver T cells belong to such a T cell inactivation/apoptosis pathway following antigen stimulation, B220$^+$TCRαβ^{lo} cells were purified from normal mouse liver. They were then fixed, rendered membrane permeable, and stained with propidium iodide (PI) to identify cells with subdiploid nuclei, a characteristic of cells undergoing apoptosis (60). As shown in Figure 2.2B, about 20% of the liver B220$^+$TCRαβ^{lo} T cells are subdiploid. Occurrence of apoptosis was also demonstrated by electrophoresis of DNA isolated from unfractionated liver MNC, which revealed characteristic nucleosomal-sized ladders of DNA fragments (60). Strikingly, apoptosis is demonstrable in neither the B220$^+$TCRαβ^{hi} cells in the liver nor T cells in the periphery, which are uniformly in the resting G_0/G_1 phase of the cell cycle (Fig. 2.2C).

Of the B220$^+$TCRαβ^{lo} cell population, 15% to 30% of the cells are in the S and G_2/M phase of the cell cycle, indicating that some of the B220$^+$TCRαβ^{lo} cells are actively proliferating. This is consistent with the findings by others that the susceptibility of a cell to apoptosis is dependent on its cell cycle status (84,85). T cells that have already entered the S phase are sensitive, whereas those in the G_1 phase are refractory to apoptosis induced by TCR ligation (84). The finding that some of the liver T cells are actively proliferating is also in line with results from earlier studies in rats. Cytogenetic analysis showed that about 9% of liver MNCs isolated from normal rats displayed mitotic activity, whereas no dividing cells were found in peripheral blood lymphocytes (86). *In vivo* labeling with 5-[^{125}I]-iododeoxyuridine showed a high rate of proliferation of Thy-1$^+$ T cells in the hepatic sinusoids, but not in the other organs of normal rats (87).

ACCUMULATION OF APOPTOTIC T CELLS IN THE LIVER

The findings described above suggest that the majority of the T cells in the liver are previously activated, end-stage T cells that are undergoing AICD in the liver. The concentration of such cells in the liver but not in the other organs suggest that liver is where T cells undergoing apoptosis *in vivo* are eliminated. To test this hypothesis, we used a line of class I MHC (K^k) restricted anti-SV40 large T antigen TCR transgenic mice to study peripheral T cell apoptosis and deletion induced by injection of one of the antigenic peptides, SV40 large T antigen peptide 562–569. Injection of the antigen peptide induces partial T cell activation, manifested by blastogenesis, onset of

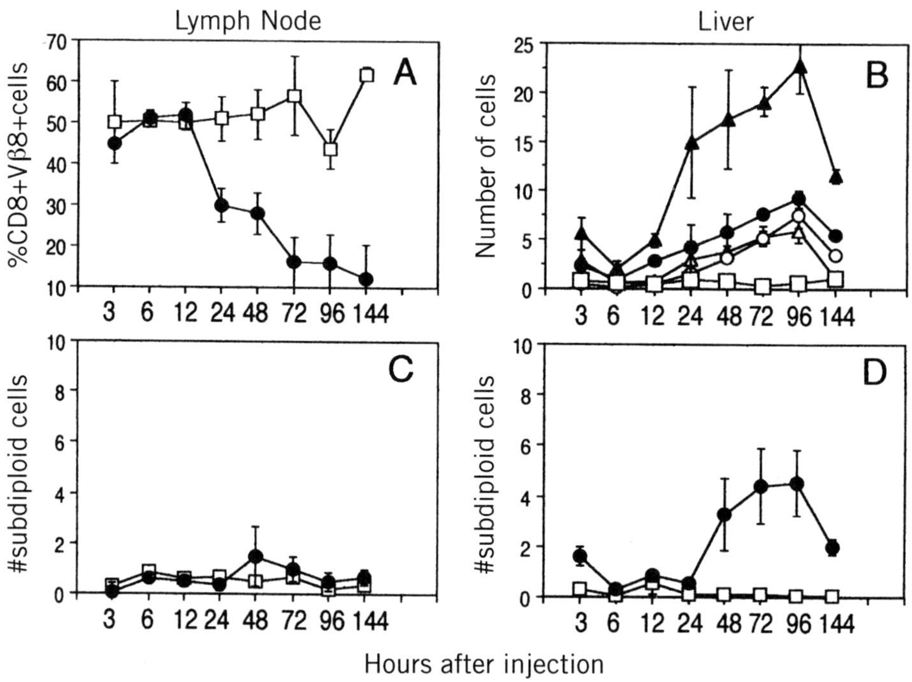

Figure 2.3. Accumulation and apoptosis of T cells in the liver during peripheral T cell deletion. (**A**): Injection of antigenic peptide causes peripheral deletion of transgenic T cells in anti-SV40 large-T antigen TCR transgenic mice (open squares: mice injected with PBS; closed circles: mice injected with antigenic peptide). (**B**): Accumulation of T cells in the liver accompanies peripheral T cell deletion in peptide-injected mice (open squares: $CD8^+$ cells in the liver of mice injected with PBS; closed triangles: mononuclear cells isolated from mice injected with peptide; closed circles: $CD4^-CD8^-$ lymphocytes in the liver of mice injected with peptide; open triangles: $CD8^{hi}$ lymphocytes in the liver of mice injected with peptide; open circles: $CD8^{lo}$ lymphocytes in the liver of mice injected with peptide). (**C**): No evidence of apoptosis in the lymph node cells. (**D**): Apoptosis of lymphocytes in the liver in mice injected with peptide. Shown are percentages and numbers of unfractionated lymphocytes in millions with subdiploid nuclei revealed by staining with PI (open squares: mice injected with PBS; closed circles: mice injected with peptide).

DNA synthesis, and the expression of a set of activation markers including B220 and CD25 (46). This is followed by gradual but profound clonal deletion of mature $CD8^+Tg^+$ cells from the lymph nodes and spleen (Fig. 2.3A). The disappearance of $CD8^+Tg^+$ cells is accompanied by a state of specific unresponsiveness to the antigen (46). One possibility for the disappearance of $CD8^+Tg^+$ cells might be that most of these cells undergo apoptosis *in situ* in the lymph nodes and spleen. However, apoptosis could not be detected in cells freshly isolated from the lymph nodes or spleen by either PI staining (Fig. 2.3C) or DNA electrophoresis (46).

As the $CD8^+Tg^+$ T cells started to disappear from the lymph nodes and the spleen 48 hours after injection, there was a massive accumulation of these cells in the liver (Fig. 2.3B). The total number of liver MNCs was dramatically increased, as were the number of $CD8^+$ T cells (Figure 2.3B). The $CD8^+Tg^+$ T cells accumulating in the liver express CD25 and B220, consistent with their activation status (46). The accumulation of T cells in the liver was accompanied by TCR and CD8 downregulations, as there was appearance of large numbers of $CD8^{lo}TCR^{lo}$ as well as $CD4^-CD8^-TCR^-$ cells that can not be accounted for by B cells, macrophages, or granulocytes (Fig. 2.3B). Many of these null cells accumulating in the liver were Thy-1^+ (data not shown), and could be TCR^- T cells that have completely downregulated TCR and CD8 molecules. The dramatic accumulation of activated T cells in the liver is a liver-specific, and antigen-specific process, as there was no parallel increase in the number of T cells in the kidneys or the lungs, nor was there any significant increase in the number of $CD4^+$ cells, most of which did not express the transgenic TCR, in the liver (46).

The hypothesis that the liver is the organ where inactivated T cells are eliminated also predicts that T cells accumulating there should be undergoing apoptosis. To this end, freshly isolated liver MNCs were stained with PI after being rendered membrane permeable. As shown in Fig. 2.3D, a large number of the isolated liver MNCs were undergoing apoptosis in the peptide-injected mice. At 96 hours and 144 hours after injection, an average of 20% of the isolated hepatic lymphocytes were subdiploid. Staining with PI also revealed that T cells are proliferating. At 48 hours after antigenic peptide injection, approximately 40% of cells were in the S phase of the cell cycle (46). Histological examination of the liver revealed the location of lymphocyte accumulation and showed further evidence of apoptosis. The number of MNCs located in the hepatic sinusoids was greatly increased in the TCR transgenic mice injected with antigenic peptide. In many sections, there were perivascular accumulations of lymphocytes, suggesting that these cells had been extracted from the circulation (46). Many of these cells are undergoing apoptosis, as indicated by very condensed nuclei sitting in a "halo" of cytoplasm, a feature characteristic of apoptotic cells (46).

ROLE OF THE LIVER IN T CELL HOMEOSTASIS AND PERIPHERAL TOLERANCE

The data discussed above clearly shows that the majority of liver $TCR\alpha\beta^{lo}$ T cells express B220 and an array of other surface markers characteristic of previously activated T cells. These cells express a low level of Fas β, and represent a population of T cells that are actively undergoing proliferation and apoptosis. The concentration of such cells in the liver of normal mice, and their accumulation during antigen-induced inactivation and deletion of mature T cells in the periphery suggest that T cells undergoing AICD *in vivo* travel to the liver, where they are eliminated. This is a liver-specific process, and not nonspecific trapping of activated T cells in tissues, as the number of T cells is not significantly increased in other major organs such as the kidneys and lungs. However, in a recently published study using mice transgenic for a TCR (F5) specific for an influenza virus nucleoprotein peptide (NP68), antigen-induced accumulation and apoptosis of T cells were observed not only in the liver, but also in the kidneys and small intestine (88). This discrepancy is likely due to the different response of the transgenic T cells in the two models. In contrast to the results obtained with the SV40-specific transgenic T cells used in our model, injection of influenza virus nucleoprotein peptide NP68 induced an initial phase of massive proliferation of transgenic T cells before deletion was observed (88). As a result, the capacity of the liver to retain and eliminate apoptotic T cells might be exceeded, leading to nonspecific trapping of activated T cells in other tissues.

The appearance of $CD8^{lo}Tg^{+}$ and $CD8^{+}Tg^{lo}$ cells in the anti-SV40 large T antigen TCR transgenic mice injected with antigenic peptide indicates that there was a TCR and coreceptor downregulation process preceding apoptosis. This is consistent with studies using superantigens or other TCR transgenic mice, where T cells may undergo TCR downregulation, coreceptor downregulation, or both upon encountering antigen (40,41,55,56). These findings suggest that the $B220^{+}CD4^{-}CD8^{-}TCR\alpha\beta^{lo}$ liver T cells found in normal unmanipulated mice are generated from mature $CD4^{+}$ or $CD8^{+}$ T cells that have downregulated the expression of their TCR and CD4/CD8 coreceptor molecules. Such a TCR and coreceptor downregulation process is also supported by the identification of minor subpopulations of cellular intermediates, namely $CD4^{lo}$-$TCR\alpha\beta^{lo}$ and $CD8^{lo}TCR\alpha\beta^{lo}$ cells that are present in the liver of normal healthy mice. It needs to be emphasized that these cellular intermediates are present only in the liver, and not in the spleen, gut, or other peripheral lymphoid tissues. Thus, *in vivo*, there appears to be an antigen-induced T cell inactivation and clearance pathway characterized by TCR and coreceptor downregulation of antigen-stimulated T cells, movement to and accumulation of such cells in the liver, and their eventual elimination via apoptosis (Fig. 2.4). This is likely to be a general T cell inactivation and clearance pathway for T cells that are programmed to undergoing apoptosis *in vivo*. Accumulation of large numbers of T cells in the liver has been described under a variety of conditions of T cell activation, such as injection of IL-2 or Con A (87,89,90), bacterial infection (91,92), and in mice bearing tumors (93). Although apoptosis was not studied in these experiments, the findings that the number of T cells is increased during T cell activation are consistent with the hypothesis that the liver is where previously activated T cells are eliminated through AICD.

Downregulation of TCR and coreceptor may be one of the normal consequences of T cell activation. While mature resting T cells express a uniformly high level of TCRαβ and CD3, T cells activated by ConA or PMA *in vitro* express significantly reduced TCRαβ and CD3 (94,95). T cell stimulation by SEA or phytohaemagglutinin (PHA) induces downregulation of both TCR and CD4 *in vitro* (96), and when activated in the presence of IL-4, $CD8^{+}$ T cells downregulate their expression of CD8 and

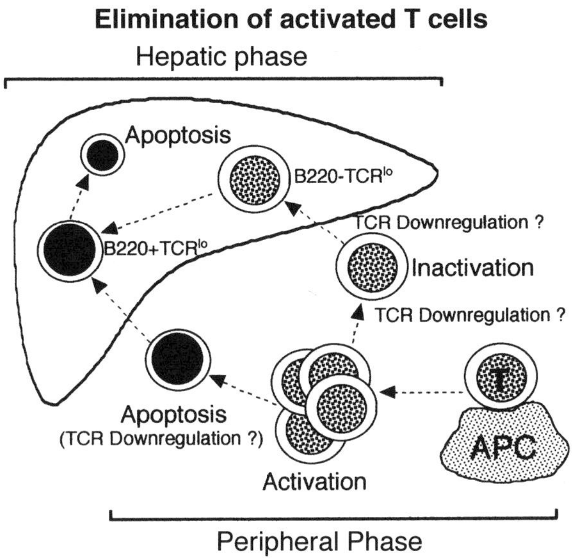

Figure 2.4. Model of T cell homeostasis. After immune response, the majority of activated T cells need to be eliminated to maintain homeostasis of the immune system. T cells may be inactivated in the periphery through TCR and/or coreceptor downregulation, and then travel to the liver to be destroyed via apoptosis. Apoptosis of activated T cells may be initiated in the periphery before, or at the time of, their migration to the liver. Alternatively, apoptosis may result from T cell interaction with cells in the liver such as the Kupffer cells and hepatocytes.

become $CD4^-CD8^-$ T cells (97). T cells with reduced expression of TCRαβ and coreceptor have also been described in local tissues in the course of acute bacterial, viral, and parasitic infection (98,99), and *in vitro* in response to peptides bound to MHC molecules expressed on antigen-presenting cells (100,101). Alternatively, downregulation of TCR and coreceptor may be a feature of T cells that are already programmed for activation-induced cell death. Downregulation of TCR/coreceptor was associated with apoptosis in mice injected with the superantigens (40,56), and in the anti-SV40 large T antigen TCR transgenic mice injected with antigenic peptide (46). However, in other experimental systems, cells that had downregulated TCR and coreceptor persisted, and reverted to a functional state upon removal to an antigen-free environment (55,56). It is not clear if the persistence of these cells represents selection of cells that are resistant to AICD.

Cell death and disposal is one of the important mechanisms for maintaining T cell homeostasis after immune stimulation. The hallmark of T cell response to foreign antigen is proliferation of antigen-specific T cells and production of cytokines. Such a response is potentially harmful to the host tissues, and needs to be terminated in a timely fashion once the offending pathogen or antigen has been successfully cleared. It is not hard to imagine that the majority of antigen stimulated T cells, with the exception of a few long-lived memory cells, need to be inactivated and eliminated. The liver is an ideal organ to carry out this function. It is a metabolically active organ, and it is the place where effete erythrocytes are destroyed and recycled. Thus by removing unwanted T cells, the liver may play an important role in maintaining the homeostasis of T cells. By eliminating potentially self-reactive T cells that are programmed for apoptosis, the liver may also be critically involved in the induction and the maintenance of peripheral T cell tolerance.

DEFECTIVE HOMEOSTASIS AND LYMPHOPROLIFERATIVE DISORDER

The importance of maintaining T cell homeostasis is most elegantly illustrated in *lpr* and *gld* mutant mice. Mice homozygous for the *lpr* or *gld* mutation have a remarkably similar lymphoproliferative disorder characterized by multisystem autoimmunity and accumulation of large numbers of T cells, mainly of the $CD4^-$-$CD8^-TCR\alpha\beta^{lo}$ phenotype (76–78). The gene defect in *lpr* mice is an insertional mutation in the second exon of the *fas* gene, while the *gld* mutation is a single amino acid substitution in the FasL, resulting in loss of its function (49). The origin of the abnormal $CD4^-CD8^-TCR\alpha\beta^{lo}$ cells in these mice is not completely understood. The $CD4^-CD8^-TCR\alpha\beta^{lo}$ cells in *lpr* and *gld* mice are $B220^+$, $CD44^+$, $Ly6C^+$, and thus are similar to the $B220^+TCR\alpha\beta^{lo}$ T cells present in the liver of normal, healthy mice (60). Such similarities have raised the possibility that the intrahepatic $B220^+TCR\alpha\beta^{lo}$ cells are the normal counterparts of the abnormal T cells found in *lpr* and *gld* mice (67,102). In *lpr* mice, cells with $CD4^-CD8^-TCR\alpha\beta^{lo}$ phenotype are increased in the liver, and if *lpr* mice are pulsed *in vivo* with [^{3}H]-thymidine, labeled T cells appeared in the liver 2 days earlier than in the lymph nodes (102). These findings have been construed as evidence that the liver is a site of extrathymic T cell differentiation, and that the accumulation of $CD4^-CD8^-TCR\alpha\beta^{lo}$ cells in *lpr* mice results from expansion of such an extrathymic T cell differentiation pathway (102).

Major support for extrathymic T cell differentiation in the liver is provided by the presence of $CD4^-CD8^-TCR\alpha\beta^{lo}$ cells in aged nude (athymic) mice (103) and AT × BM mice (104), and the expression of recombination-activation genes (RAG) detected by polymerase chain reaction (PCR) (104,105). However, we were unable to detect mRNA or RAG-1 or RAG-2 in liver MNCs by Northern blotting analysis (106). In the study where RAG-1 and RAG-2 gene expression was detected in liver T cells by PCR, RAG-1 and RAG-2 activity was also detected in the T cells isolated from the Peyer's patches and spleen at the same level of sensitivity (105). Therefore, the positive result probably represents oversensitivity of the PCR assay. The presence of relatively large numbers of $CD4^-CD8^-TCR\alpha\beta^{lo}$ cells in the livers of nude and AT × BM mice is indeed consistent with the idea that these cells are generated extrahymically in the liver (103,104). However, the possibility that liver T cells originated at some other site, such as the gastrointestinal epithelium, is not excluded. It is now clear that intestinal intra-epithelial lymphocytes (IEL) develop extrathymically *in situ* in the intestinal epithelium, and thus are present in both nude and AT × BM mice (107). Antigen-activated IELs that are programmed for apoptosis may leave the gastrointestinal epithelium, and travel to the liver to be eliminated. The similarities between some liver T cells and intestinal IELs, including the expression of IL-2 receptor β chain, CD44, and ICAM-1, as well as the usage of CD8αα (108,109), are compatible with the suggestion that some of the liver T cells might have been derived from the gut epithelium. The recent finding that TCRγδ T cells of intestinal type are preferentially expanded in the periphery of TCRα-knockout *lpr* mice (110) indicates that there is migration of IELs from the gut to the systemic lymphoid tissues, but their accumulation there is normally limited by the expression of the *fas* gene. The portal vein drains the gastrointestinal tract, and the liver is the first organ to interact with T cells that have entered the blood circulation from the gastrointestinal tract. It is possible that most of these cells are eliminated through apoptosis in the liver under normal conditions.

Accumulating evidence has shown that most of the abnormal $CD4^-CD8^-TCR\alpha\beta^{lo}$ cells found in *lpr* and *gld* mice are previously activated, end-stage T cells that fail to be appropriately eliminated in the periphery (47,54,79). In addition to the expression of a variety of surface markers associated with prior activation, *lpr* cells have been shown to have hyperphosphorylated CD3ζ chains (110), consistent with an activation status. Despite their phenotype indicative of prior activation, *lpr* and *gld* cells are functionally incompetent. They do not respond to TCR-mediated stimulation *in vitro*, and quickly die off through accelerated apoptosis in culture (111), indicating that they are end-stage cells. It is now clear that Fas–FasL interaction is critically involved in the apoptosis of activated T cells, although an alternative mechanism involving TNF exists (47,48). Antigen-driven peripheral T cell deletion is abrogated in *lpr* mice after injection of staphylococcal enterotoxin B (54), and in a line of TCR transgenic *lpr* mice after injection of antigenic peptide (47). It is possible, therefore, that in the absence of Fas or FasL, antigen-induced expression of B220 and downregulation of TCR/coreceptor is not affected, nor is their ability to migrate to the liver, but that the delivery of the apoptosis-inducing signal is blocked. This results in accumulation of $B220^+CD4^-CD8^-TCR\alpha\beta^{lo}$ T cells in the liver and their eventual return to the periphery. This may explain the phenotype of T cells accumulating in *lpr* mice, and the time delay between the appearance of ^{3}H-labeled T cells in the liver and the lymph nodes after *in vivo* pulsing with ^{3}H-thymidine. A defect in this T cell inactivation and clearance pathway would also result in failure to eliminate potentially self-reactive T cells, leading to breakdown of T cell tolerance and multisystem autoimmunity.

THE LIVER–T CELL INTERACTION

The interaction between circulating T cells and the liver may be facilitated by the unique characteristics of the intrahepatic vascular bed, notably the widely fenestrated sinusoidal endothelium, the numerous Kupffer cells anchored in the sinusoids, the low perfusion pressure, and the lack of a basement membrane separating the endothelium and the liver parenchyma. These unique features maximize the physical contact between circulating T cells and the liver, and make it possible for the circulating lymphocytes to directly interact not only with the endothelial cells and Kupffer cells, but also with the hepatocytes.

It is well known that the mammalian liver has sophisticated sugar recognition systems with receptors capable of recognizing and binding specific carbohydrate residues (112). By far the most widely studied is the asialoglycoproteins receptor (ASGP-R) (112). Expressed specifically on the plasma membrane of hepatocytes, ASGP-R is known to be responsible for the clearance of circulating biologically reactive glycoproteins, such as antigen-antibody complexes (112). Most recent studies have shown that ASGP-R is also involved in the recognition and removal of hepatocytes that are undergoing apoptosis (113). Interestingly, the expression of B220 determinant on activated T cells is increased by treatment with neuraminidase, indicating the presence of sialic acid moieties on the extracellular domain of the molecule (70). It is tempting to speculate that B220 mediates homing and retention of apoptotic T cells in the liver by interacting with the ASGP-R expressed on hepatocytes.

Lymphocyte trafficking is typically regulated by adhesion molecules, membrane glycoproteins that mediate cell–cell or cell–matrix interaction (114). Interaction of T cells with hepatocytes may also be mediated by interaction between lymphocyte-associated antigen 1 (LFA-1) expressed on T cells and intercellular adhesion molecule 1 (ICAM-1) on hepatocytes (115). Primary cultured murine hepatocytes express ICAM-1 and bind T cells *in vitro* (115). Interestingly, T cell activation by phorbol myristic acid (PMA) significantly increased the adhesion of T cells to hepatocytes (115). In addition to the interaction between LFA-1 and ICAM-1, other adhesion interactions are likely to exist, as antibodies directed against LFA-1 and ICAM-1 could only partially inhibit the adhesion between T cells and hepatocytes (115).

Tissue-selective migration of T cells is often mediated by endothelial adhesion molecules that are preferentially expressed in the particular tissue. Examples include mucosa addressin cell adhesion molecule expressed on intestinal endothelium, which mediates migration of T cells expressing α4β7 integrin to the gut (116). Trafficking and retention of apoptotic T cells in the liver may be governed by a similar mechanism. However, no liver-specific adhesion molecules have been described. Several conventional adhesion molecules, including ICAM-1, ICAM-2, VCAM-1, and the newly described vascular adhesion protein 1 (VAP-1) appear to be constitutively expressed on sinusoidal endothelium in normal, noninflamed human liver (117–119). It is not clear if these conventional adhesion molecules are sufficient to mediate selective migration and retention of apoptotic T cells in the liver. It is also important to note that Kupffer cells make up about 15% of the total number of cells in the liver (64). Due to their anatomic location in the sinusoids, they may be the predominant cell type in the liver to interact with circulating T cells. However, the adhesion molecules expressed on Kupffer cells, and their interaction with T cells have not been studied.

It is not clear if the liver is directly involved in the induction of apoptosis of previously activated T cells. It is fairly clear that both Fas-mediated and TNF-mediated apoptosis can contribute to AICD and the deletion of activated peripheral T cells (47,48,54). However, the types of cells involved in the induction of apoptosis of activated T cells is not understood (120). Although Fas is constitutively expressed in normal hepatocytes, neither FasL nor TNF is expressed on hepatocytes under normal conditions. However, the liver may be involved in the induction of T cell apoptosis through other mechanisms. The liver expresses galectin-1, a protein that can cause apoptosis of human T cells (121). In addition, a 70- to 80-kD protein that can induce apoptosis of thymoma EL-4 cells *in vitro* has been isolated from murine liver (122). The role of these novel proteins in the induction of T cell apoptosis *in vivo* is not clear. It is also possible that apoptosis of previously activated T cells may result from their interaction with Kupffer cells residing in the hepatic sinusoids. It has been reported that presentation by APCs may lead to apoptosis of antigen-specific T cells. Examples include $CD8^+$ dendritic cells isolated from murine spleen (123), and astrocytes in rat central nervous system (124). The former induces apoptosis of antigen-specific T cells through interaction of Fas on activated T cells and FasL on $CD8^+$ dendritic cells (123). The question remains as to whether Kupffer cells express FasL, and if so, whether they are involved in the induction of apoptosis of activated T cells.

CONCLUDING REMARKS

The object of this discussion has been to summarize the available data leading to the hypothesis that the majority of $TCR\alpha\beta^{lo}$ T cells in the liver are previously activated, end-stage cells belonging to an *in vivo* T cell inactivation and clearance pathway. The concentration of such cells in the liver suggests that the liver is a special organ where these cells are eventually eliminated. By removing postactivation T cells that are undergoing apoptosis, the liver may be actively involved in establishing T cell homeostasis and peripheral T cell tolerance. It is not clear how the liver and circulating T cells interact, and whether the liver is involved in the induction of apoptosis of T cells. Nor is it clear whether, and how, the liver and gut immune system interact.

Studying the dynamic interaction between the liver and T cells will certainly help us to better understand the pathogenesis of certain autoimmune liver diseases that are characterized by T cell infiltration of the liver parenchyma. For example, some immune-mediated liver diseases may not be due to immune response specifically directed against the liver, but may rather be a type of "bystander" liver damage due to accumulation of large numbers of T cells and subsequent leakage of cytokines and intracellular proteolytic enzymes. *In vivo* injection of ConA, a potent stimulator of T cell activation, causes hepatocellular damage with massive intrahepatic T cell accumulation (90). The liver damage is clearly mediated by activated T cells, as injection of ConA to mice with T cell deficiency such as severe combined immunodeficient (SCID) and athymic *nude* mice, or mice in which T cell activation was blocked using FK506, or antibodies against CD4 and Thy1, caused no liver damage (90). Histological evidence of focal liver damage was observed, along with massive intrahepatic T cell accumulation, in the anti-SV40 large T antigen TCR transgenic mice injected with antigenic peptide (46). Such a bystander effect may also explain liver function abnormalities often seen clinically in cases of severe infection such as sepsis and bacteremia. One may wonder why such a T cell clearance mechanism exists if it can cause liver damage. It is less surprising, however, when considered in light of the tremendous capacity of the liver to recycle and regenerate. Damage to other tissues and organs may be more detrimental, and may even be fatal to the host.

The hypothesis that liver is involved in establishing peripheral T cell tolerance by deleting potentially self-reactive T cells may also explain the well-known observations that have been collectively called "hepatic tolerogenecity" in the organ transplantation field. The liver is the most tolerogenic of all transplanted organs. Liver allografts or xenografts are accepted relatively easily (125–129). In fact, liver allografts can be accepted across most MHC barriers in mice without the need for immunosuppressive therapy (130). The mechanism underlying these observations is not understood, but may be related to the ability of the liver to induce tolerance by eliminating activated T cells.

REFERENCES

1. Clevers, H., Alarcon, B., Wileman, T., and Terhorst, C. 1988. The T cell receptor/CD3 complex: a dynamic protein ensemble. *Annu. Rev. Immunol.* 6:629–662.
2. Adkins, B., Mueller, C., Okada, C.Y., Reichert, R.A., and Weissman, I.L. 1987. Early events of T-cell maturation. *Annu. Rev. Immunol.* 5:325–365.
3. Fowlkes, B.J., and Pardoll, D.M. 1989. Molecular and cellular events of T cell development. *Annu. Rev. Immunol.* 44:207–220.
4. Littman, D.R. 1987. The structure of the CD4 and CD8 genes. *Annu. Rev. Immunol.* 5:561–584.
5. Leahy, D.J. 1995. A structural view of CD4 and CD8. *FASEB J.* 9:17–25.
6. Rocha, B., Vassalli, P., and Guy-grand, D. 1991. The Vβ repertoire of mouse homodimeric a CD8+ intraepithelial lymphocytes reveals a major extrathymic pathway of T cell differentiation. *J. Exp. Med.* 173:483–491.
7. Lefrancois, L. 1991. Phenotypic complexity of intraepithelial lymphocytes of the small intestine. *J. Immunol.* 147:1746.
8. Gay, D., Buus, S., Pasternak, J., Kappler, J., and Marrack, P. 1988. T cell accessory molecule CD4 recognizes a monomorphic determinant on isolated Ia. *Proc. Natl. Acad. Sci. U.S.A.* 85:5629–5633.
9. Connolly, J.M., Potter, T.A., Wormstall, E.-M., and Hansen, T.H. 1988. The Lyt-2 molecule recognises residues in the class I alpha-3 domain in allogeneic cytotoxic T cell responses. *J. Exp. Med.* 168:325–341.
10. Salter, R.D., Benjamin, R.J., Wesley, P.K., Buston, S.E., Garrett, T.P.J., Clayberger, C., Krensky, A.M., Norment, A.M., Littman, D.R., and Parham, P. 1990. A binding site for the T-cell co-receptor CD8 on the alpha-3 domain of HLA-A2. *Nature* 345:41–46.
11. Janeway, C.A. Jr. 1992. The T cell receptor as a multicomponent signaling machine: CD4/CD8 coreceptors and CD45 in T cell activation. *Annu. Rev. Immunol.* 10:645–674.
12. Eisen, H.N., Sykuleve, Y., and Tsomides, T.J. 1996. Antigen-specific T-cell receptors and their reactions with complexes formed by peptides with major histocompatibility complex proteins. *Adv. Prot. Chem.* 49:1–56.
13. Robey, E., and Allison, J.P. 1995. T-cell activation: Integration of signals from the antigen receptor and costimulatory molecules. *Immunol. Today* 16:307–310.
14. Chan, A.C., Iwashima, M., Turck, C.W., and Weiss, A. 1992. ZAP-70: A 70 kd protein-tyrosine kinase that associates with the TCR zeta chain. *Cell* 71:649–662.

15. Elder, M.E., Lin, D., Clever, J., Chan, A.C., Hope, T.J., Weiss, A., and Parslow, T.G. 1994. Human severe combined immunodeficiency due to a defect in ZAP-70, a T cell tyrosine kinase. *Science* 264:1596–1598.
16. Chan, A., Kadlecek, T.A., Elder, M.E., Pilipovich, A.H., Kuo, W., Iwashima, M., Parslow, T.G., and Weiss, A. 1994. ZAP-7 deficiency in an autosomal recessive form of severe combined immunodeficiency. *Science* 264:1599–1602.
17. Straus, D., and Weiss, A. 1992. Genetic evidence for the involvement of the *lck* tyrosine kinase in signal transduction through the T cell antigen receptor. *Cell* 70:585–593.
18. Veillette, A., Bookman, M.A., and Horak, E.M. 1989. Signal transduction through the CD4 receptor involves the activation of the internal membrane tyrosine-protein kinase P56lck. *Nature* 338:257–258.
19. Barber, E.K., Dasgupta, J.D., Schlossman, S.F., Trevillyan, J.M., and Rudd, C.E. 1989. The CD4 and CD8 antigens are coupled to a protein-tyrosine kinase (p56lck) that phosphorylates the CD3 complex. *Proc. Natl. Acad. Sci. U.S.A.* 86:3277–3281.
20. Janeway, C.A., and Bottomly, K. 1994. Signals and signs for lymphocyte responses. *Cell* 76:275–285.
21. Koulova, L., Clark, E.A., Shu, G., and Dupont, B. 1991. The CD28 ligand B7/BB1 provides costimulatory signal for alloactivation of CD4+ T cells. *J. Exp. Med.* 173:759–762.
22. Linsley, P., Brady, W., Grosmaire, L., Aruffo, A., Damle, N.K., and Ledbetter, J.A. 1991. Binding of the B cell activation antigen B7 to CD28 costimulates T cell proliferation and interleukin 2 mRNA accumulation. *J. Exp. Med.* 173:721–730.
23. Freeman, P.S., Gribben, J.G., Boussiotis, V.A., Ng, J.W., Restivo, V.A.J., Lombard, L.A., Gray, G.S., and Nadler, L.M. 1993. Cloning of B7.2: a CTLA-4 counter receptor that costimulates human T cell proliferation. *Science* 262:909–911.
24. Shahinian, A., Pfeffer, K., Lee, K.P., Kundig, T.M., Kishihara, K., Wakeham, A., Kawai, K., Ohashi, P.S., Thompson, C.B., and Mak, T.W. 1993. Differential T cell costimulatory requirements in CD28-deficient mice. *Science* 261:609–612.
25. King, C.L., Xianli, J., June, C.H., Abe, R., and Lee, K.P. 1996. CD28-deficient mice generate an impaired Th2 response to Schistosoma mansoni infection. *Eur. J. Immunol.* 26:2448–2455.
26. Linsley, P.S., Wallace, P.M., Johnson, J., Gibson, M.G., Greene, J.L., Ledbetter, J.A., Singh, C., and Tepper, M.A. 1992. Immunosuppression in vivo by a soluble form of the CTLA-4 T cell activation molecule. *Science* 257:792–795.
27. Wallace, P.M., Rodgers, J.N., Leytze, G.M., Johnson, J.S., and Linsley, P.S. 1995. Induction and reversal of long-lived specific unresponsiveness to a T-dependent antigen following CTLA4Ig treatment. *J. Immunol.* 154:5885–5895.
28. Lenschow, D.J., Zeng, Y., Thistlethwaite, J.R., Montag, A., Brady, W., Gibson, M.G., Linsley, P.S., and Bluestone, J.A. 1992. Long-term survival of xenogeneic pancreatic islet grafts by CTLA4Ig. *Science* 257:789–792.
29. Schwartz, R.H. 1996. Models of T cell anergy: Is there a common molecular pathway. *J. Exp. Med.* 184:1–8.
30. Jenkins, M.K., and Schwartz, R.H. 1987. Antigen presentation by chemically modified splenocytes induces antigen-specific T cell unresponsiveness in vitro and in vivo. *J. Exp. Med.* 165:302–308.

31. Quill, H., and Schwartz, R.H. 1987. Stimulation of normal inducer T cell clones with antigen presented by purified Ia molecules in planar lipid membranes: specific induction of a long-lived state of proliferation nonresponsiveness. *J. Immunol.* 183:3704–3712.

32. Kang, S., Beverly, B., Tran, A., Brorson, K., Schwartz, R.H., and Lenardo, M.J. 1992. Transactivation by AP-1 is a molecular target of T cell clonal anergy. *Science* 257:1134–1136.

33. Harding, F.A., McArthur, J.G., Gross, G.A., Raulet, D.H., and Allison, J.P. 1992. CD-28 mediated signaling co-stimulates murine T cells and prevents induction of anergy in T cell clones. *Nature* 356:607–609.

34. Groux, H., Bigler, M., de Vries, J.E., and Roncarolo, M.G. 1996. Interleukin-10 induces a long-term antigen-specific anergic state in human CD4+ T cells. *J. Exp. Med.* 184:19–29.

35. Sloan-Lancaster, J., Evavold, B.D., and Allen, P.M. 1993. Induction of T cell anergy by altered T-cell-receptor ligand on liver antigen-presenting cells. *Nature* 363:156–159.

36. Green, D.R., and Scott, D.W. 1994. Activation-induced apoptosis in lymphocytes. *Curr. Opin. Immunol.* 6:476–487.

37. Kabelitz, D., Phol, T., and Pechhold, K. 1995. T cell apoptosis triggered via the CD3/T cell receptor complex and alternative activation pathways. *Curr. Top. Microbiol. Immunol.* 200:1–14.

38. Kawabe, Y., and Ochi, A. 1991. Programmed cell death and extrathymic reduction of Vβ8+ CD4+ T cells in mice tolerant to Staphylococcus aureus enterotoxin B. *Nature* 349:245–247.

39. Webb, S., Morris, C., and Sprent, J. 1990. Extrathymic tolerance of mature T cells: clonal elimination as a consequence of immunity. *Cell* 63:1249–1256.

40. Huang, L., and Crispe, I.N. 1993. Superantigen-driven peripheral deletion of T cells: apoptosis occurs in cells that have lost the α/β T cell receptor. *J. Immunol.* 151:1844–1851.

41. Rocha, B., and von Boehmer, H. 1992. Peripheral selection of the T cell repertoire. *Science* 251:1225–1228.

42. Mamalaki, C., Tanaka, Y., Corbella, P., Chandler, P., Simpson, E., and Kioussis, D. 1993. T cell deletion follows chronic antigen specific T cell activation in vivo. *Int. Immunol.* 5:1285–1292.

43. Liblau, R.S., Tisch, R., Shokat, K., Yang, X., Dumont, N., Goodnow, C.C., and McDevitt, H.O. 1996. Intravenous injection of soluble antigen induces thymic and peripheral T-cell apoptosis. *Proc. Natl. Acad. Sci. U.S.A.* 93:3031–3036.

44. Miethke, T., Wahl, C., Heeg, K., and Wagner, H. 1995. Superantigens: the paradox of T-cell activation versus inactivation. *Int. Arch. Allergy. Immunol.* 106:3–7.

45. Kyburz, D., Aichele, P., Speiser, D.E., Hengartner, H., Zinkernagel, R.M., and Pircher, H. 1993. T cell immunity after a viral infection versus T cell tolerance induced by soluble viral peptides. *Eur. J. Immunol.* 23:1956–1962.

46. Huang, L., Soldevila, G., Leeker, M., Flavell, R., and Crispe, I.N. 1994. The liver eliminates T cells undergoing antigen-triggered apoptosis in vivo. *Immunity* 1:741–749.

47. Singer, G.G., and Abbas, A.K. 1994. The FAS antigen is involved in peripheral but not thymic deletion of T lymphocytes in T cell receptor transgenic mice. *Immunity* 1:365–372.

48. Sytwu, H.K., Liblau, R.S., and McDevitt, H.O. 1996. The roles of Fas/APO-1 (CD95) and TNF in antigen-induced programmed cell death in T-cell receptor transgenic mice. *Immunity* 5:17–30.

49. Nagata, S., and Suda, T. 1995. Fas and Fas ligand: *lpr* and *gld* mutations. *Immunol. Today* 16:39–43.

50. Ju, S.T., Panka, D.J., Cui, H., Ettinger, R., El-Khatib, M., Sherr, D.H., Stanger, B.Z., and Marshak-Rothstein, A. 1995. Fas (CD95)/FasL interactions required for programmed cell death after T-cell activation. *Nature* 373:444–448.

51. Boshell, M., McLeod, J., Walker, L., Hall, N., Patel, Y. and Sansom, D. 1996. Effects of antigen presentation on superantigen-induced apoptosis mediated by Fas/Fas ligand interactions in human T cells. *Immunology* 87:586–592.

52. Watanabe-Fukunaga, R., Brannan, C.I., Copeland, N.G., Jenkins, N.A., and Nagata, S. 1992. Lymphoproliferation disorder in mice explained by defects in Fas antigen that mediates apoptosis. *Nature* 356:314–356.

53. Takahashi, T., Tanaka, M., Brannan, C.I., Jenkins, N.A., Copeland, N.G., and Nagata, S. 1994. Generalized lymphoproliferative disease in mice, caused by a point mutation in the Fas ligand. *Cell* 76:969–976.

54. Scott, D.E., Kisch, W.J., and Steinberg, A.D. 1993. Studies of T cell deletion and T cell anergy following in vivo administration of SEB to normal and lupus-prone mice. *J. Immunol.* 150:664–672.

55. Schonrich, G., Kalinke, U., Momberg, F., Malissen, M., Schmitt-Verhulst, A.-M., Malissen, B., Hammerling, G.J., and Arnold, B. 1991. Downregulation of T cell receptors on self-reactive T cells as a novel mechanism for extrathymic tolerance induction. *Cell* 65:293–304.

56. Miethke, T., Wahl, C., Gaus, H., Heeg, K., and Wagner, H. 1994. Exogenous superantigens acutely trigger distinct levels of peripheral tolerance/immunosuppression: dose-response relationship. *Eur. J. Immunol.* 24:1893–1900.

57. Mori, T., Nishikawa, K., Saito, S., Enomoto, M., Ito, A., Kurai, N., Shimoyama, T., Ichijo, M., and Narita, N. 1993. T-cell receptors are expressed but down-regulated on intradecidual T lymphocytes. *Am. J. Reprod. Immunol.* 29:1–4.

58. Ferber, I., Schonrich, G., Schenkel, J., Mellor, A., Hammerling, G., and Arnold, B. 1994. Levels of peripheral T cell tolerance induced by different doses of tolerogen. *Science* 263:674–676.

59. Itoh, H., Abo, T., Sugawara, S., Kanno, A., and Kumagai, K. 1988. Age-related variation in the proportion and activity of murine liver natural killer cells and their cytotoxicity against regenerating hepatocytes. *J. Immunol.* 141:315.

60. Huang, L., Sye, K., and Crispe, I.N. 1993. Proliferation and apoptosis of B220+CD4-CD8-TCRα/β^{int} T cells in the liver of normal adult mice: implication for *lpr* pathogenesis. *Int. Immunol.* 6:533–540.

61. Hata, K., Zhang, X.R., Iwatsuki, S., Van Thiel, D., Herberman, R.B., and Whiteside, T. 1990. Isolation, phenotyping and functional analysis of lymphocytes from human liver. *Clin. Immunol. Immunopathol.* 56:401–419.

62. Seki, S., Kono, D.H., Balderas, R.S., and Theofilopoulos, A.N. 1994. Vβ repertoire of murine hepatic T cells: implication for selection of double negative $\alpha\beta$+ T cells. *J. Immunol.* 153:637–646.

63. Mosley, R.L., Styre, D., and Klein, J.R. 1990. Differentiation and functional maturation of bone marrow-derived intestinal epithelial T cells expressing membrane T cell receptor in athymic radiation chimeras. *J. Immunol.* 145:1369–1375.

64. Bioulac-Sage, P., Kupier, J., van Berkel, T.J.C., and Balabaud, C. 1996. Lymphocyte and macrophage populations in the liver. *Hepato-Gastrolenterology* 43:4–14.

65. Winnock, M., Lafon, M.E., Boulard, A., Ferrer, A.M., Saric, J., Dubuisson, L., Bioulac-Sage, P., and Balabaud, C. 1991. Characterization of liver-associated natural killer cells in patients with liver tumors. *Hepatology* 13:676–682.

66. Bouwens, L., Remels, L., Baeekeland, M., Van Bossuyt, H., and Wisse, E. 1987. Large granular lymphocytes or "pit cells" from rat liver: isolation, ultrastructural characterization and natural killer activity. *Eur. J. Immunol.* 17:37–42.

67. Ohteki, T., Seki, S., Abo, T., and Kumagai, K. 1990. Liver is a possible site for the proliferation of abnormal CD3+4-8- double-negative lymphocytes in autoimmune MRL-*lpr/lpr* mice. *J. Exp. Med.* 172:7–12.

68. MacDonald, H.R. 1995. NK1.1+ T cell receptor-a/b+ cells: new clues to their origin, specificity, and function. *J. Exp. Med.* 182:633–638.

69. Coffman, R.L., and Weissman, I.V. 1981. B220: a B cell specific member of T220 glycoprotein family. *Nature* 289:681–683.

70. Watanabe, Y., and Akaike, T. 1994. Activation signal induces the expression of B cell-specific CD45R epitope (6B2) on murine T cells. *Scand. J. Immunol.* 39:419–425.

71. Guehler, S.R., Bluestone, J., and Barrett, T.A. 1996. Immune deviation of 2C transgenic intraepithelial lymphocytes in antigen-bearing hosts. *J. Exp. Med.* 184:493–503.

72. De Bruijn, M.L., Peterson, P.A., and Jackson, M.R. 1996. Induction of heat-stable antigen expression by phagocytosis is involved in in vitro activation of unprimed CTL by macrophages. *J. Immunol.* 156:2686–2692.

73. Giese, T., and Davidson, W.F. 1995. The accumulation of B220+CD4-CD8- (DN) T cells in C3H-lpr/lpr mice is not accelerated by the stimulation of CD8+ cells or B220+ DN T cells with staphylococcal enterotoxin B and occurs independently of Vbeta8+ T cells. *Int. Immunol.* 7:1213–1223.

74. Ballas, Z.K., and Rasmussen, W. 1993. Lymphokine-activated killer cells. VII. IL-4 induces an NK1.1+CD8α+β– TCR-α/β B220+ lymphokine-activated killer subset. *J. Immunol.* 150:17–30.

75. Koyasu, S. 1994. CD3+CD16+NK1.1+B220+ large granular lymphocytes arise from both α/βTCR+CD4-CD8- and γ/δTCR+CD4-CD8- cells. *J. Exp. Med.* 179:1957–1972.

76. Davidson, W.F., Dumont, F.J., Bedigian, H.G., Fowlkes, B.J., and Morse, H.C., III. 1986. Phenotypic, functional, and molecular genetic comparisons of the abnormal lymphoid cells of C3H-lpr/lpr and C3H-gld/gld mice. *J. Immunol.* 136:4075–4084.

77. Dixon, F.J. 1987. Basic elements of murine systemic lupus erythematosus. *J. Rheumatol.* 14:3.

78. Theofilopoulos, A.N., and Dixon, F.J. 1985. Murine models of systemic lupus erythyematosus. *Adv. Immunol.* 37:269–390.

79. Gillette-Ferguson, I., and Sidman, C.L. 1994. A specific intercellular pathway of apoptotic cell death is defective in the mature peripheral T cells of autoimmune lpr and gld mice. *Eur. J. Immunol.* 24:1181–1185.

80. Zanders, E.D., Lamb, J.R., Feldman, M., Green, N., and Beverley, P.C.L. 1983. Tolerance of T-cell clones is associated with membrane antigen changes. *Nature* 303:625–627.

81. Boyer, C., Auphan, N., Luton, F., Malburet, J.M., Barad, M., Bizozzero, J.P., Reggio, H., and Schmitt-Verhulst, A.M. 1991. T cell receptor (CD3) complex internalization following activation of a cytotoxic T cell clone: evidence for a protein kinase C-dependent staurosporine-sensitive step. *Eur. J. Immunol.* 21:1623–1634.

82. Valitutti, S., Muller, S., Dessing, M., and Lanzavecchia, A. 1996. Different responses are elicited in cytotoxic T lymphocytes by different levels of T cell receptor occupancy. *J. Exp. Med.* 183:1917–1921.

83. Hughes, D.P.M., and Crispe, I.N. 1995. A naturally occurring soluble isoform of murine fas generated by alternative splicing. *J. Exp. Med.* 182:1395–1401.

84. Boehme, S.A., and Lenardo, M.J. 1993. Propriocidal apoptosis of mature T lymphocytes occurs at S phase of the cell cycle. *Eur. J. Immunol.* 23:1552–1556.

85. Nishioka, W., and Welsh, R. 1994. Susceptibility to cytotoxic T lymphocyte-induced apoptosis is a function of the proliferative status of the target. *J. Exp. Med.* 179:769–774.

86. Lukomska, B., Pienkowska, B., Andrzejewski, W., and Olszewski, W. L. 1991. Liver sinusoidal cytotoxic cells are recruited from blood and divide locally. *J. Hepatol.* 12:332–335.

87. Ettinghausen, S.E., Lipford, E.H., Mule, J.J., and Rosenberg, R.A. 1985. Systemic administration of recombinant interleukin 2 stimulates in vivo lymphoid cell proliferation in tissues. *J. Immunol.* 135:1488–1497.

88. Wack, A., Corbella, P., Harker, N., Crispe, I.N., and Kioussis, D. 1997. Multiple sites of post-activation CD8+ T cell disposal. *Eur. J. Immunol.* 27:577–583.

89. Bouwens, L., Marinelli, A., and Kuppen, P.J.K. 1990. Electron microscopic observation on the accumulation of large granular lymphocytes (pit cells) and Kupffer cells in the liver of rats treated with continuous infusion of interleukin-2. *Hepatology* 12:1365–1370.

90. Tiegs, G., Hentschel, J., and Wendel, A. 1992. A T cell-dependent experimental liver injury in mice inducible by concanavalin A. *J. Clin. Invest.* 90:196–203.

91. Abo, T., Ohteki, T., Seki, S., Koyamada, N., Yoshikai, Y., Masuda, T., Rikiishi, H., and Kumagai, K. 1991. The appearance of T cells bearing self-reactive T cell receptor in the livers of mice injected with bacteria. *J. Exp. Med.* 174:417.

92. Matsuzaki, G., Li, X., Kadena, T., Song, F., Hiromatsu, K., Yoshida, H., and Nomoto, K. 1995. Early appearance of T cell receptor α/β+ CD4-CD8- T cells with a skewed variable region repertoire after infection with *Listeria monocytogenes*. *Eur. J. Immunol.* 25:1985–1991.

93. Seki, S., Abo, T., Sugiura, K., Ohteki, T., Kobata, T., Yagita, H., Okumura, K., Rikiishi, H., Osuda, T.M., and Kumagai, K. 1991. Reciprocal T cell response in the liver and thymus of mice injected with syngeneic tumor cells. *Cell Immunol.* 137:46–55.

94. Strickland, D., Kees, U.R., and Holt, P.G. 1996. Regulation of T-cell activation in the lung: isolated lung T cells exhibit surface phenotypic characteristics of recent activation including down-modulated T-cell receptors, but are locked into the G0/G1 phase of the cell cycle. *Immunology* 87:242–249.

95. Cantrell, D.A., Verbi, W., Davies, A., Parker, P., and Crumpton, M.J. 1988. Evidence that protein C kinase differentially regulates the human T lymphocyte CD2 and CD3 surface antigens. *Eur. J. Immunol.* 18:1931–1940.

96. Bodo, I., Vloka, J.D., and Cleveland, W.L. 1993. CD4 but not CD8 is comodulated with the T-cell antigen receptor (TCR) after activation of a CD4+CD8+ human leukemia line with staphylococcal enterotoxin. *Immunol. Lett.* 37:53–62.

97. Erard, F., Wild, M.T., Garcia-Sanz, J.A., and le Gros, G. 1993. Switch of CD8+ T cells to noncytolytic CD4-CD8- cells that make Th2 cytokines and help B cells. *Science* 260:1802–1805.

98. Kawakami, K., Teruya, K., Tohyama, M., Kudeken, N., Yonamine, Y., and Saito, A. 1995. Mac1 discriminates unusual CD4-CD8- double-negative T cells bearing α/β antigen re-

ceptor from conventional ones with either CD4 of CD8 in murine lung. *Immunol. Lett.* 46:143–152.

99. Faure, P., Marussig, M., Gossens, P., Miltgen, F., and Mazier, D. 1994. Characterization of liver lymphomyeloid cells in mice infected with Plasmodium yoelli sporozoites. *Immunology* 82:645–650.
100. Valitutti, S., Muller, S., Cella, M., Padovan, E., and Lanzavechia, A. 1995. Serial triggering of many T cell receptors by a few peptide-MHC complexes. *Nature* 375:148–151.
101. Viola, A., and Lanzavecchia, A. 1996. T cell activation determined by T cell receptor number and turnable thresholds. *Science* 273:104–106.
102. Seki, S., Abo, T., Ohteki, T., Sugiura, K., and Kumagai, K. 1991. Unusual α/β-T cells expanded in autoimmune lpr mice are probably a counterpart of normal T cells in the liver. *J. Immunol.* 147:1214–1221.
103. Iiai, T., Watanabe, S., Seki, S., Sugiura, K., Hirokawa, K., Utsuyama, M., Takahashi-Iwanaga, H., Iwanaga, T., Ohteki, T., and Abo, T. 1992. Ontogeny and development of extrathymic T cells in mouse liver. *Immunology* 77:556–563.
104. Sato, K., Ohtsuka, K., Hasegawa, K., Yamagiwa, S., Watanabe, H., Asakura, H., and Abo, T. 1995. Evidence for extrathymic generation of intermediate T cell receptor cells in the liver revealed in thymectomized, irradiated mice subjected to bone marrow transplantation. *J. Exp. Med.* 182:759–769.
105. Makino, Y., Yamagata, N., Sasho, T., Adachi, Y., Kanno, R., Koseki, H., Kanno, M., and Taniguchi, M. 1993. Extrathymic development of Vα14-positive T cells. *J. Exp. Med.* 177:1399.
106. Crispe, I.N., and Huang, L. 1994. Neonatal, moribund and undead T cells: the role of the liver in T cell development. *Semin. Immunol.* 6:39–41.
107. Poussier, P., and Julius, M. 1994. Thymus independent T cell development and selection in the intestinal epithelium. *Annu. Rev. Immunol.* 12:521–553.
108. Ohtsuka, K., Iiai, T., Watanabe, H., Tanaka, T., Miyasaka, M., Sato, K., Asakura, H., and Abo, T. 1994. Similarities and differences between extrathymic T cells residing in mouse liver and intestine. *Cell. Immunol.* 153:52–66.
109. Ohtsuka, K., Hasegawa, K., Sato, K., Arai, K., Watanabe, H., Asakura, H., and Abo, T. 1994. A similar expression pattern of adhesion molecules between intermediate TCR cells in the liver and intraepithelial lymphocytes in the intestine. *Microbiol. Immunol.* 38:677–683.
110. Hughes, D.P.M., Hayday, A., Craft, J.E., Owen, M.J., and Crispe, I.N. 1995. T cells with γ/δ T cell receptor (TCR) of intestinal type are preferentially expanded in TCR-α-deficient lpr mice. *J. Exp. Med.* 182:233–241.
111. van Houten, N., and Budd, R.C. 1992. Accelerated programmed cell death of MRL-*lpr*/*lpr* lymphocytes. *J. Immunol.* 149:2513–2517.
112. Ashwell, G., and Harford, J. 1982. Carbohydrate-specific receptors of the liver. *Ann. Rev. Biochem* 51:531–554.
113. Dini, L., Autuori, F., Lentini, A., Oliverio, S., and Piacentini, M. 1992. The clearance of apoptotic cells in the liver is mediated by the asialoglycoprotein receptor. *FEBS Lett.* 296:174–178.
114. Springer, T.A. 1994. Traffic signals for lymphocyte recirculation and leukocyte emigration: a multistep paradigm. *Cell* 76:301–305.

115. Morita, M., Watanabe, Y., and Akaike, T. 1994. Inflammatory cytokines up-regulate intercellular adhesion molecule-1 expression on primary cultured mouse hepatocytes and T-lymphocyte adhesion. *Hepatology* 19:426–431.

116. Picker, L.J., and Butcher, E.C. 1992. Physiologic and molecular mechanisms of lymphocyte homing. *Annu. Rev. Immunol.* 10:561–591.

117. Steinhoff, G., Behbrend, M., Schrader, M., Duijvestijn, A.M., and Wonigeit, K. 1993. Expression patterns of leukocyte adhesion ligand molecules on human liver endothelia-lack of ELAM-1 and CD62 inducibility on sinusoidal endothelia and distinct distribution of VCAM-1, ICAM-1, ICAM-2 and LFA-3. *Am. J. Path.* 142:481–488.

118. Volpes, R., van den Oord, J.J., and Desmet, V.J. 1992. Vascular adhesion molecules in acute and chronic liver disease. *Hepatology* 15:269–275.

119. McNab, G., Reeves, J.L., Salmi, M., Hubscher, S., Sirpa, J., and Adams, D.A. 1996. Vascular adhesion protein 1 mediates binding of T cells to human hepatic endothelium. *Gastroenterology* 110:522–528.

120. Crispe, I.N. 1994. Fatal interactions: Fas-induced apoptosis of mature T cells. *Immunity* 1:1–3.

121. Perillo, N.L., Pace, K.E., Seihamer, J.J., and Baum, L.G. 1995. Apoptosis of T cells mediated by galectin-1. *Nature* 378:736–739.

122. Kazansky, D.B., Agranovich, I.V., Azhipa, O.Y., Shtil, A.A., Anosova, N.G., Chernyshova, A.D., and Brondz, B.D. 1995. Immunosuppressive factor from liver induces apoptosis in thymoma EL-4 cells but not normal MHC class II-specific T lymphocytes. *Immunol. Lett.* 45:5–11.

123. Suss, G., and Shortman, K. 1996. A subclass of dendritic cells kills CD4 T cells via Fas/Fas-ligand induced apoptosis. *J. Exp. Med.* 183:1789–1796.

124. Gold, R., Schmied, M., Tontsch, U., Hartung, H.P., Wekerle, H., Toyka, K.V., and Lassmann, H. 1996. Antigen presentation by astrocytes primes rat T lymphocytes for apoptotic cell death: a model for T-cell apoptosis in vivo. *Brain* 119:651–659.

125. Calne, R.Y., Sells, R.A., Pena, J.R., and Davis, D.R. 1969. Induction of immunological tolerance by liver allografts. *Nature* 223:472–476.

126. Starzl, T.E., Marchioro, T.L., Porter, K.A., Taylor, P.D., Faris, T.D., Herrmann, T.J., Hlad, C.J., and Waddell, W.R. 1965. Factors determining short- and long-term survival after orthotopic liver homotransplantation in the dog. *Surgery* 58:131–155.

127. Murase, N., Demetris, A.J., Kim, D.G., Todo, S., Fung, J.J., and Starzl, T.E. 1990. Rejection of the multivisceral allograft in rats: a sequential analysis with comparison to isolated orthotopic small bowel and liver grafts. *Surgery* 108:880–890.

128. Kamada, N., Davies, H.F.F.S., and Roser, B. 1981. Reversal of transplantation immunity by liver grafting. *Nature* 292:840–842.

129. Valdivia, L.A., Fung, J.J., Demetris, A.J., and Starzl, T.E. 1991. Differential survival of hamster-to-rat liver and cardiac xenografts under FK506 immunosuppression. *Transplant Proc.* 23:3269–3271.

130. Qian, S., Demetris, A.J., Murase, N., Rao, A.S., Fung, J.J., and Starzl, T.E. 1994. Murine liver allograft transplantation: tolerance and donor cell chimerism. *Hepatology* 19:916–924.

CHAPTER 3

γδ CELLS ARE ACTIVE IN THE LIVER

L. WEN
Yale University School of Medicine, New Haven, CT

Y. MA and D. VERGANI
King's College Medical School, London, United Kingdom

A. C. HAYDAY
Yale University, New Haven, CT

INTRODUCTION

Weighing over 1 kg in humans, the liver is the largest solid organ in the body. It has a dual blood supply—the hepatic artery and the hepatic portal vein that forms from the mesenteric and splenic veins. The total liver blood flow is about one quarter of the resting cardiac output. The liver acts akin to a large biochemical factory, synthesizing and metabolizing a vast number and array of specialized proteins, carbohydrates, and lipids. It is also a major excretory pathway for large and particularly hydrophobic metabolites, foreign substances, and many drugs.

Conceptually, the lavish blood supply, the linkage to the gut, and the handling of large amounts of foreign materials might establish a special role for the liver in immunity. In reality, the immune status of the liver has proved a contentious area for many years, and we remain largely uncertain of the phenotypes and functions of lymphocyte populations that are genuinely localized to the liver. Interestingly, some of the information that we have about lymphocytes in the liver has been provided by studies of γδ T cells, a third class of lymphocyte after B cells and αβ T cells, that is conserved in all vertebrate immune systems studied to date. While that information has so far failed to clarify the origins, antigen specificities, and long-term fate of γδ T cells in the liver, it has nonetheless strongly indicated that γδ T cells are functionally active in the liver. Experiments that implicate hepatic γδ cells in the regulation of transplant rejection, autoimmune liver disease, liver infection, and liver malignancy are the focus of this brief review. These broad activities of γδ T cells confirm that an improved understanding of liver T cells is likely to provide useful and important information with regard to liver pathophysiology.

T Lymphocytes in the Liver: Immunobiology, Pathology, and Host Defense, Edited by I. Nicholas Crispe
ISBN 0-471-19218-X

EXTRATHYMIC γδ T CELL DEVELOPMENT

Of one thing we are certain: the liver acts as a major source of lymphocytes. In mice, both T and B lymphocytes derive from fetal liver hematopoietic stem cells up until approximately 2 days postpartum. Humans, by contrast, are viewed as being born more "immunologically mature," and the switchover from liver-derived to bone-marrow-derived progenitors occurs during fetal ontogeny. From either site of ontogeny, T cell precursors migrate at a very early stage of development to the thymus, where the specialized microenvironment facilitates critical T cell maturation events, including T cell receptor gene rearrangement and selection events (1), before the cells emigrate to recirculate as mature T cells from the bloodstream through peripheral lymphoid tissues.

Although the majority of T cells require the specialized thymic environment for maturation and selection, the possibility has for some time been raised that some "T cells" might complete their maturation in the liver. Numerous observations underlie this suggestion. For example, primitive chordates such as hagfish are claimed to develop an adaptive cellular immune system in the absence of an overt thymus. In addition, it is clear that some T cell populations develop in athymic animals such as the *nude* mouse (2–4). Because such T cell populations seem to be enriched in subsets of γδ cells (5,6), it has been considered for some time that γδ T cells might complete their development in the liver.

There were attractive components to this idea. First, many subsets of γδ T cells develop early in fetal ontogeny when hematopoiesis in the liver is active (5–7). Second, the majority of γδ cells are "double negative" (DN) cells, expressing neither CD4 nor CD8 coreceptors. Consistent with this they rarely if ever recognize processed peptide antigen presented by polymorphic class I and class II major histocompatibility complex (MHC) molecules (8–10). Not surprisingly then, γδ cells do not undergo MHC-dependent selection events of the kind that are critical to the development of $CD4^+$ and $CD8^+$ αβ T cells (11). Hence, it can be fairly argued that γδ cell maturation has less dependence than conventional αβ T cells on the specialized anatomy of the thymus. (The same might be proposed for rare subsets of mature αβ T cells, that are also DN, and that may not recognize primarily peptide antigens presented by MHC molecules).

Data seemingly supportive of liver T cell development have been provided by numerous studies, including our own detection of T cell receptor (TCR) V_γ-J_γ gene rearrangements in the livers of fetal mice prior to the development of the thymus (6). Likewise, liver samples from humans and from athymic mice show expression of recombinase activating genes (RAG-1 and RAG-2) responsible for antigen receptor gene rearrangements, and of preTα, a surrogate TCR α chain gene that is implicated solely in T cell development (12). Moreover, T cells, including γδ T cells, can be isolated from the fetal liver.

These data notwithstanding, there exists little substantial evidence linking liver γδ T cells to the "developmental observations" of gene rearrangement, RAG gene expression, and preTα expression, and it remains plausible that the latter observations reflect nothing other than abortive attempts at T cell development. At the same time, studies of other sites of extrathymic T cell development have continued, and by now the consensus is that in species where T cells can develop extrathymically, the cells most likely complete their maturation in the gut and possibly the skin, rather than in the liver (13–15). Those arguments have been laid out previously in other reviews (16–19). In summary, there is as yet no clear evidence that subsets of γδ T cells develop from start to finish in the liver of either fetal or adult animals (20).

THE PECULIAR LOCALIZATIONS OF MATURE γδ T CELLS IN ADULT ANIMALS

αβ T cells can be distinguished from γδ T cells in numerous ways. Among these is anatomic localization. While αβ T cells comprise the major T cell compartment in the blood and lymphoid tissues, γδ T cells comprise a variable and usually low percentage of splenic and lymph node lymphocytes. Moreover, while splenic B cells and αβ T cells are mostly confined to the white pulp, splenic γδ T cells are "dotted" throughout the organ, in red and white pulp alike (21). Because lymphoid anatomy is such a critical component of lymphoid function, in particular antigen sampling, such observations on the localizations of γδ T cells have fueled speculation that γδ T cells reside within tissues to perform functions that are distinct from the conventional, pathogen-specific responses that physiologically define αβ T cells and B cells (22).

Such speculation has been further fueled by the study of intraepithelial lymphocytes (IELs), among which the representation of γδ T cells can be very high (1,5,7). This was first noticed in animals as widely diverged as chickens and mice, and in the latter, essentially all resident lymphocytes in the epidermis are $TCR\gamma\delta^{+}$ (23,24). Although there is great variability in the numbers of γδ T cells in epithelial sheets of humans (e.g., humans mostly lack resident epidermal T cells), the numbers of $\gamma\delta^{+}$ IELs in some individuals, under certain conditions, can be very high. Thus, γδ T cells dominate the gut IEL repertoire of humans suffering from celiac disease (CD), an allergic reaction in the gut to the ingestion of wheat gliadin, which develops a complicating autoimmune component (25–27). Moreover, biopsy specimens from individuals with CD show that the representation of γδ T cells in the epithelium far exceeds that in the adjoining systemic compartment, the lamina propria, that by contrast, is enriched in αβ T cells (25). Hence, the "epithelial-tropism" of γδ T cells is a phenomenon that is apparently conserved across a broad evolutionary span, and as such is a subject of much investigation.

The most extensive studies of $\gamma\delta^{+}$ IELs have been in the mouse, in which large numbers of γδ cells populate the skin, uterine, tongue, and intestinal epithelia, as well as the lung at or around birth (1,5,7). Given the "epithelial constitution" of the liver, there has naturally been much interest in whether the liver too is a site of a resident γδ T cell population. The data currently available do not dispell this possibility.

γδ T CELLS IN LIVER

Numerous studies in both adult mice and humans have shown that up to 30% of hepatic mononuclear cells may be $\gamma\delta^{+}$, whereas γδ T cells compose only a very small proportion of mononuclear cells detected in fetal liver. Consistent with this, it was noted both in humans and mice that soon after birth the number of hepatic γδ T cells can increase significantly (28–30). Parallel observations characterize the intestinal γδ T cell populations. The expanding hepatic γδ T cells have a lymphoblastic morphology, adhering to the sinusoidal endothelial cells, and when freshly isolated, they commonly show spontaneous proliferation in culture (28). These strong indications of biological activity have led to the proposal that antigen-mediated expansion in the postnatal period plays a major role for the elevation of the hepatic γδ T cells. This would in turn be consistent with the physiologic and anatomic features of liver described at the beginning of this chapter. Blood from the small intestine, traveling directly to the liver via the hepatic portal vein, is consequently rich in digested food products. The liver is also an early site of contact for ingested or invasive bacteria and toxic products derived from either microorganisms or chemical compounds that arrive from the gut.

Nonetheless, despite the seemingly intimate association between gut and liver, hepatic γδ T cells can be distinguished from the more widely studied intestinal intraepithelial γδ T cells. Indeed, in their somewhat limited phenotypic comparison of γδ T cells from within different organs (spleen, thymus, gut and liver), Sato et al. (31) found distinguishing organ-specific properties, as summarized in Table 3.1.

Many molecular characterizations of γδ TCR have revealed signatory V gene usages in different organs, such as Vγ5 with Vδ1 in the skin; Vγ6 with Vδ1 in the reproductive organs; Vγ7 or Vγ1 with Vδ4, Vδ5, or Vδ6 in the intestine; and Vγ4 or Vγ1 with Vδ4, Vδ5, or Vδ6 in the thymus, spleen and lymph nodes (1). The underlying biological reason for these distinct subsets of limited diversity has been a focus of controversy. However, recent studies from our own laboratory strongly indicate that γδ T cells expressing the "appropriate" TCR in a particular tissue are enriched *in situ* by contact with some type of selecting ligand (32). More specifically, we found that mutation of the Vγ5 gene, ordinarily used by almost all skin lymphocytes, results in the development of "replacement" skin γδ T cells, many of which continue to react with a clonotypic antibody ordinarily specific for conformational determinants on the $V\gamma5^+$ TCR of epidermal T cells. Hence, although the linear gene segment was disrupted, the TCR conformation was retained, compatible with selection of epithelial γδ T cells based on TCR-mediated interactions in the respective tissues. The "select-

TABLE 3.1 Phenotypic Characterization of γδ T Cells from Different Organs by Flow Cytometry

	Spleen	Thymus	Liver	Intestine
1. $IL\text{-}2R_\beta$*	+/–†	+/–	+	+/–
2. Nature of CD8 expression on γδ T cells	CD8αβ	CD8αβ	CD8αα	CD8αα
3. Representation of DN γδ cells compared to $CD8^+$ γδ cells	Many more	Many more	Similar numbers	Fewer

*Surface expression of IL-2 receptor β chain.

†Some positive and some negative.

ing antigens" may be derived either from exogenous agents (notably microorganisms), or (perhaps more likely) from endogenous antigens such as stress-induced proteins, low-molecular-weight phosphorylated moieties, or nucleotide derivatives, all of which have been shown to stimulate γδ T cells (33–36).

Complying with this paradigm, murine hepatic γδ Tcells appear to be enriched in cells bearing a particular TCR, in this case, Vγ1 with Vδ6 (34,37). Because this limited TCR usage is not an unique one, being shared with other subsets of γδ T cells in the thymus, the lymphoid circulation, and the gut, one cannot conclude that hepatic cells are unique, rather than infiltrates of subsets of γδ T cells from one or more other sites. Notwithstanding this, the observations that hepatic γδ T cells can be distinguished from other γδ T cell subsets by a combination of defined cellular and molecular criteria (Table 3.1) lay a foundation for the idea that, beginning shortly after birth, the liver may be an important anatomic site for the proliferation of a distinct subset of $\gamma\delta^+$ lymphocytes. This presents a valid and important area for further study.

A direct approach to such study would be to use clones of such hepatic γδ T cells, and/or the TCRs cloned therefrom, as reagents to determine the cells' antigen specificities. The potential reconciliation of such specificities with the physiology of the liver offers a promising way to understand the biology of at least one population of liver lymphocytes. Alternatively, the infiltration of a specific subset of γδ Tcells into the liver from other sites might reflect the imminent destruction of such cells after activation, a phenomenon that is considered elsewhere in this monograph. Whether or not the latter is true, a number of studies, reviewed below, indicate that liver γδ cells are biologically active.

IMMUNOREGULATION BY HEPATIC γδ CELLS

For decades, myriad observations have been interpreted as evidence for the existence of immunoregulatory (i.e., suppressor) T cells. The description of $CD4^+$ TR1 cells, that produce interleukin-10 (IL–10), and that downregulate immune responses is one recent such observation (38). Over the past 2 years, a number of independent studies have strongly indicated that γδ T cells *de facto* downregulate αβ T cell responses *in vivo*. For example, $TCR\delta^{-/-}$ mice responding to infection by a natural murine-tropic coccidial parasite of the gut show significantly enhanced immunopathology compared with the regulated response of normal, γδ-cell bearing mice (39). Entirely consistent with this, the αβ T-cell-dependent autoimmune, lupus-like disease in MRL/lpr mice is significantly worsened in $TCR\delta^{-/-}$ variants of the same strain (40). Focusing on the αβ T cell response, itself, Kaufmann and colleagues reported that αβ T cells in mice depleted of γδ T cells by use of anti-γδ T cell monoclonal antibodies, showed uncharacteristically vigorous spontaneous proliferation and IL-2 production (41).

While the mechanism(s) by which γδ cells effect such regulation of αβ T cells remain(s) to be described, it is conceivable that at least some part is played by cytokine production. Thus, it has been well established that $CD4^{(+)}$ αβ T cells secretingT helper type 3 (Th2)-cytokines, such as IL–4 and IL–10, inhibit the development and function of αβ(⁺) Th1 cells that are responsible for T cell–mediated inflammatory responses. Moreover, the reverse also appears to be true. Since we and others have shown that clones of γδ cells can comply with the Th1 and Th2 paradigm (42), one can envisage down-regulation of αβ T cell responses by one or other type of γδ cell.

This issue has been examined with regard to hepatic γδ T cells by Gorczynski and his colleagues (43). They reported that mice primed with allogeneic lymphocytes via the portal vein showed significantly delayed rejection of subsequent allogeneic skin grafts. Similar delayed rejection was also observed if hepatic γδ T cells were used, via the tail vein, for priming (43). Delayed rejection was associated with preferential production of Th2-cytokines, such as IL-4 and IL-10. In a key observation, the investigators noted that treatment of the mice *in vivo* with anti-γδ TCR monoclonal antibodies abolished the increased graft survival and reversed the bias toward Th2-cytokine production (43–45). In short, these studies provide clear evidence for a regulatory capacity of γδ T cells in the liver.

Nonetheless, two important qualifications should probably be attached to these studies. First, not all hepatic γδ T cells are likely to be Th2 cells: indeed, our own studies have pointed to a predominance of Th1 γδ cells in the liver, mirroring a likely predominance of Th1 γδ cells over Th2 γδ cells in the lymphoid circulation (Wen and Hayday, unpublished data). Second, the immunoregulatory phenotype exerted by hepatic γδ cells may reflect a secondary consequence rather than the raison d'être of γδ T cell function. The primary function of the cells may be to respond with a particular effector function to as-yet-unelucidated ligands, as a secondary result of which, coincident αβ T cell responses may be downregulated, directly or indirectly, by the particular cytokines produced by the effector γδ cells.

This view readily accommodates the evidence that γδ T cells can both downregulate and promote immune responses. For example, while the autoimmune, lupus-like disease in γδ T cell–deficient MRL/lpr mice is more severe than that in γδ-bearing littermates, γδ T cells can also promote autoimmunity, measured both by the development of autoreactive immunoglobulin G (IgG) in αβ T cell–deficient MRL/lpr mice (46), and by the direct functional interactions of γδ T cells and B cells both *in vivo*, and *in vitro* (42,46–48). Hence, under different circumstances, yet to be defined, γδ T cells can be seen as either regulating or promoting autoimmune disease. Such considerations apply to the involvement of γδ T cells in autoimmune liver disease.

HEPATIC γδ T CELLS IN AUTOIMMUNITY

Autoimmune liver disorders are a group of self-perpetuating diseases with inflammation of either intra- and extrahepatic bile ducts (such as primary sclerosing cholangitis, PSC, and primary biliary cirrhosis, PBC), or hepatocytes (such as chronic active hepatitis, CAH). Inflammation is followed by cirrhosis, and eventually liver failure. Patients with PSC and CAH also exhibit hypergammaglobulinemia, with high titers of both organ-specific and non-organ-specific autoantibodies (49–52). As with essentially all autoimmune diseases, the etiology of autoimmune liver disease is unelucidated, and may feature a microbial component. Indeed, nearly 70% of patients with

PSC also suffer from inflammatory bowel disease, a severe and chronic inflammation primarily of the colon, that almost certainly has a microbial component to its etiology. Furthermore, a significant fraction of patients with CAH additionally suffer from autoimmune thyroiditis. These observations suggest that in both examples of autoimmune liver disease, a dysregulation of lymphocytes in the liver is one component of a more generalized susceptibility to organ-specific autoimmunity. By this view, the targeting of the liver in both cases may reflect damage to the liver (for example inflicted by a pathogen or a toxin), the local immune response to which becomes deregulated because of genetic factors predisposing toward autoimmunity.

The notable histopathological feature of autoimmune liver disease is a heavy portal lymphocyte infiltrate, mainly comprising $CD3^+$ cells. Our studies have investigated the contribution of γδ T cells to such infiltrates. First, we reported that significantly increased levels of γδ T cells were present in the circulation of juvenile patients with autoimmune liver diseases, compared to control cohorts (53–55). The monoclonal antibodies BB3 and A13, that were used in the study, identify two distinct, non-overlapping subsets of γδ T cells that together represent essentially all γδ T cells in the peripheral blood of healthy individuals (53). BB3 recognizes disulphide-linked γδ TCR heterodimers that predominantly use the Cγ1/Vδ2 genes, whereas A13 identifies non-disulphide-linked γδ TCR heterodimers that employ the Cγ2/Vδ1 genes (56,57).

In the peripheral blood of healthy individuals, $BB3^+$ γδ T cells comprise over two thirds of the circulating γδ T cells, whereas the elevated γδ T cells in patients with autoimmune liver diseases are largely $A13^+$. This suggests that the $C\gamma2/V\delta1^+$ γδ T cells have undergone specific clonal expansion. Provocatively, the $A13^+$ subtype of γδ T cells is also overrepresented in the peripheral blood, synovial membrane and synovial fluid of rheumatoid arthritis patients (58–60), in the gastrointestinal tract of patients with CD (61,62), and in the circulation of HIV-infected individuals and AIDS patients (63–65). These findings suggest that under these various circumstances, there is a "TCR-ligand" specific activation of $A13^+$ γδ cells, in response to either endogenous stimuli, such as autoantigens, and/or exogenous stimuli, such as microbial antigens. Consistent with this, $A13^+$ γδ T cells, isolated from the blood of patients with autoimmune liver disease, expressed the activation marker, HLA-DR, and the memory-associated marker, $CD45R0^+$ (53). A more recent study by Martins et al. (55) described similar findings.

To characterize further the nature of γδ T cell involvement in autoimmune liver diseases, several hundred T cell clones were generated from both the peripheral blood and liver parenchyma of patients with autoimmune liver diseases. The use of IL-2 in the cloning protocol ensured that only cells actively involved in immune responses, and therefore expressing the IL-2 receptor (IL-2R), were expanded. The high frequency of $CD4^+$ αβ T cells among clones generated from peripheral blood reflects our previous report of an high percentage of $CD4^+$ αβ T cells among the $IL2\text{-}R^+$ population in the circulation of patients with autoimmune liver diseases (66). However, in contrast to the clones derived from the peripheral blood, a large proportion of clones derived from liver biopsies were either γδ T cells or $CD8^+$ αβ T cells (Fig. 3.1). Approximately 80% of the liver-derived γδ T cell clones were also $A13^+$, the non-disulphide-linked γδ TCR heterodimers, reflecting the high concentration of those cells found in the circulation of the same patients.

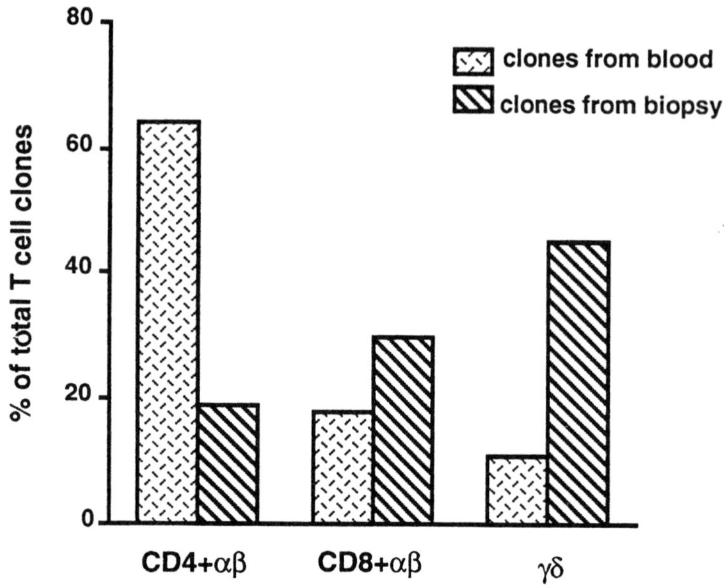

Figure 3.1. Phenotype distribution of T cell clones derived from peripheral blood and liver biopsis of patients with autoimmune liver disease. The surface phenotype of T cell clones was determined by two-colour cytofluorometric analysis using a FACScan (Becton Dickinson). The following monoclonal antibodies (mAbs) conjugated with fluorescein isothiocyanate (FITC) or phycoerythrin (PE) were used at the suggested manufacturer's concentrations in a direct immunofluorescence technique: anti-CD3, -CD4, -CD8, -TCR αβ, -TCR γδ (Becton Dickinson). An unrelated mAb, anti-keyhole limpet haemocyanin (Becton Dickinson), was used as negative control.

The reason for the conspicuous accumulation of $A13^+$ γδ T cells in the liver remains to be resolved. As we considered above, a spectrum of possibilities exist. It may reflect an antigen-driven expansion of resident hepatic γδ cells; it may reflect a functional spread into the liver of a subset of γδ cells initially activated at other sites; or it may reflect the imminent destruction of such cells, following hyperactivation at other sites. Nonetheless, the pathological features of autoimmune liver disease indicate that for some period of time, at least, the hepatic lymphocytes are active and causative of a liver cell destruction akin to cytolysis toward infected cell targets in conventional assays of immune function. Furthermore, the high representation of a subset of γδ T cells in the livers of patients with autoimmune liver disease is specific, since it is not seen under other circumstances, notably in liver biopsies either of liver transplant patients or individuals with chronic hepatitis virus B (HBV) infection (L. Wen and A. Hayday, unpublished data). The fact that virtually all the T cell clones generated from the liver of autoimmune liver disease patients express the memory marker CD45R0 on their surface is consistent with the proposal that the cells recognize antigens specific to this condition (as opposed to HBV infection) and are active *in situ*.

Consistent with this hypothesis, approximately one quarter of the cloned T cells tested, including γδ T cell clones, showed proliferative responses to liver membrane preparations. Blocking assays using monoclonal antibodies suggested that the γδ T cell clones, like the reactive αβ T cells, recognized the liver antigens via their respective TCR-CD3 complexes, and that the cells' manifest response to antigen recognition was dependent on an autocrine activity of IL-2 (L. Wen and A. Hayday, unpublished data).

Likewise, assessments of cytolytic activity of the T cell clones towards liver-derived and non-liver-derived cell lines demonstrated that γδ T cells preferentially lysed the liver derived target cells, suggesting that the target(s) of cytotoxicity is expressed, either solely or at higher density, on cells of liver origin (Fig. 3.2). The relatively strong reactivity of the γδ cell clones toward various targets, as opposed to the rather negligible activities αβ T cell clones, shown in Figure 3.2, most likely reflects an MHC-independence of the γδ T cells that is consistent with our general understanding of TCR γδ specificities, outlined at the beginning of this review (1,10). Currently, the TCRs of the γδ clones are being analyzed as a means of estimating the potential diversity of their antigen recognition. Early evidence, comparing one clone with another, suggests that the TCRs are polyclonal, rather than oligoclonal, but more extensive analyses are required before firm conclusions can be drawn. In summary, at least some cases of autoimmune liver disease are characterized by an enrichment for hepatic γδ T cells that show both recognition and biological activity toward liver cells.

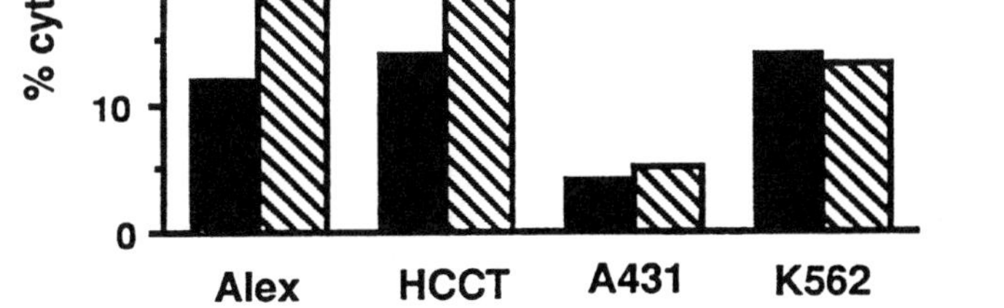

Figure 3.2. Cytolytic activity of αβ and γδ T cell clones derived from liver biopsis of patients with autoimune liver disease. Cytotoxicity was evaluated in a modified 4 hour ^{51}Cr-release assay. Four cell lines were used as target: Alexander and HCCT, human hepatoma cell lines, were used as organ-specific targets; A431, a human epithelial carcinoma was used as non-liver derived target and K562, a human erythroleukaemia cell line was employed as not only another non-liver derived target but also a natural killer (NK)-sensitive cell line. Cytotoxicity assays were performed at effector/target (E:T) ratio of 20:1, 10:1 and 5:1 and showed a linear response over the 3 ratios (data not shown). The intermediate 10:1 ratio was used in the Figure. Specific lysis was calculated according to the standard formula.

HEPATIC γδ T CELLS IN INFECTION

γδ T cells, particularly those stationed within epithelia, have been proposed by us and our colleagues to constitute the first line of defense against infection (22). This hypothesis has been tested recently, by use of mycobacteria, eubacteria, viruses, and protozoa to infect mutant mice that lack either γδ T cells, αβ T cells, or both. The clear consensus of these experiments is that αβ T cells are both necessary and sufficient to mount pathogen-specific protective responses (39,67). Nonetheless, another common finding seems to be that the immunodeficiency of mice that lack αβ T cells is less than that of mice that lack both αβ T cells and γδ T cells, clearly demonstrating that γδ T cells can respond to myriad infectious agents, and, as a result, provide a measure of immunoprotective effector function (39,67). The molecular interactions underlying such responses of γδ T cells are now the focus of much study. In this regard, one intensively studied system is the infection of mice by *Listeria monocytogenes*, an intracellular pathogen that replicates inside mononuclear phagocytes and hepatocytes of infected hosts.

Several reports have noted that absolute numbers of γδ T cells in the liver increase significantly following infection with *Listeria monocytogenes* (68–70). Moreover, Belles et al. (70) reported that the liver γδ T cell response showed a dose-dependent relationship to the titer of the infectious inoculum. At low doses of infection, the γδ T cell response occurred late in the course of the disease, while at higher doses, the response of hepatic γδ T cells was earlier and of greater magnitude.

A functional involvement of hepatic γδ T cells in the control of the immune response to *Listeria* was tested directly, both by use of antibody to deplete γδ T cells *in vivo* (68), and by use of gene-targeted γδ T cell–deficient mice (67). In the livers of mice lacking αβ T cells, bacteria grew to large numbers within hepatocytes, reflecting a serious deficiency in the immune response to infected cells. By contrast, the livers of mice lacking γδ T cells contained many extracellular bacteria. Most conspicuously, however, liver lesions in γδ T cell–deficient mice were far more extensive than those in either normal or αβ T cell–deficient mice (71). The most likely explanation for these data is that they manifest immunoregulation by hepatic γδ T cells. Ferrick and his colleagues (72,73) demonstrated that γδ T cells could "discriminate" between different pathogens early in infections, and, as a result, produce different cytokines (Th1 vs. Th2). Hence, as was discussed in the context of γδ T cell regulation of graft rejection, it is possible that the downregulatory effects of γδ T cells toward the immune response to *Listeria* are a secondary effect of the production by γδ T cells of a distinct set of effector cytokines in response to infection.

Such responses in the liver are not confined to *Listeria*. After infection by *Leishmania major*, expanded, actively cycling γδ T cells were found in both the lymph nodes and the liver (74). Together, these results strongly indicate that hepatic γδ T cells respond to infection, either *in situ*, or as infiltrates from other sites, and that the presence of such activated cells in the liver has clear phenotypic effects in the liver. Moreover, it is conceivable that the major effects of γδ T cells in the response to hepatocyte infection have not yet been accurately assessed, because the most appropriate animal model systems have not yet been employed.

HEPATIC γδ T CELLS IN MALIGNANCY

Inherent in the concept of tumor surveillance is the hypothesis that cells of the acquired and/or innate immune response recognize tumor cells in the early phase of malignancy and eliminate them. Putative "tumor antigens" are on the one hand, peptides derived from mutated or ectopically expressed autologous proteins, which are recognized by αβ T cells and, on the other hand, "activation" antigens, expressed by hyperactive cells, that might be recognized by γδ T cells. Such antigens might include heat shock proteins (hsps) (33); isopentenyl pyrophosphate and related intermediates in the farnosylation of activated *ras* proteins (36,75); ceramides and gangliosides that can be characteristic of transformed cells (76); and nucleotide derivatives used in purine and pyrimidine salvage pathways that characterize periods of very active DNA synthesis and cell division (35). There are established examples of γδ T cells responding to many of these antigens (10). Some myco-bacterial heat-shock proteins are strongly homologous to mammalian proteins, and γδ T cells reactive with the myco-bacterial proteins were able to respond to various tumor cells (77–83).

Consistent with the reactivity of γδ T cells toward tumor antigens, are the many reports that a significant portion of tumor-infiltrating lymphocytes (TILs) are γδ T cells (83–86). Moreover, those $\gamma\delta^+$ TILs usually exhibit strong cytolytic effects towards autologous tumor cells. Additionally, mice transgenic for a $V\gamma1^+$ TCR showed substantially increased resistance to various T cell leukemias (87), and some of our own work has contributed to finding that B cell lymphomagenesis is actively downregulated by γδ T cells *in vivo* (88).

In studying the potential involvement of hepatic γδ cells in tumor surveillance, Seki and colleagues (89) observed that livers obtained from cancer patients (gastric, intestinal, or pulmonary cancers) who had no apparent hepatic metastasis, contained a significantly larger proportion of hepatic γδ T cells. By morphologic appearance, these hepatic, tumor-associated γδ T cells were large lymphoblasts that proliferated spontaneously *in vitro*, whereas the bulk of γδ T cells harvested from other organs, such as spleen and peripheral blood, were small resting cells (89). When tumor cell lines were injected into laboratory mice, essentially the same findings were obtained (90). These results strongly indicate that the liver, in both human and murine systems, can act as a reservoir of activated γδ T cells with *de facto* tumor surveillance capacity in tumor-bearing hosts.

SUMMARY AND PERSPECTIVES

The study of hepatic γδ T cells can provide a fruitful pathway into liver lymphocyte function. We have reviewed a number of diverse, independent experimental studies in both humans and mice, that describe the presence in the liver of activated γδ T cells. In each species, hepatic γδ T cells comprise primarily a limited subset of γδ T cells that is significantly expanded under some but not all conditions of liver dysregulation. There is essentially no firm evidence that the liver γδ T cells developed *in situ* via a pathway of extrathymic T cell development in the liver, although this is difficult to rule out. More likely, the cells matured elsewhere and then either homed to the liver directly (to take up positions as resident hepatic lymphocytes) or infiltrated the liver following antigen-mediated activation in other anatomical sites, such as the spleen and gut. Possibly, such activated γδ T cells home to the liver, destined to be culled. Nonetheless, whatever the origin and long-term fate of such hepatic γδ T cells, the experiments that we have reviewed indicate that the cells can exert conspicuous immune effects while in the liver. Specifically, hepatic γδ T cells appear to regulate alloreactive and pathogen-reactive αβ T cell responses; exert an effector function in the development of autoimmune liver disease; and, possibly by the same mechanism, show antitumor activity. Thus, hepatic γδ T cells may either influence or be responsible for significant components of both liver immunity and liver pathophysiology. Therefore, increasingly detailed studies of the antigenic stimuli for hepatic γδ T cells, and of the cells' origins are a potentially effective approach to clarifying T cell function in the liver.

Given that the prime expansion of γδ T cells in the liver occurs shortly after birth, at a time when αβ T cell functions are still not fully developed, it is conceivable that the major immunoprotective functions of hepatic γδ T cells are most evident in newborn animals. Indeed, this may be equally true for other subsets of $\gamma\delta^+$ IELs. In all vertebrates examined, γδ T cells are disproportionately abundant in the neo- and perinatal periods (1,5–7). To test this hypothesis requires an improved animal model system, namely one in which infections and other challenges to the liver are undertaken and measured over the very first weeks of life. This is the period of the most extreme confrontation with the environment that any animal experiences. The host responses that are mounted during this period can then be compared for mice that either have or lack γδ T cells. By this means, the still-open possibility that there is an important resident population of immunoprotective γδ T cells in the liver will be tested.

ACKNOWLEDGMENTS

A.C.H. acknowledges support from the NIH (AI27855 and AI38932) and from the Yale Liver Center for a Pilot Project Grant. We thank our close colleagues for all sorts of help and support.

REFERENCES

1. Bell, J.I., Owen, M.J., and Simpson, E., eds. 1995. *T Cell Receptor*. Oxford, UK: Oxford University Press.
2. Pardoll, D., Fowlkes, B.J., Lew, A.M., Maloy, W.L., Weston, M.A., Bluestone, J.A., Schwartz, R.H., Coligan, J.E., and Kruisbeek, A.M. 1988. Thymus dependent and thymus independent developmental pathways for peripheral T cell receptor γδ-bearing lymphocytes. *J. Immunol.* 140:4091–4096.
3. Pereira, P., Gerber, D., Huang, S.Y., and Tonegawa, S. 1995. Ontogenetic development and tissue distribution of Vγ-1 expressing γδ T lymphocytes in normal mice. *J. Exp. Med.* 182:1921–1930.

4. Makino, Y., Yamagata, N., Sasho, T., et al. 1993. Extrathymic development of Valpha 14-positive T cells. *J. Exp. Med.* 177:1399–1408.
5. Haas, W., Pereira, P., and Tonegawa, S. 1993. γδ cells. *Annu. Rev. Immunol.* 11:637–685.
6. Carding, S.R., Kyes, S., Jenkinson, E., Kingston, R., Bottomly, K., Owen, J.J.T., and Hayday, A.C. 1990. Developmentally regulated fetal thymic and extrathymic expression of T cell receptor γδ gene expression. *Genes Dev.* 4:1304–1315.
7. Havran, W., and Allison, J.P. 1988. Developmentally ordered appearance of thymocytes expressing different T cell antigen receptors. *Nature* 335:443–445.
8. Brenner, M.B., McLean, J., Dialynas, D., Strominger, J.L., Smith, J.A., Owen, F.L., Seidman, J.G., Ip, S., Rosen, F., and Krangel, M.S. 1986. Identification of a putative second T cell receptor. *Nature* 322:145–149.
9. Jones, B., Carding, S., Kyes, S., Mjolsness, S., Janeway, C.A., and Hayday, A. 1988. Molecular analysis of T cell receptor gamma gene expression in allo-activated splenic T cells of adult mice. *Eur. J. Immunol.* 18:1907–1915.
10. Chien, Y.-H., Jores, R., and Crowley, M.P. 1996. Recognition by γδ T cells. *Annu. Rev. Immunol.* 14:511–532.
11. Passoni, L., Hoffman, E., Kim, S., Crompton, T., Pao, W., Dong, M.-Q., Owen, M.J., and Hayday, A.C. 1997. Intrathymic δ selection events in γδ T cell development. *Immunity* 7:83–95.
12. Bruno, L., Rocha, B., Rolink, A., von Boehmer, H., and Rodewald, H.-R. 1995. Intra- and extra-thymic expression of the preT cell receptor α gene. *Eur. J. Immunol.* 25:1877–1882.
13. Lynch, S., Kelleher, D., McManus, R., and O'Farrelly, C. 1995. Rag1 and Rag2 expression in human intestinal epithelium: Evidence of extrathymic T cell differentiation. *Eur. J. Immunol.* 25:1143–1147.
14. Kanamori, Y., Ishimaru, K., Nanno, M., Maki, K., Ikuta, K., Nariuchi, H., and Ishikawa, H. 1996. Identification of novel lymphoid tissues in murine intestinal mucosa where clusters of c-kit$^+$ IL7-R$^+$ Thy1$^+$ lymphohemopoietic progenitors develop. *J. Exp. Med.* 184:1449–1459.
15. Elbe, A., Kilgus, O., Strohal, R., Payer, E., Schreiber, S., and Stingl. G. 1992. Fetal skin: A site of dendritic epidermal T cell development. *J. Immunol.* 149:1694–1701.
16. Klein, J.R. 1995. T-lymphopoietic capacity of the mouse intestinal epithelium. *Semin. Immunol.* 7:291–297.
17. Lefrancois, L., and Puddington, L. 1995. Extrathymic intestinal T-cell development: Virtual reality? *Immunol. Today* 16:16–21.
18. Poussier, P., and Julius, M. 1994. Thymus independent T cell development and selection in the intestinal epithelium. *Ann. Rev. Immunol.* 12:521–553.
19. Hayday, A.C. 1993. Not in the thymus. *Curr. Biol.* 3:525–528.
20. Crispe, I.N., and Huang, L. 1994. Neonatal, moribund and undead T cells: The role of the liver in T cell development. *Semin. Immunol.* 6:39–41.
21. Bucy, P., Chen, C.L., Cihak, J., Loaxh, U., and Cooper, M.D. 1988. Avian T cells expressing γδ receptors localize in the splenic sinusoids and the intestinal epithelium. *J. Immunol.* 141:2200–2205.
22. Janeway, C.A., Jr., Jones, B., and Hayday, A.C. 1988. Specificity and function of T cells bearing γδ receptors. *Immunol. Today* 9:73–76.
23. Kuziel, W.A., Takashima, A., Bonyhadi, M., Bergstrasser, J., Allison, J.P., Tigelaar, R.E., and Tucker, P.W. 1987. Regulation of T cell receptor γ chain RNA expression in murine thy1(+) dendritic epidermal cells. *Nature* 328:263–266.

24. Stingl, G., Koning, F., Yamada, H., Yokoyama, W.M., Tschachler, E., Bluestone, J.A., Steiner, G., Samelson, L.E., Lew, A.M., Coligan, J.E., and Shevach, E.M. 1987. Thy1(+) dendritic epidermal cells express T3 antigen and the T cell receptor γ chain. *Proc. Natl. Acad. Sci. U.S.A.* 84:4586–4589.
25. Halstensen, T.S., Scott, H., and Brandtzaeg, P. 1989. Intraepithelial T cells of the TCR γδ (+) CD8(–) and Vδ1,Jδ1(+) phenotype are increased in coeliac disease. *Scand. J. Immunol.* 30:665–672.
26. Maki, M., Holm, K., Collin, P., Savilahti, E. 1991. Increase in γδ T cell receptor bearing lymphocytes in normal small bowel mucosa in latent coeliac disease. *Gut* 32:1412–1414.
27. Hayday, A.C., Roberts, S.J., and Smith, A.L. 1997. γδ cells in coeliac disease. In *Coeliac Disease*, Maki, M., Collin, P., Visakorpi, J.K., eds. Coeliac Disease Study Group.
28. Ohteki, T., Abo, T., Seki, S., et al. 1991. Predominant appearance of gamma/delta T lymphocytes in the liver of mice after birth. *Eur. J. Immunol.* 21:1733–1740.
29. Witherden, D.A., Kimpton, W.G., Abernethy, N.J., and Cahill, R.N. 1994. Changes in thymic export of gamma delta and alpha beta T cells during fetal and postnatal development. *Eur. J. Immunol.* 24:2329–2336.
30. Tsukahara, A., Seki, S., Iiai, T., et al. 1997. Mouse liver T cells: Their change with aging and in comparison with peripheral T cells. *Hepatology* 26:301–309.
31. Sato, K., Ohtsuka, K., Watanabe, H., Asakura, H., and Abo, T. 1993. Detailed characterization of gamma delta T cells within the organs in mice: Classification into three groups. *Immunology* 80:380–387.
32. Mallick-Wood, C.A., Lewis, J., Richie, L.I., Owen, M.J., Tigelaar, R.E., and Hayday, A.C. 1998. Conservation of T cell receptor conformation in epidermal γδ cells with disrupted primary Vγ gene usage. *Science* 279:1729–1733.
33. Haregewoin, A., Soman, G., Hom, R.C., and Finberg, R.W. 1989. Human gamma delta+ T cells respond to mycobacterial heat-shock protein. *Nature* 340:309–312.
34. Roark, C.E., Vollmer, M.K., Cranfill, R.L., Carding, S.R., Born, W.K., and O'Brien, R.L. 1993. Liver gamma delta T cells. TCR junctions reveal differences in heat shock protein-60-reactive cells in liver and spleen. *J. Immunol.* 150:4867–4875.
35. Constant, P., Davodeau, F., Peyrat, M.A., Poquet, Y., Puzo, G., Bonneville, M., and Fournie, J.J. 1994. Stimulation of human γδ T cells by nonpeptidic mycobacterial ligands. *Science* 264:267–270.
36. Tanaka, Y., Sano, S., Nieves, E., et al. 1994. Nonpeptide ligands for human gamma delta T cells. *Proc. Natl. Acad. Sci. U.S.A.* 91:8175–8179.
37. Kodaira, Y., Yokomuro, K., Tanaka, S., Miyazaki, J.I., and Ikuta, K. 1996. Developmental heterogeneity of V gamma 1.1 T cells in the mouse liver. *Immunology* 87:213–219.
38. Groux, H., O'Garra, A., Bigler, M., Rouleau, M., Antonenko, S., de Vries, J.E., and Roncarlo, M.G. 1997. A CD4(+) T cell subset inhibits antigen-specific T-cell responses and prevents colitis. *Nature* 389:737–742.
39. Roberts, S.J., Smith, A.L., West, A.B., Wen, L., Findly, R.C., Owen, M.J., and Hayday, A.C. 1996. T cell receptor αβ(+) and γδ(+) deficient mice display abnormal but distinct phenotypes toward a natural infection of the intestinal epithelium. *Proc. Natl. Acad. Sci. U.S.A.* 93:11774–11779.
40. Peng, S.L., Madaio, M.P, Hayday, A.C., and Craft, J. 1996. Propagation and regulation of systemic autoimmunity by γδ cells. *J. Immunol.* 157:5689–5698.

41. Kaufmann, S.H., Blum, C., and Yamamoto, S. 1993. Crosstalk between alpha/beta T cells and gamma/delta T cells in vivo: Activation of alpha/beta T-cell responses after gamma/delta T-cell modulation with the monoclonal antibody GL3. *Proc. Natl. Acad. Sci. U.S.A.* 90:9620–9624.

42. Wen, L., Barber, D.F., Pao, W., Wong, F.S., Owen, M.J., and Hayday, A. 1998. Primary γδ cell clones can be defined phenotypically and functionally as Th1/Th2 cells, and illustrate the association of CD4 with Th2 differentiation. *J. Immunol.* 160:1965–1974.

43. Gorczynski, R.M. 1994. Adoptive transfer of unresponsiveness to allogeneic skin grafts with hepatic gamma delta + T cells. *Immunology* 81:27–35.

44. Gorczynski, R.M., Chen, Z., Hoang, Y., and Rossi, B.B. 1996. A subset of gamma delta T-cell receptor-positive cells produce T-helper type-2 cytokines and regulate mouse skin graft rejection following portal venous pretransplant preimmunization. *Immunology* 87:381–389.

45. Gorczynski, R.M., Cohen, Z., Fu, X.M., Hua, Z., Sun, Y., and Chen, Z. 1996. Interleukin-13, in combination with anti-interleukin-12, increases graft prolongation after portal venous immunization with cultured allogeneic bone marrow-derived dendritic cells. *Transplantation* 62:1592–1600.

46. Wen, L., Roberts, S.J., Viney, J.L., Wong, F.S., Mallick, C., Peng, Q., Craft, J., Findly, R.C., Owen, M.J., and Hayday, A.C. 1994. Immunoglobulin synthesis and generalised autoimmunity in mice congenitally deficient in αβ T cells. *Nature* 369:654–658.

47. Wen, L., Pao, W., Wong, F.S., Peng, Q., Craft, J., Zheng, B., Kelsoe, G., Dianda, L., Owen, M.J., and Hayday, A.C. 1996. Germinal center formation, immunoglobulin class switching, and autoantibody production driven by non-αβ T cells. *J. Exp. Med.* 181:2141–2152.

48. Pao, W., Wen, L., Smith, A.L., Gulbranson-Judge, A., Zheng, B., Kelsoe, G., Owen, M.J., MacLennan, I., and Hayday, A.C. 1996. γδ T cell help for B cells is stimulated by repeated parasitic infection. *Curr. Biol.* 6:1317–1325.

49. Czaja, A.J. 1995. Autoantibodies. *Baillieres Clin. Gastroenterol.* 9:723–744.

50. Gregorio, G.V., Davies, E.T., Mieli, V.G., and Vergani, D. 1995. Significance of extractable nuclear antigens in childhood autoimmune liver disease. *Clin. Exp. Immunol.* 102:308–313.

51. Ma, Y., Gaken, J., McFarlane, B.M., et al. 1997. Alcohol dehydrogenase: A target of humoral autoimmune response in liver disease. *Gastroenterology* 112:483–492.

52. Manns, M.P., and Obermayer, S.P. 1997. Cytochromes P450 and uridine triphosphate-glucuronosyltransferases: Model autoantigens to study drug-induced, virus-induced, and autoimmune liver disease. *Hepatology* 26:1054–1066.

53. Wen, L., Peakman, M., Mieli, V.G., and Vergani, D. 1992. Elevation of activated gamma delta T cell receptor bearing T lymphocytes in patients with autoimmune chronic liver disease. *Clin. Exp. Immunol.* 89:78–82.

54. Niehues, T., Gulwani, A.B., Goldman, I.S., McKinley, M.J., and Silver, J. 1994. Marked gamma delta T-cell decrease in peripheral blood of patients with primary biliary cirrhosis (PBC). *Autoimmunity* 18:267–273.

55. Martins, E.B., Graham, A.K., Chapman, R.W., and Fleming, K.A. 1996. Elevation of gamma delta T lymphocytes in peripheral blood and livers of patients with primary sclerosing cholangitis and other autoimmune liver diseases. *Hepatology* 23:988–993.

56. Ferrini, S., Zarcone, D., Viale, M., et al. 1989. Morphologic and functional characterization of human peripheral blood T cells expressing the T cell receptor gamma/delta. *Eur. J. Immunol.* 19:1183–1188.

57. Ferrini, S., Prigione, I., Bottino, C., et al. 1989. Monoclonal antibodies which react with the T cell receptor gamma/delta recognize different subsets of CD3+WT31– T lymphocytes. *Eur. J. Immunol.* 19:57–61.

58. Smith, M.D., Broker, B., Moretta, L., et al. 1990. T gamma delta cells and their subsets in blood and synovial tissue from rheumatoid arthritis patients. *Scand. J. Immunol.* 32:585–593.

59. Meliconi, R., Pitzalis, C., Kingsley, G.H., and Panayi, G.S. 1991. Gamma/delta T cells and their subpopulations in blood and synovial fluid from rheumatoid arthritis and spondyloarthritis. *Clin. Immunol. Immunopathol.* 59:165–172.

60. Lunardi, C., Marguerie, C., Walport, M.J., and So, A.K. 1992. T gamma delta cells and their subsets in blood and synovial fluid from patients with rheumatoid arthritis. *Br. J. Rheumatol.* 31:527–530.

61. Spencer, J., Isaacson, P.G., Diss, T.C., and MacDonald, T.T. 1989. Expression of disulfide-linked and non-disulfide-linked forms of the T cell receptor gamma/delta heterodimer in human intestinal intraepithelial lymphocytes. *Eur. J. Immunol.* 19:1335–1338.

62. Rust, C., Kooy, Y., Pena, S., Mearin, M.L., Kluin, P., and Koning, F. 1992. Phenotypical and functional characterization of small intestinal TcR gamma delta + T cells in coeliac disease. *Scand. J. Immunol.* 35:459–468.

63. Kozbor, D., Hyjek, E., Wiaderkiewicz, R., Kurzawski, G., and Lischner, H.W. 1993. Analysis of gamma delta+ T cells in peripheral blood of children with perinatal human immunodeficiency virus (HIV) infection. *J. Clin. Immunol.* 13:193–203.

64. Boullier, S., Cochet, M., Poccia, F., and Gougeon, M.L. 1995. CDR3-independent gamma delta V delta 1+ T cell expansion in the peripheral blood of HIV-infected persons. *J. Immunol.* 154:1418–1431.

65. Poccia, F., Boullier, S., Lecoeur, H., et al. 1996. Peripheral V gamma 9/V delta 2 T cell deletion and anergy to nonpeptidic mycobacterial antigens in asymptomatic HIV-1-infected persons. *J. Immunol.* 157:449–461.

66. Wen, L., Peakman, M., Lobo, Y.A., et al. 1990. T-cell-directed hepatocyte damage in autoimmune chronic active hepatitis. *Lancet* 336:1527–1530.

67. Mombaerts, P., Arnoldi, J., Russ, F., Tonegawa, S., and Kaufmann, S.H. 1993. Different roles of alpha beta and gamma delta T cells in immunity against an intracellular bacterial pathogen. *Nature* 365:53–56.

68. Fu, Y.X., Roark, C.E., Kelly, K., et al. 1994. Immune protection and control of inflammatory tissue necrosis by gamma delta T cells. *J. Immunol.* 153:3101–3115.

69. Roark, C.E., Vollmer, M.K., Campbell, P.A., Born, W.K., and O'Brien, R.L. 1996. Response of a gamma delta+ T cell receptor invariant subset during bacterial infection. *J. Immunol.* 156:2214–2220.

70. Belles, C., Kuhl, A.K., Donoghue, A.J., et al. 1996. Bias in the gamma delta T cell response to Listeria monocytogenes. V delta 6.3+ cells are a major component of the gamma delta T cell response to Listeria monocytogenes. *J. Immunol.* 156:4280–4289.

71. Fu, Y.X., Roark, C.E., Kelly, K., et al. 1994. Immune protection and control of inflammatory tissue necrosis by gamma delta T cells. *J. Immunol.* 153:3101–3115.

72. Ferrick, D.A., Schrenzel, M.D., Mulvania, T., Hsieh, B., Ferlin, W.G., and Lepper, H. 1995. Differential production of interferon-gamma and interleukin-4 in response to Th1- and Th2-stimulating pathogens by gamma delta T cells in vivo. *Nature* 373:255–257.

73. Hsieh, B., Schrenzel, M.D., Mulvania, T., Lepper, H.D., DiMolfetto, L.L., and Ferrick, D.A. 1996. In vivo cytokine production in murine listeriosis. Evidence for immunoregulation by gamma delta+ T cells. *J. Immunol.* 156:232–237.

74. Rosat, J.P., Schreyer, M., Ohteki, T., Waanders, G.A., MacDonald, H.R., and Louis, J.A. 1994. Selective expansion of activated V delta 4+ cells during experimental infection of mice with Leishmania major. *Eur. J. Immunol.* 24:496–499.

75. Tanaka, Y., Morita, C.T., Tanaka, Y., Nieves, E., Brenner, M.B., and Bloom, B.R. 1995. Natural and synthetic non-peptide antigens recognized by human gamma delta T cells. *Nature* 375:155–158.

76. Kawano, T., Cui, J., Koezuka, Y., Toura, I., Kaneko, Y, Motoki, K., Ueno, H., Nakagawa, R., Sato, H., Kondo, E., Koseki, H., and Taniguchi, M. 1997. CD1d-restricted and T cell receptor mediated activation of Vα14 NKT cells by glycosylceramides. *Science* 278:1626–1630.

77. Bukowski, J.F., Morita, C.T., Tanaka, Y., Bloom, B.R., Brenner, M.B., and Band, H. 1995. V gamma 2V delta 2 TCR-dependent recognition of non-peptide antigens and Daudi cells analyzed by TCR gene transfer. *J. Immunol.* 154:998–1006.

78. Morita, C.T., Beckman, E.M., Bukowski, J.F., et al. 1995. Direct presentation of nonpeptide prenyl pyrophosphate antigens to human gamma delta T cells. *Immunity* 3:495–507.

79. Kim, H.T., Nelson, E.L., Clayberger, C., Sanjanwala, M., Sklar, J., and Krensky, A.M. 1995. Gamma delta T cell recognition of tumor Ig peptide. *J. Immunol.* 154:1614–1623.

80. Wei, Y., Zhao, X., Kariya, Y., Fukata, H., Teshigawara, K., and Uchida, A. 1996. Induction of autologous tumor killing by heat treatment of fresh human tumor cells: Involvement of gamma delta T cells and heat shock protein 70. *Cancer Res.* 56:1104–1110.

81. Fisch, P., Malkovsky, M., Kovats, S., Sturn, E., Braakman, E., Klein, B.S., Voss, S.D., Morrissey, L.W., DeMars, R., Welch, W.J., Bolhuis, R.L.H., and Sondel, P. 1990. Recognition by human Vγ9/Vδ2 T cells of a GroEL homolog on Daudi Burkitts lymphoma cells. *Science* 250:1269–1273.

82. Zocchi, M.R., Ferrarini, M., and Rugarli, C. 1990. Selective lysis of the autologous tumor by delta TCS1+ gamma/delta+ tumor-infiltrating lymphocytes from human lung carcinomas. *Eur. J. Immunol.*; 20:2685–2689.

83. Ferrarini, M., Pupa, S.M., Zocchi, M.R., Rugarli, C., and Menard, S. 1994. Distinct pattern of HSP72 and monomeric laminin receptor expression in human lung cancers infiltrated by gamma/delta T lymphocytes. *Int. J. Cancer* 57:486–490.

84. Chin, K., Morise, K., Kanayama, K., and Nagura, H. 1995. Immunohistochemical study of gamma delta T cell receptor-positive cells in the capsular region of hepatocellular carcinoma: Possible role in defense against expansion of carcinoma in the liver. *J. Gastroenterol.* 30:330–337.

85. Zhao, X., Wei, Y.Q., Kariya, Y., Teshigawara, K., and Uchida, A. 1995. Accumulation of gamma/delta T cells in human dysgerminoma and seminoma: Roles in autologous tumor killing and granuloma formation. *Immunol. Invest.* 24:607–618.

86. Choudhary, A., Davodeau, F., Moreau, A., Peyrat, M.A., Bonneville, M., and Jotereau, F. 1995. Selective lysis of autologous tumor cells by recurrent gamma delta tumor-infiltrating lymphocytes from renal carcinoma. *J. Immunol.*; 154:3932–3940.

87. Penninger, J.M., Wen, T., Timms, E., et al. 1995. Spontaneous resistance to acute T-cell leukaemias in TCRV gamma 1.1J gamma 4C gamma 4 transgenic mice. *Nature* 375:241–244.

88. Peng, S.L., Robert, M.E., Hayday, A.C., and Craft, J. 1996. A tumor-suppressor function for fas (CD95) revealed in T cell deficient mice. *J. Exp. Med.* 184:1149–1154.

89. Seki, S., Abo, T., Masuda, T., et al. 1990. Identification of activated T cell receptor gamma delta lymphocytes in the liver of tumor-bearing hosts. *J. Clin. Invest.* 86:409–415.

90. Seki, S., Abo, T., Sugiura, K., et al. 1991. Reciprocal T cell responses in the liver and thymus of mice injected with syngeneic tumor cells. *Cell Immunol.* 137:46–60.

CHAPTER 4

EXTRATHYMIC T CELLS IN THE LIVER

TORU ABO, ANURA WEERASINGHE, and HISAMI WATANABE
Niigata University, School of Medicine, Niigata, Japan

INTRODUCTION

In a series of recent studies (1–5), we have demonstrated that the liver is an important immune organ that produces extrathymic T cells in mice and humans. It is well known that the liver comprises pluripotent stem cells at fetal stages. However, the liver seems to keep such stem cells even after birth, and the stem cells consistently give rise to extrathymic T cells in the liver throughout life (6). Kanamori et al. (7) recently reported that c-kit$^+$ stem cells are also present in the cryptopatches of the small intestine in mice. These stem cells may give rise to another population of extrathymic T cells in the intestine. Since the liver originated from a diverticulum of the intestine in phylogeny (8), it is likely that both stem cells and extrathymic T cells in the intestine and liver originated from common progenitors. There has been speculation that the stem cells and extrathymic T cells in the intestine and liver may have a longer phylogenetic history than the stem cells in the bone marrow, and conventional T cells in the thymus.

Considering the incompleteness of the negative selection for self-reactive forbidden clones in extrathymic pathways of T cell differentiation (9), extrathymic T cells might be important for the recognition and elimination of abnormal self cells generated in the body. On the other hand, thymus-derived T cells might be associated with the recognition and elimination of foreign antigens. Thus, self-reactive T cell clones are rarely seen in these T cells in the periphery. This is true even in immunosuppressive states (10). In other words, extrathymic T cells and conventional T cells have different (possibly reciprocal) physiological roles in immunological surveillance of the body. As will be shown in this chapter, extrathymic T cells are responsible for many immunological responses of aging, autoimmune diseases, intracellular infections, pregnancy, malignancy, and chronic graft-versus-host disease (GVHD), etc. Without

T Lymphocytes in the Liver: Immunobiology, Pathology, and Host Defense, Edited by I. Nicholas Crispe
ISBN 0-471-19218-X

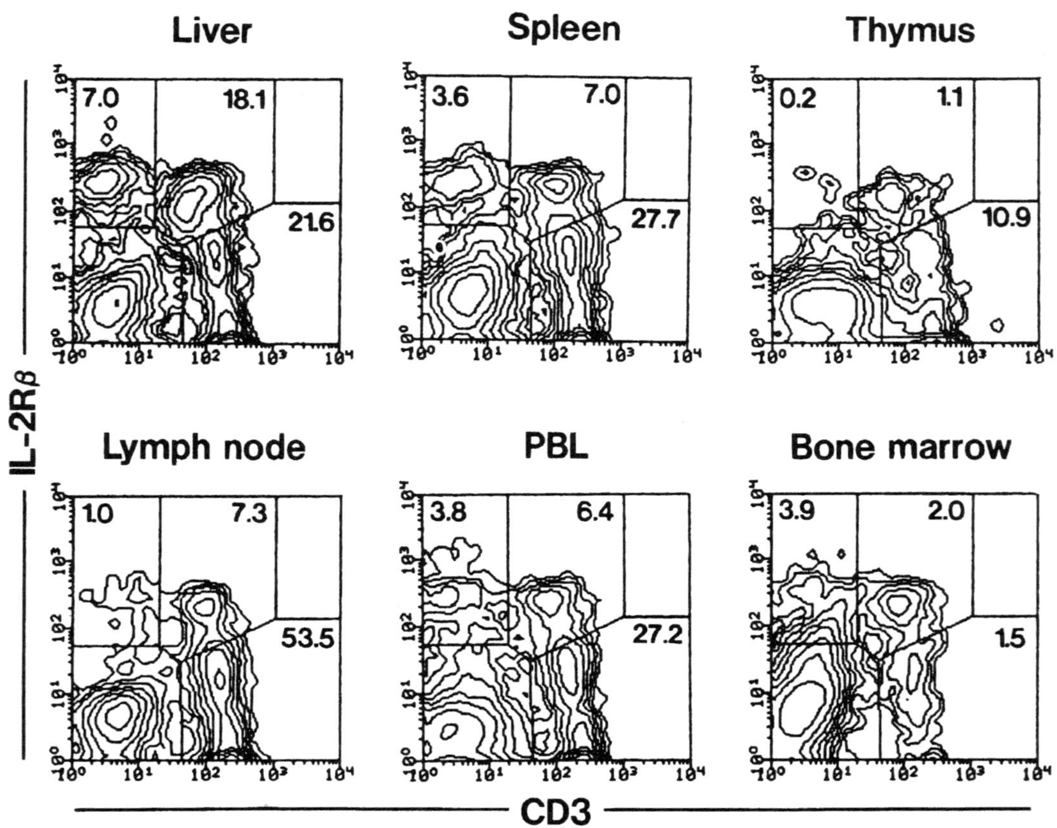

Figure 4.1. Identification of TCR^{int} cells in various immune organs by two-color staining for CD3 and IL-2Rβ. MNC were isolated from various organs of adult mice. This staining simultaneously identifies $CD3^-IL\text{-}2R\beta^+$NK cells, $CD3^{int}IL\text{-}2R\beta^+$ cells (i.e., $CD3^{int}$ cells of extrathymic origin), $CD3^{high}IL\text{-}2R\beta^-$ cells (i.e., $CD3^{high}$ cells of thymic origin), and $CD3^-IL\text{-}2R\beta^-$ B cells.

involving the concept of extrathymic T cells, the immunological responses in above-mentioned conditions could not be properly understood.

IDENTIFICATION OF TCR^{int} CELLS IN THE LIVER OF MICE

Reflecting the primordial features of extrathymic T cells, there are many properties of extrathymic T cells by which they can be distinguished from thymus-derived T cells. Some of these properties include the intermediate density of the TCR-CD3 complex on their surface (therefore, we term them intermediate T cell receptor cells or TCR^{int} cells) (2) and the constitutive expression of interleukin-2R β-chain (IL-2Rβ) (11–13). In this regard, we applied two-color immunofluorescence staining for CD3 (or TCR) and IL-2Rβ to identify TCR^{int} cells in various immune organs of mice (Fig. 4.1). This staining is also very useful for identification of other lymphocyte populations, TCR^{high} cells, NK cells and B cells: namely, NK cells are CD3^{-}IL-2Rβ^{+}, CD3^{int} cells (i.e., extrathymic T cells) are CD3^{int}IL-2Rβ^{+}, CD3^{high} cells (i.e., thymus-derived T cells) are CD3^{high}IL-2Rβ^{-}, and B cells are CD3^{-}IL-2Rβ^{-}.

The constitutive expression of IL-2Rβ on CD3^{int} cells indicates one of the primordial properties for this population. Because of this property, CD3^{int} cells respond immediately to corresponding antigens. For example, after intracellular infection with *Listeria monocytogenes*, lymphocyte activation occurs in the order NK cells, extrathymic T cells, thymus-derived T cells (14). Although CD3^{int} cells express IL-2Rβ under resting conditions, they usually do not acquire the expression of IL-2α *in vivo*. In other words, they have only a limited ability to express the intermediate affinity of IL-2R (i.e., IL-2Rα^{-}β^{+}) (15). This property also indicates one of their primordial properties in phylogenetic development. They have, however, an ability to express IL-2Rα in long-term cultures in the presence of IL-2 (16). In contrast, conventional T cells are IL-2Rα^{-}β^{-} under resting conditions. After antigenic stimulation, they acquire the high affinity of IL-2R (i.e., IL-2Rα^{+}β^{+}). Reflecting this situation, they respond to corresponding antigens at relatively late stages of stimulation (e.g., day 7 or

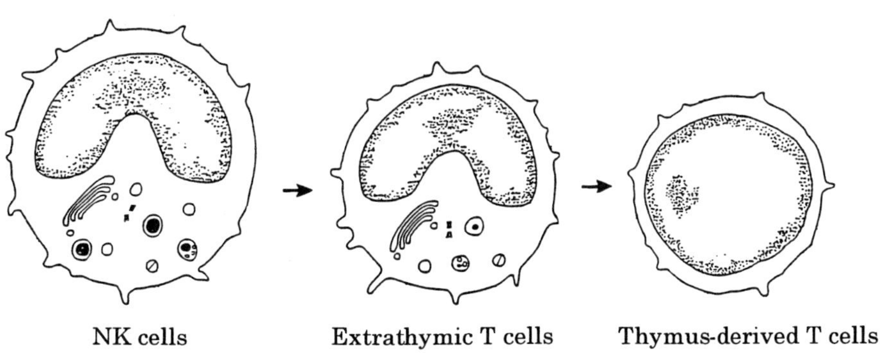

Figure 4.2. Phylogenetic development of NK/T lineage lymphocytes. A sequential change of the morphology in NK cells, extrathymic T cells, and thymus-derived T cells suggests a route of their phylogenetic development.

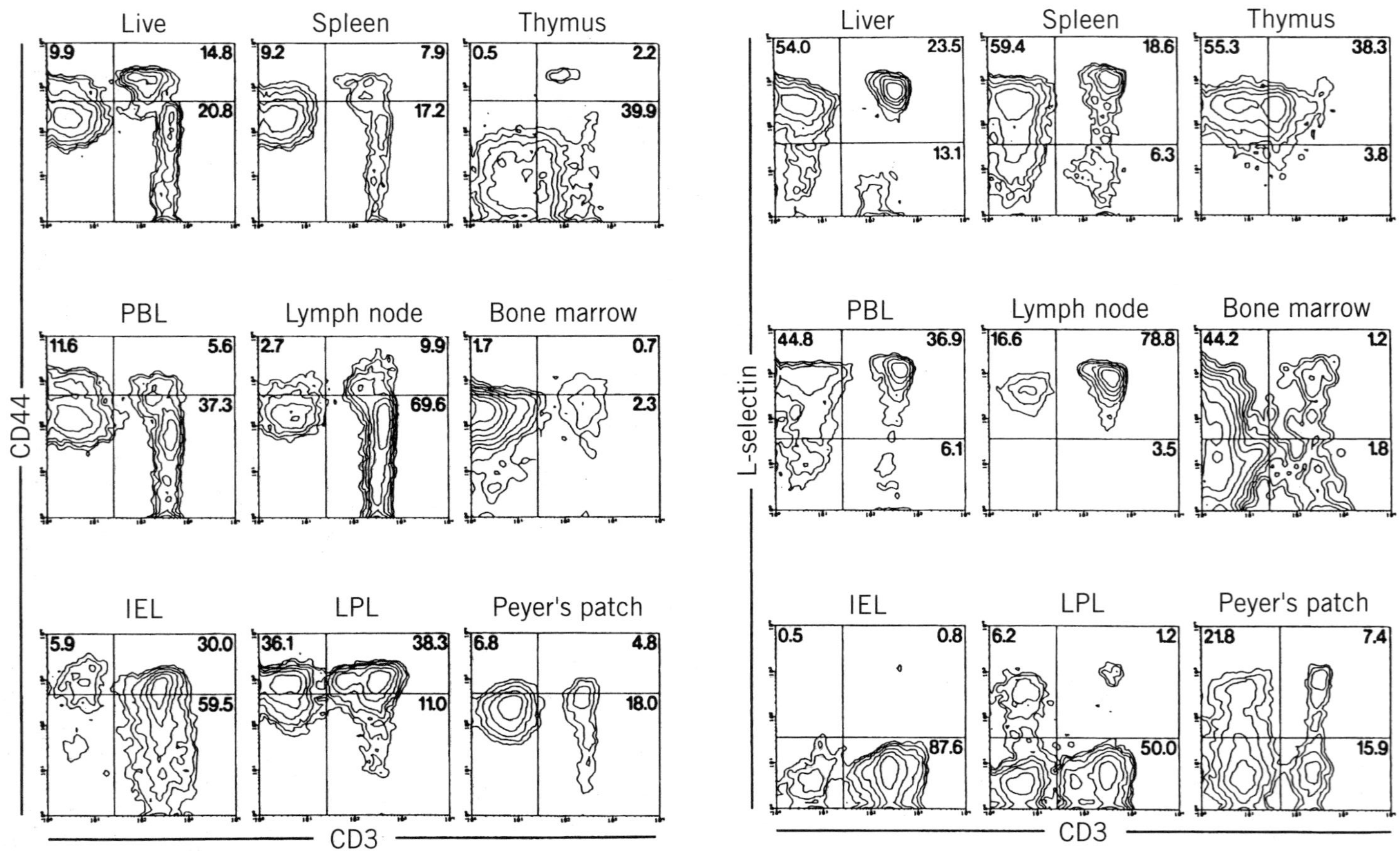

Figure 4.3. Adhesion molecules expressed on extrathymic T cells. Two-color staining for CD3 and CD44 and that for CD3 and L-selectin were performed in various immune organs of adult mice. $CD3^{int}$ cells have the phenotype of $CD44^{+}$L-selectin^{-}, whereas $CD3^{high}$ cells have inversely the phenotype of $CD44^{-}$L-selectin^{+}. The staining pattern of intestinal T cells resembles that of $CD3^{int}$ cells in the liver. Axes show fluorescence intensity. Numbers show percentages of cells in each sub-population.

later after listerial infection) (14). However, their responses are ultimately greater than those of NK cells and extrathymic T cells.

TCR^{high} cells never contain double-negative (DN) CD4$^-$8$^-$ cells in the periphery. However, TCR^{int} cells always comprise up to 30% of DN CD4$^-$8$^-$ (5). At least in adulthood, γδ T cells are rarely generated through the intrathymic pathway of T cell differentiation. On the other hand, such γδ T cells are preferentially generated through the extrathymic pathways in the liver and in the intestine (13,17). γδ T cells usually have the CD8$^+$ phenotype.

It is known that NK and T cells share common precursors in ontogeny and at an early stage of differentiation (18). Therefore, these lymphocytes are sometimes referred to as a NK/T lineage. If we observe their morphology, a sequential route of phylogenetic development is suggested (Fig. 4.2). It is presumed that extrathymic T cells are at an intermediate position between NK cells and thymus-derived T cells in this route. This scheme indicates phylogenetic events only, and NK/T cells do not switch their phenotype after differentiation in our body. Although conventional T cells have the morphology of small resting lymphocytes, they acquire the morphology of lymphoblasts after antigenic stimulation and have the highest responses of any lymphocytes.

The adhesion molecules expressed on extrathymic T cells are unique, namely, they are CD44$^+$L-selectin$^-$ (Fig. 4.3). In sharp contrast, thymus-derived T cells are CD44$^-$L-selectin$^+$. This inverted expression of adhesion molecules might be associated with their unique homing to the immune organs (19,20). Extrathymic T cells localize to the sinusoidal walls in the liver, whereas thymus-derived T cells home to the lymph nodes and the white pulp of the spleen. CD44 antigens are ligands for hyaluronic acid and others; therefore, CD44 antigens may interact with hyaluronic acid (extracellular matrix) of sinusoidal walls in the liver. On the other hand, L-selectin is known to be the lymph node homing receptor. Accordingly, L-selectin$^-$ extrathymic T cells do not home this organ and usually stay at the liver. Figure 4.3 includes the data for intestinal T cells, including IELs (intraepithelial lymphocytes), LPLs (lamina propria lymphocytes), and Peyer's patch lymphocytes. The staining pattern of these intestinal T cells resembles that of extrathymic T cells in the liver. The expression level of LFA-1 antigens on extrathymic T cells is higher than that on thymus-derived T cells (13).

RELATIONSHIP BETWEEN NK1.1$^+$ AND NK1.1$^-$ SUBSETS AMONG TCR^{int} CELLS

As previously mentioned, TCR^{int} cells are most abundant in the liver. However, a minor population of TCR^{int} cells are also present in other immune organs, including the spleen, bone marrow, lymph nodes, and even thymus (21–28). There are two subsets among TCR^{int} cells: NK1.1$^+$ and NK1.1$^-$ (5). Depending on the organ in which they are located, the ratios of NK1.1$^+$ and NK1.1$^-$ subsets among TCR^{int} cells are varied. The proportions of NK1.1$^+$ subsets are higher in the liver and thymus (up to 70%) than those in the spleen, bone marrow, and lymph nodes (less than 30%) (Table 4.1).

TABLE 4.1 A Comparison of the Relationship Between IL-2Rβ^{+} int CD3 Cells and NK1.1^{+} Cells in Various Organs[a]

	% NK1.1^{+} Cells Among IL-2Rβ^{+} int CD3 Cells		
Organs	B6	SJL	NZB
Liver	69.6 ± 11.9	50.9 ± 7.2	56.9 ± 1.9
Spleen	15.8 ± 4.7	22.0 ± 4.3	35.5 ± 0.3
Thymus	56.9 ± 9.2	60.3 ± 8.9	52.6 ± 7.6
Lymph nodes	4.9 ± 2.0	ND	ND
Bone marrow	27.2 ± 6.3	ND	ND

[a]B6, SJL, and NZB mice at the age of 18 wk were used. The values were obtained by three-color staining for CD3 (FITC), IL-2Rβ (PE), and NK1.1 (Red 613). Mean and 1 SD were produced from six mice of each strain.

NK1.1^{+} subsets of TCR^{int} cells have been identified by many investigators and are referred to as NK-T cells or natural T cells (29–32).

Like the liver, the thymus is the site of a minor pathway of TCR^{int} cell differentiation. This pathway is called an alternative intrathymic pathway (29–32) (Fig. 4.4). On the other hand, a major pathway for conventional T cells, which are generated by passing through a double-positive (DP) CD4^{+}8^{+} stage, is called the mainstream pathway. Although many investigators have focused their attention only on NK-T cells (i.e.,

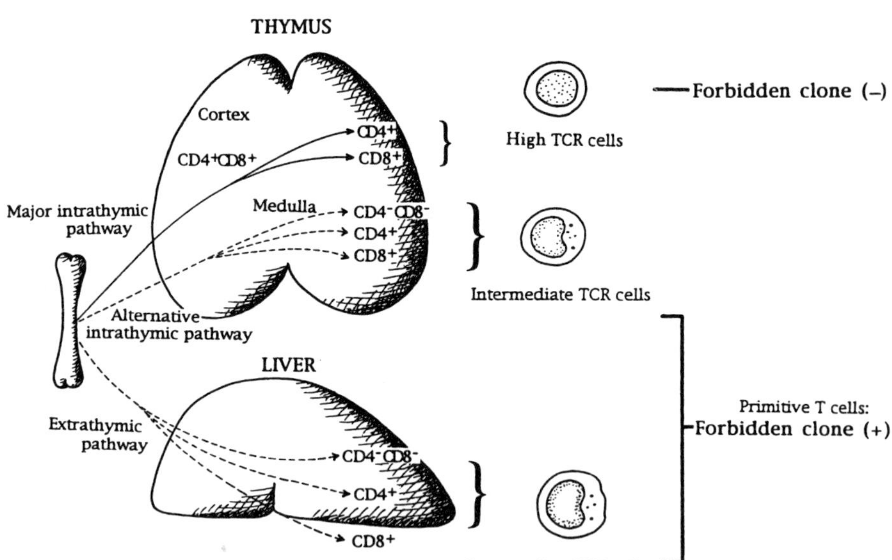

Figure 4.4. Pathways of T cell differentiation. There is a major pathway of T cell differentiation in the thymus, which produce TCR^{high} cells (i.e., the mainstream in the thymus). TCR^{int} cells (i.e., primitive or primordial T cells) are generated by the primordial pathways in the liver and thymic medulla. The primordial pathway in the thymus (mainly in the thymic medulla) is also referred to as an alternative intrathymic pathway of T cell differentiation.

NK1.1$^+$ subsets of TCR^{int} cells), at least 20% to 30% of TCR^{int} cells in the thymus are the NK1.1$^-$ subsets (5). The NK1.1$^+$ subsets consist mainly of DN CD4$^-$8$^-$ and CD4$^+$ cells. On the other hand, the NK1.1$^-$ subsets of TCR^{int} cells are mainly CD8$^+$ (5).

It is well established that NK-T cells preferentially use an invariant Vα14Jα281 chain for TCR$\alpha\beta$ (33–35). However, there is no such invariance of Vα for TCR$\alpha\beta$ in the NK1.1$^-$ subset (5). It is conceivable that the NK1.1$^-$ subsets have a well-developed form in the phylogenetic development of TCR^{int} cells.

The cytotoxic activity against YAC-1 cells (an NK-sensitive target) and syngeneic thymocytes has recently been compared in the purified NK1.1$^+$ and NK1.1$^-$ subsets of TCR^{int} cells (36,37). Both cytotoxic activities are prominently seen in the NK1.1$^+$ subset. They have cytotoxic mechanisms of both Fas ligand/Fas molecules and perforin. However, we could not deny the possibility that the NK1.1$^-$ subset acquires potent cytotoxicity after some antigenic stimulations. This speculation arises from the fact that the clonal diversity of the NK1.1$^-$ subset is greater than that of the NK1.1$^+$ subset (manuscript submitted for publication), so that they can undergo clonal expansion when stimulated.

It was reported that NK-T cells preferentially produce IL-4, which induces a switch from T helper type 1 (Th1) to Th2 cells (38,39). However, a recent study by Arase (personal communication) et al. has indicated that it depends on the kinds of stimulations for NK-T cells. Thus, some stimulations induce interferon-γ (IFNγ) rather than IL-4 in this population. We have also found that the profile for cytokine production in TCR^{int} cells is similar to that of Th0, i.e., the simultaneous production of IFNγ and IL-4 (T. Abo et al., unpublished observations).

A COMPARISON BETWEEN THE PROPERTIES OF HEPATIC T CELLS AND IEL IN THE INTESTINE

It had been suspected in earlier studies that some Thy-1$^+$ cells might be generated at intraepithelial sites of the intestine in a thymus-independent manner (40–42). After identification of the TCR genes, and using monoclonal antibodies (mAb) against TCR, it was confirmed that such cells eventually comprise T cells and are generated extrathymically (43–46). Subsequently, T cells existing in the lamina propria were also determined to be of extrathymic origin, whereas T cells in Peyer's patches were found to be of thymic origin. In this section, we directly compare the phenotypes of TCR^{int} cells in the liver, and IELs and lamina propria lymphocytes (LPLs) in the intestine (Fig. 4.5). Mononuclear cells (MNCs) isolated from the liver are examined in parallel.

As already mentioned, TCR^{int} cells are clearly demonstrated to exist in the liver, but generally not in the spleen and thymus. However, MNCs in the intestine showed rather unique patterns of staining, depending on the sites of isolation. Two-color staining for CD3 and IL-2Rβ is applied in these experiments. In the case of IELs, major populations are CD3^{superhigh}IL-2Rβ^+ and CD3^{high}IL-2Rβ^-. Both of them are of extrathymic origin as shown elsewhere. On the other hand, the staining pattern of LPLs slightly mimicks that of liver MNCs, although these CD3^{int} cells have a lower density of IL-2Rβ. As expected, all CD3$^+$ cells in Peyer's patches are regular CD3^{high}

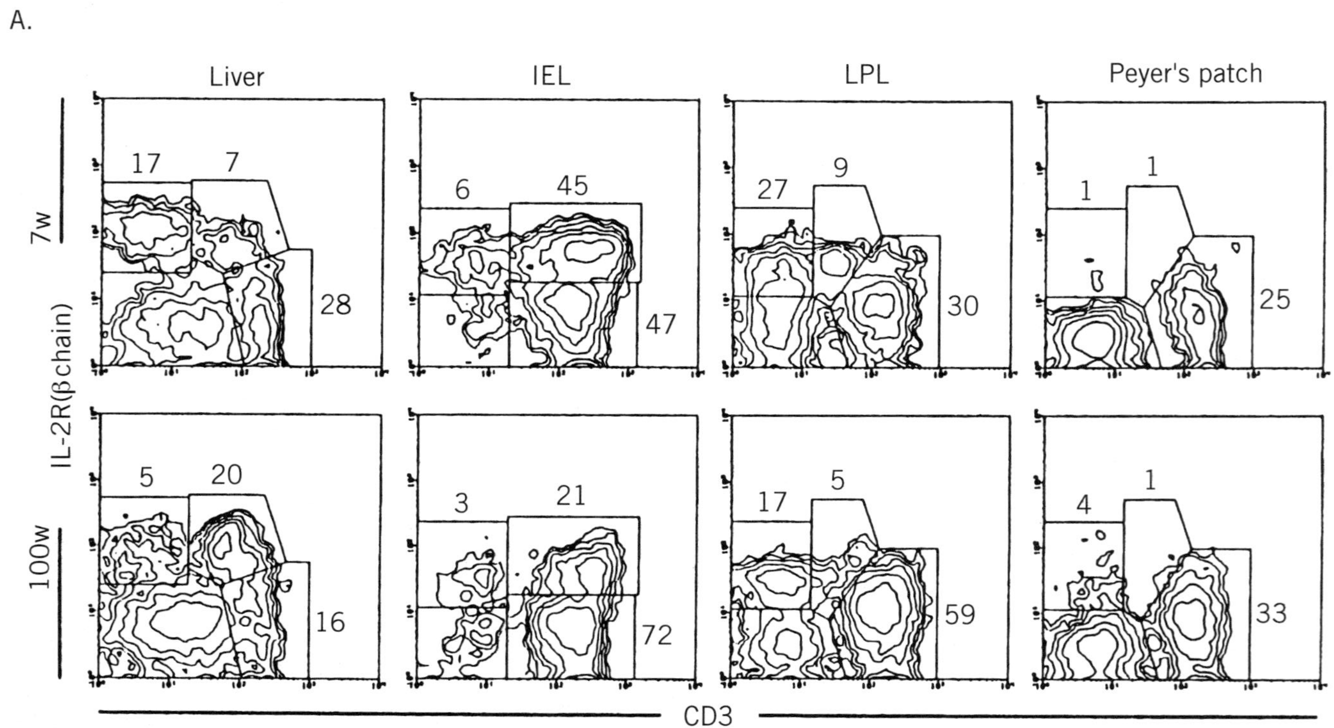

Figure 4.5. (continued)

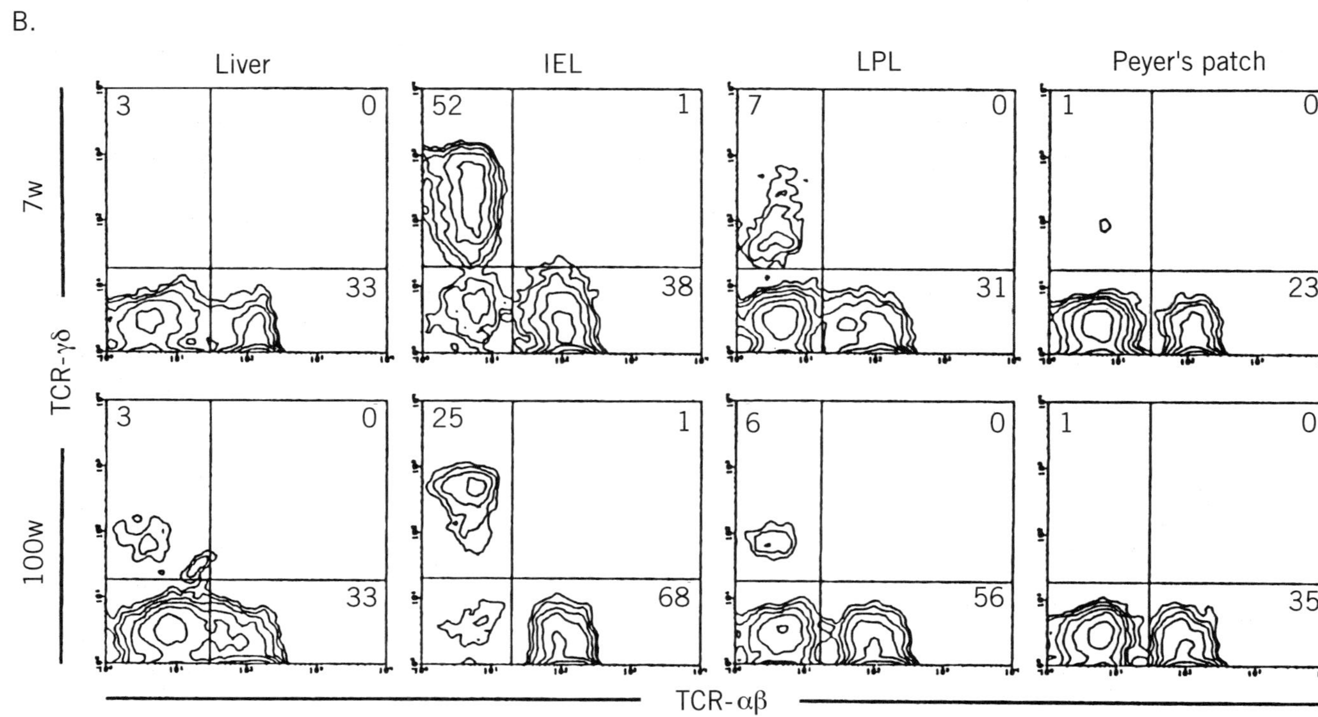

Figure 4.5. (continued)

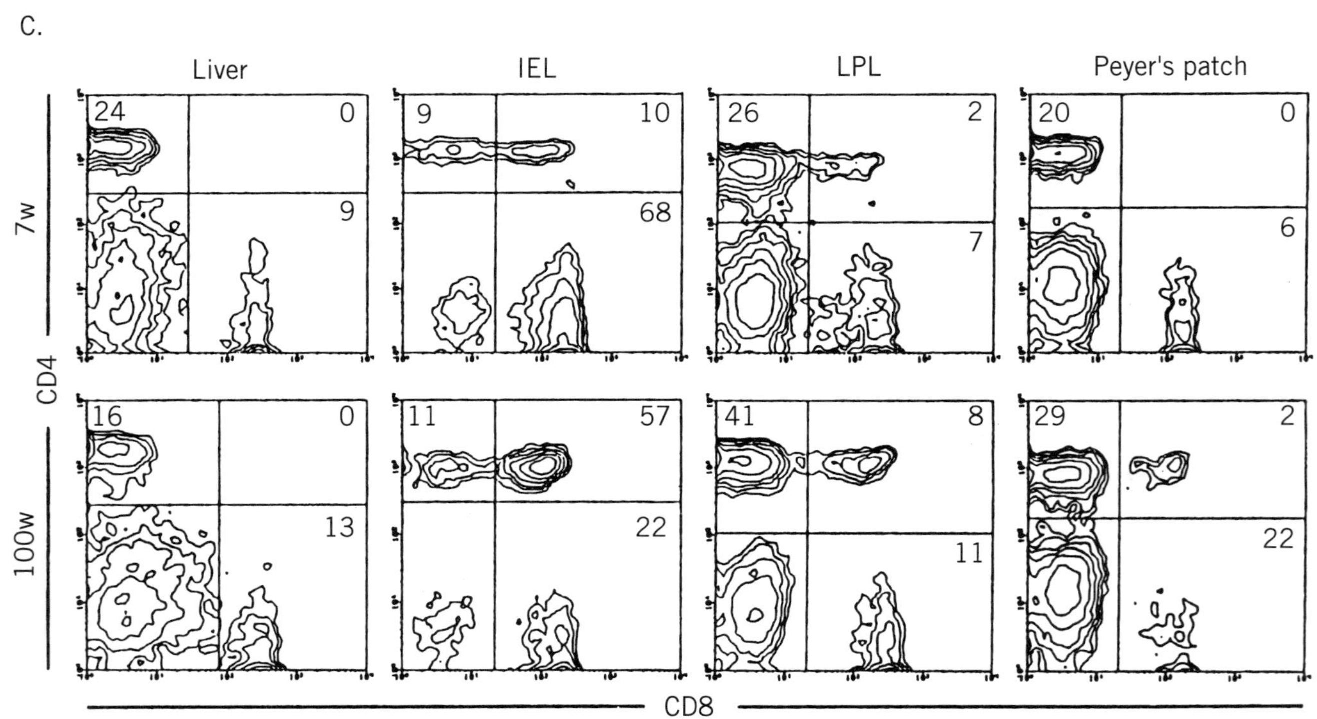

Figure 4.5. Comparisons of the phenotypes among mononuclear cells (MNC) isolated from the various immune organs in mice. (**A**). Two-color staining for CD3 and IL-2Rβ, (**B**). Two-color staining for TCRαβ and TCRγδ, (**C**). Two-color staining for CD4 and CD8. IEL showed a unique staining pattern, showing both IL-2Rβ$^+$ and IL-2Rβ$^-$ populations. The staining pattern of LPL was similar to that of liver MNC. γδTcells were mainly present in hepatic MNC and IEL in the intestine. Units as in Figure 4.1.

TABLE 4.2 Similarities and Differences Between Intermediate TCR Cells in the Liver and IEL in the Intestine

Intermediate TCR Cells/IEL
A. Similarities:
1. LGL morphology in some populations
2. Expansion with aging
3. Preponderance of $\gamma\delta$ T cells
4. A significant proportion of autoreactive forbidden T cell oligoclones
5. IL-2Rβ expression
6. Acquisition of CD4 and CD8 antigens without thymic microenvironments
7. $\alpha\alpha$ homodimer of CD8
8. Low response to T cell mitogens (e.g., phytohemagglutinin and concanavalin A)
9. Radioresistant
10. Lacking in scid mice
B. Differences:
1. Intermediate TCR/High TCR
2. Some DN $CD4^-8^-$ cells/Some DP $CD4^+8^+$ cells
3. All IL-2Rβ^+/IL-2Rβ^+ and IL-2Rβ^-
4. CD4 dominant/CD8 dominant
5. Vγ1, 2/Vδ6/Vγ4,6
6. Migrate to the periphery/Function at the site where they are generated

cells lacking IL-2Rβ. Two-color staining for TCR$\alpha\beta$ and TCR$\gamma\delta$ demonstrated that $\gamma\delta$ T cells are abundant only in the liver and at intraepithelial sites of the intestine.

The results of two-color staining for CD4 and CD8 are interesting, in that not only thymocytes but also IELs consist of DP $CD4^+8^+$ T cells. As already established, DP thymocytes are immature T cells with TCR^{dull}, while those of IELs are mature T cells with TCR^{high} (47–49). With aging, $CD3^{int}$ cells in the liver and $\alpha\beta$ T cells in the intestine tend to increase. DP $\alpha\beta$ T cells become abundant in the intestine while $\gamma\delta$ T cells become rare in mice at the age of 100 weeks. It is conceivable that both $CD3^{int}$ cells in the liver and T cells in the intestine are generated as primordial T cells in early phylogeny. However, they may subsequently develop by independent processes at their respective sites. A comparison of the properties of hepatic T cells and IELs in the intestine is presented in Table 4.2.

Why are extrathymic T cells generated both in the liver and the intestine? Phylogenetically, a primitive liver is known to develop as projections from the intestinal tissue (Fig. 4.6). Reflecting this situation, IELs and submucosal lymphocytes, which may originally develop from macrophages or NK cells existing at the sites of endodermal cells, are common to the liver and intestine in early phylogeny.

Since extrathymic T cells in the liver are located under but not on, the sites of endodermal cells (i.e., parenchymal hepatocytes), it is quite possible that the properties of extrathymic T cells in the liver are more similar to those of LPLs than to those of IELs. LPLs are located under the epithelial cells, while IELs are situated on the epithelial cells. It is known that sinusoidal lumens are open to the peritonal cavity in in-

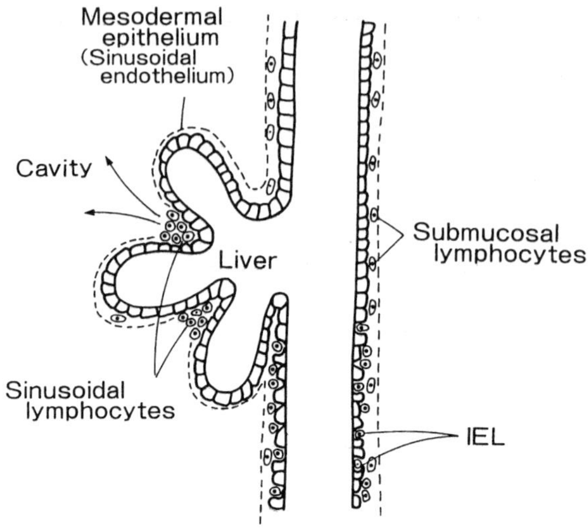

Figure 4.6. A scheme showing why IEL in the intestine and sinusoidal lymphocytes in the liver have certain properties in common. The liver was developed as a diverticulum from the intestine in phylogeny.

vertebrates with an open vessel system, and it is suspected that extrathymic T cells produced in the hepatic sinusoids previously functioned in the peritoneal cavity to survey atypical cells generated *in vivo* at those phylogenetic stages. In fact, we were able to obtain numerous lymphoid cells from the peritoneal cavity in arthropods (e.g., crab and shrimp) (50).

GENERATION OF TCR^{int} CELLS FROM c-kit$^+$ STEM CELLS WHICH EXIST IN THE LIVER

Do the c-kit$^+$ stem cells seen in the liver and intestine originate from the bone marrow? To answer this question, we have recently produced a parabiosis of B6.Ly5.1 and B6.Ly5.2 mice (S. Suzuki et al., unpublished observations). Within 3 days, the parabiotics share a circulation system. The origins of mixed lymphocytes through the circulation are identified by mAbs against Ly5.1 and Ly5.2 antigens in conjunction with immunofluorescence tests. By 14 days after parabiosis, all lymphocytes in the blood, spleen, and lymph nodes in each partner become a half-and-half mixture of Ly5.1$^+$ and Ly5.2$^+$ cells. On the other hand, extrathymic T cells in the liver and intestine hardly mixed. These results suggest that extrathymic T cells, both in the liver and the intestine, arise from their own stem cells. If c-kit$^+$ stem cells seen in the liver and intestine are supplied from the bone marrow, extrathymic T cells should have been derived from both parabiotic mice.

This interpretation seems to be reasonable, because c-kit$^+$ stem cells exist in the parenchymal space of the liver and in the cryptopatches of the small intestine. When mice are injected with estrogen, c-kit$^+$ stem cells and the generation of extrathymic T cells become predominant in the liver. At that time, many lymphoid and myeloid cells are proliferating in the parenchymal space in the liver (Fig. 4.7).

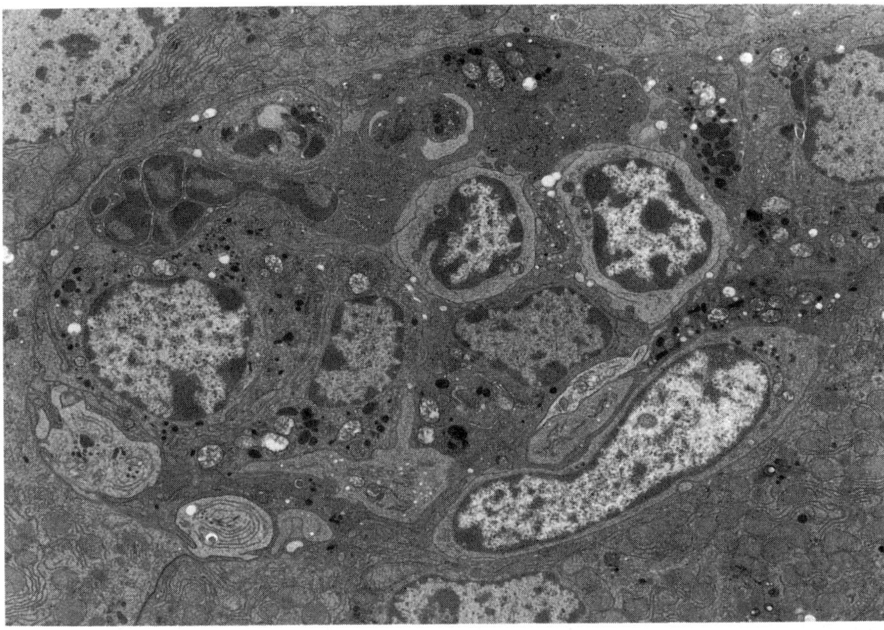

Figure 4.7. Electron microscopy of the liver in mice treated with estrogen (×3,500). The liver specimen was obtained on day 3 after estrogen administration. Many nonparenchymal cells were estimated to be both lymphoid cells and myeloid cells.

Since hepatocytes in the liver and epithelial cells in the intestine share the same origin, these epithelial cells function as stroma cells which support the differentiation of extrathymic T cells. Indeed, it is known that hepatocytes and epithelial cells in the intestine produce many cytokines in common (51–55). One of these is IL-7 (56).

Among the lymphocyte population in the liver and intestine, TCR cells in the liver and lymphocytes in the Peyer's patches become a half-and-half mixture by 2 weeks after parabiosis. Therefore, these lymphocytes have originated from the other places (e.g., the thymus). TCR^{int} cells in the liver are generated in the parenchymal space and then move to hepatic sinusoidal lumen. Even under this situation, TCR^{int} cells, especially NK1.1^{+} subset, rarely mix in the parabiotics. This result also suggests that NK-T cells work in the place where they are generated. In contrast, the NK1.1^{-} subset of TCR^{int} cells shows an intermediate pattern between NK-T cells and TCR^{high} cells. It is speculated that the NK1.1^{+} subset seen in the liver is of hepatic origin, while some NK1.1^{-} subsets seen in the liver originate in other organs (e.g., the bone marrow). Possibly, c-kit^{+} cells in the digestive tract have a longer history than do those in the bone marrow. Thus, the bone marrow may have developed from a more primordial hematopoietic organ early in the evolution of land vertebrates.

SELF-REACTIVE FORBIDDEN CLONES ARE CONFINED TO THE PATHWAYS OF TCR^{int}-CELL DIFFERENTIATION

Extrathymic T cells carry many primordial properties that differ from those of conventional T cells. Some of the most important features ascribed to extrathymic T cells are the composition of forbidden clones in the Minor lymphocyte stimulating (Mls) system (9,10,57) and the actual self-reactivities (36,58). These features and functions might be the result of the intermediate density of TCR-CD3 complex on the surface. Due to the limited density of TCR-CD3 complex, negative selection for eliminating self-reactive clones is incomplete. Although another population of extrathymic T cells in the intestine (i.e., intraepithelial lymphocytes, IELs) also contains forbidden clones, the levels of such clones are relatively higher in extrathymic T cells of the liver than in IELs of the intestine. As already mentioned, the density of TCR-CD3 complex on IELs in the intestine is comparable to that on conventional T cells (i.e., TCR^{high} cells).

When self-reactive forbidden clones are estimated in the Mls system, we usually use BALB/c or C3H/He mice. Both mice carry Mls-1^b2^a, and V$\beta 3^+$ and V$\beta 11^+$ cells are forbidden clones. Thus, Mls antigens are minor histocompatibility antigens (originated from retrovirus genes), acting as endogenous superantigens, and therefore eliminate specific Vβ^+ cells. The mainstream of T cell differentiation efficiently eliminates such self-reactive forbidden clones at a DP CD4$^+$8$^+$ stage (9) (see Fig. 4.8). This is true under severe immunosuppressive conditions (1). If this is so, a question then arises as to why self-reactive clones appear in the periphery. In a recent study, we have demonstrated that this is due to the resistance of TCR^{int} cell differentiation to the immunosuppressive conditions (10). In other words, the relative dominance of TCR^{int} cells in the periphery after immunosuppressive therapy induces the above-mentioned conditions. At that time, there is no leakage of forbidden clones into TCR^{high} cells.

In B6 mice and some other mice, there is no expression of MHC class II, region E (I–E) antigens. Since Mls antigens are presented by I–E antigens, these B6 mice do not have self-reactive forbidden clones based on Vβ^+ expression. When we estimate NK-T cells (i.e., NK1.1$^+$ T cells), only B6 mice and some others carry NK1.1 alloantigens. In this case, we have to use F_1 mice (e.g., [B6 × BALB/c] F_1 mice) to simultaneously identify NK-T cells and forbidden clones. Our previous studies have indicated that both NK1.1$^+$ and NK1.1$^-$ subsets of TCR^{int} cells consist of forbidden clones at almost the same levels (5).

TCR^{int} cells not only contain forbidden clones but also mediate self-reactivity against rapidly proliferating self cells and malignant cells (36,58). Such target cells include thymocytes, hepatocytes, intestinal epithelial cells, and established tumor cell lines. Concerning the existence of TCR^{int} cells in the thymus, liver, intestine, and tumor sites, TCR^{int} cells may play important roles *in vivo* for the regulation of cell proliferation and the surveillance of malignant cells.

What kinds of self-antigens or tumor antigens are recognized by TCR^{int} cells? The information about this subject is limited. If there are such antigens, they might be rep-

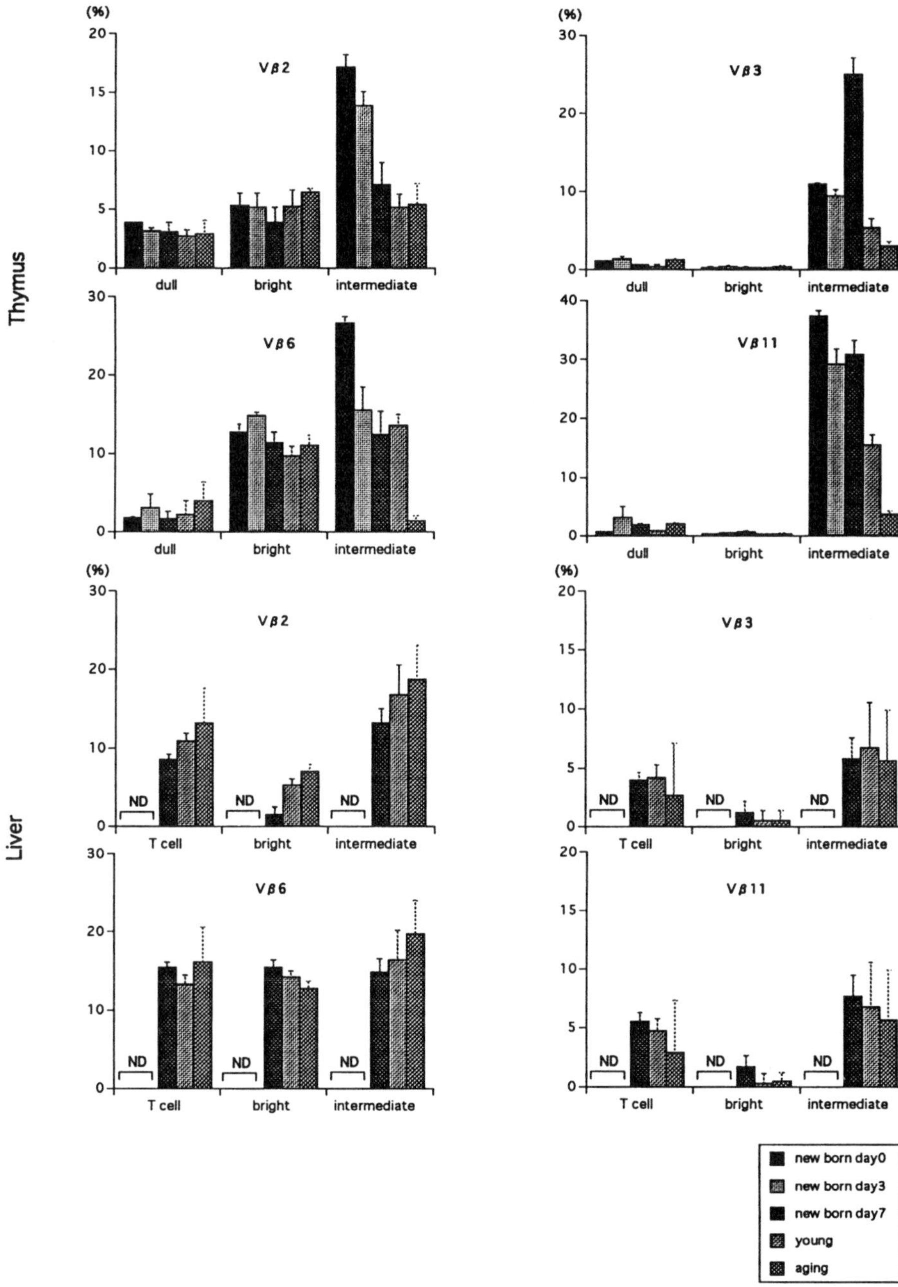

Figure 4.8. *(continued)*

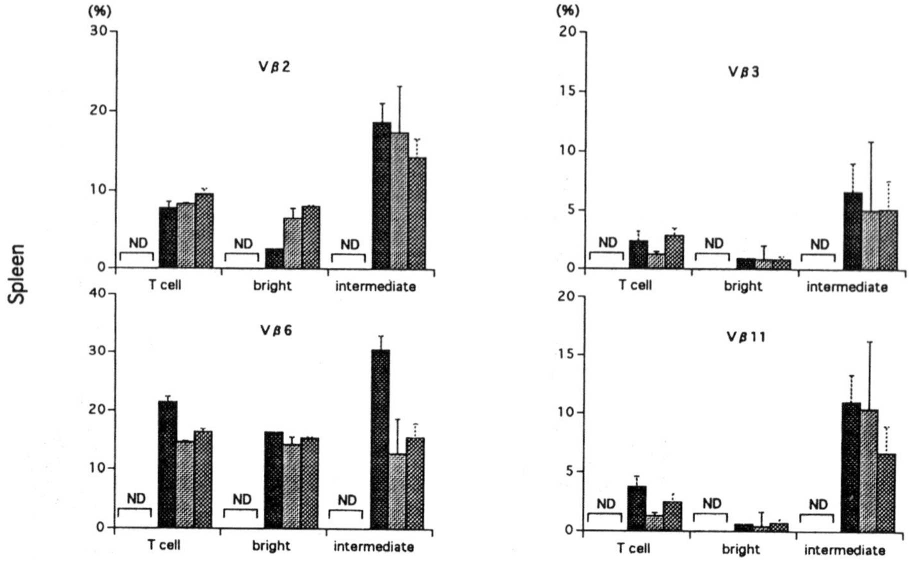

Figure 4.8. Self-reactive forbidden clones estimated in the Mls system are confined to CD3^{int} cells in all tested organs. Age-dependent variation in the proportion of self-reactive clones in CD3^{int} cells in the thymus, liver, and spleen was examined. In these experiments, six C3H/He mice at the ages indicated in the figure (young = 8 weeks old, aging = 50 weeks old) were used to produce the mean and one SD. In the case of C3H/He mice (Mls-1^{b}2^{a}), Vβ3^{+} and Vβ11^{+} cells are self-reactive forbidden clones. The proportion of forbidden clones tended to decrease as a function of age in the CD3^{int} population, especially in the thymus. Since CD3^{int} cells appeared from day 4 after birth, the proportion of Vβ^{+} cells among CD3^{int} cells was not detectable (ND) in newborn mice day 0 and day 3.

resented to TCR^{int} cells in the context with some monomorphic MHC antigens such as CD1 and TL antigens (59–62). We have demonstrated that TL-transgenic mice show the expansion of TCR^{int} cells in the generalized sites of these mice (62). However, the representation of some antigens for TCR^{int} cells seems not to be confined to monomorphic MHC antigens. The disparity of polymorphic MHC antigens, including both class I and class II MHC antigens, influences the phenotype of expanding TCR^{int} cells (63). This is true even in the disparity of allogenic MHC antigens (T. Abo et al., unpublished observation), leading to the conclusion that TCR^{int} cells can recognize a wider range of MHC antigens than initially believed.

In the case of humans, monomorphic MHC antigens include not only CD1 antigen but also HLA-E, F, G antigens (64–69). Interestingly, HLA-E is mainly expressed on intestinal epithelial cells, HLA-F is on hepatocytes, and HLA-G is on decidual membrane. All these sites are estimated to be those where extrathymic T cells exist. It is speculated that primordial T cells recognize some self-antigens in the context of these monomorphic MHC antigens. After the phylogenetic development of conventional

T cells and polymorphic MHC antigens, such primordial T cells and primordial MHC antigens remain at specific sites in our body.

OTHER PRIMITIVE LYMPHOCYTES, NK CELLS AND $CD5^+B$ CELLS

The description thus far has shown that phylogenetically extrathymic T cells might be more primordial than thymus-derived T cells. In this respect, NK cells seem to be the most primitive lymphocytes that have arisen during T cell development. NK cells and extrathymic T cells share many common properties such as LGL (large granular lymphocyte) morphology and constitutive expression of IL-2Rβ. NK cells have already acquired a primitive form of CD3 complex, which is activated via CD16 molecules on the cell surface (70,71). There is a possibility that some cells carrying primitive TCR-like molecules other than CD16 might exist somewhere in animals.

It is well established that $CD5^+B$ cells, which preferentially produce autoantibodies, exist in the peritoneal cavity and the spleen of autoimmune NZB/W F_1 mice (72–75). These $CD5^+B$ cells have also been found in the thymic medulla and the hepatic sinusoids of normal and diseased living bodies (76). This pattern of localization is quite similar to that of primordial T cells. Moreover, it is reported that some DN $CD4^-8^-$ αβ T cells mediate help to $CD5^+B$ cells (77,78). This raises the possibility that $CD5^+B$ cells, together with extrathymic T cells, comprise a primitive immune system. If this is the case, more highly developed T cells (thymus-derived T cells) may comprise a higher immune system together with regular $CD5^-B$ cells. Further investigation is required.

RECIPROCAL REGULATION OF INTRA- AND EXTRATHYMIC T CELL DIFFERENTIATION

Extrathymic pathways of T cell differentiation are activated with aging and under conditions of malignancies, pregnancy, and bacterial infections. Interestingly, thymic involution or atrophy always accompanies these conditions. We feel that intra- and extrathymic pathways of T cell differentiation are reciprocally regulated by certain factors. Tumor necrosis factor (TNF) α and β, and estrogen, are possibly such factors (79–82). Our previous findings showed that lymphotoxin (TNFβ) simultaneously induces the activation of TCR^{int} cells in the liver and the inactivation of intrathymic T cell differentiation (showing profound thymic atrophy). This reciprocal response induced by TNFβ is quite transient in duration (a few days). On the other hand, administration of estrogen induces a long-lasting effect (a few weeks) of the reciprocal response. We speculate that TNFβ (and TNFα) and estrogen may be the actual mediators for the reciprocal responses seen under conditions of malignancies, bacterial infections, and pregnancy, respectively.

Steroid hormones, such as glucocorticoids, are known to induce profound thymic atrophy and subsequent suppression of intrathymic T cell differentiation when injected into humans and animals. In the case of glucocorticoids, the simultaneous suppression of extrathymic T cell differentiation is induced (81). As a result, with regard to the intrathymic pathway, glucocorticoids are estimated to be completely immunosuppressive drugs, whereas TNFβ and estrogen are considered to be selective immunosuppressive drugs.

As already mentioned, extrathymic T cells and thymus-derived T cells seem to have separate functions in protecting the living body (i.e., a dichotomy of functions). For example, extrathymic T cells survey atypical cells generated *in vivo* by virtue of their autoreactivity, whereas T cells of thymic origin act to eliminate foreign antigens in the context of self-MHC antigens. Consequently, their reciprocal activation may be very important in the appropriate accomplishment of their own functions.

BIOLOGICAL FUNCTION OF TCR^{int} CELLS

Aging

In youth, the levels of TCR^{int} cells in the liver (i.e., one of the extrathymic pathways) and thymus (i.e., an alternative intrathymic pathway) are very low, but these levels increase as a function of age (12,13). In other words, the immune system in youth is highly dependent on the mainstream of T cell differentiation in the thymus. The homing sites for these thymus-derived T cells are the lymph nodes, the white pulp in the spleen, and the Peyer's patches in the intestine. It is conceivable that conventional T cells processing foreign antigens are much more important in youth, namely, in the most active stages of life. On the other hand, in parallel with age-associated thymic involution, the number and proportion of TCR^{int} cells increase in the liver and all other immune organs. Infected cells and atypical cells whose numbers increase with aging might be surveyed by such TCR^{int} cells. In the case of mice, the proportions of TCR^{int} cells overcome those of TCR^{high} cells in all immune organs at more than 100 weeks of age (13). This is true even in the thymus; that is, the alternative intrathymic pathway becomes more prominent than the mainstream.

It is well established that lymphocytes infiltrate various organs such as the lacrimal glands and salivary glands in aged mice and humans. In a recent study, we demonstrated that the majority of such lymphocytes belong to TCR^{int} cells (T. Abo et al., unpublished observations). In the case of *aly/aly* mice, which genetically lack the formation of lymph nodes and Peyer's patches, lymphocyte infiltration into the salivary gland is accelerated, and these mice therefore show Sjögren syndrome-like signs as a function of age. The majority of these infiltrating lymphocytes are also estimated to be TCR^{int} cells, including both the $NK1.1^+$ and $NK1.1^-$ subsets (T. Abo et al., unpublished observations). In other words, the underlying mechanisms in aging and some autoimmune diseases have some similarities.

Autoimmune Diseases

Responses of the autoreactivity medicated by TCR^{int} cells are usually beneficial for immunological surveillance. However, the overactivation of TCR^{int} cells seems to be responsible for the onset of certain autoimmune diseases (83–85). In this respect, we would like to propose one possible mechanism involved in the induction of autoimmune diseases. In recent studies, we have focused attention on adrenergic and cholinergic receptors on leukocytes. In the cases of phagocytic cells such as granulocytes and macrophages, adrenergic receptors are much more dominant than cholinergic receptors on the surface (86–89). In contrast, conventional T and B cells carry cholinergic receptors more predominantly (90) (see Fig. 4.9). Possibly reflecting this situation, granulocytes tend to increase in number and activate in function during sympathetic stress. On the other hand, under physical conditions showing parasympathetic stress, conventional T and B cells increase in number and become activated (91,92). Interestingly, NK cells and extrathymic T cells (i.e., primordial lymphocytes) carry far more adrenergic receptors than cholinergic receptors.

When humans and animals are exposed to severe mental or physical stresses, both granulocytes and extrathymic T cells increase in number as a generalized response in

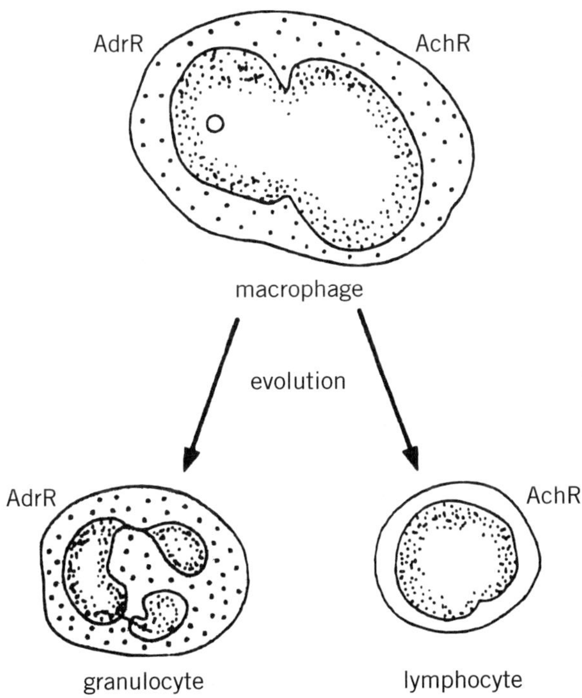

Figure 4.9. Surface receptors that accept stimuli from the autonomic nervous system, on leukocytes. Macrophages or ancestor macrophages carry both adrenergic receptors (AdrR) and acetylcholine receptors (AchR) on the surface. At a subsequent stage in evaluation, granulocytes and lymphocytes developed. At that time, granulocytes mainly acquired AdrR and acted in response to sympathetic nerve stimuli, whereas lymphocytes mainly acquired AchR and acted in response to parasympathetic nerve stimuli. This is because granulocytes must process bacteria by their phagocytotic function, whereas lymphocytes must process small antigens by their recognition system under resting conditions.

the body. As already known and shown in our recent studies (89), the production of granulocytes and extrathymic T cells occurs very quickly. This is due to their short life span (e.g., the life span of granulocytes is only 2–3 days). It is known that granulocytes release free radicals and superoxides when they undergo apoptosis (93,94). On the other hand, extrathymic T cells have a potential to mediate autoreactivity (37). As a result, activated granulocytes and extrathymic T cells induced under sympathetic nerve strain might be responsible for the induction of tissue damage and for the subsequent onset of autoimmune diseases. Many clinicians empirically know that patients have often experienced severe infections (e.g., a common cold due to viral infection) just before the onset of autoimmune diseases.

Genetic backgrounds in humans and animals may also be associated with the above-mentioned mechanisms involved in autoimmune diseases. We have recently found that patients with autoimmune diseases (e.g., rheumatoid arthritus, multiple sclerosis, and systemic lupus erythematosus) and mice of autoimmune models (e.g., MRL-*lpr/lpr* mice and NZB/WF$_1$ mice) have higher levels of granulocytes and extrathymic T cells just before and after the onset of disease.

Infection by Intracellular Pathogens

Virus, rickettsia, some bacteria (e.g., *Listeria* and *Salmonera*) and many protozoa are known to act as intracellular pathogens. Since they grow in the cytoplasm of some cells in the body, it is easy to speculate that antibodies and conventional T cells hardly attack these pathogens. On the other hand, NK cells and extrathymic T cells may attack abnormal cells infected with these pathogens. Based on this working hypothesis, we have investigated the immune responses in mice infected with *Listeria monocytogenes* (14) and *Herpes simplex* virus (95). Mice with either infection show a prominent expansion of TCR^{int} cells in the liver and other organs. A unique order of lymphocyte activation is also seen in these mice, i.e., NK cells, extrathymic T cells, conventional T cells. An induction of conventional T cells at the late stage of infections suggests that disseminated pathogens might be finally processed by these T cells. In recent studies, we have intensively investigated how murine and human immune systems are activated during malaria infection (T. Abo et al., unpublished observation). Surprisingly, one of the most prominent expansions of extrathymic T cells in the liver occurs in mice infected with *Plasmodium*. Further experiments and clinical studies remain to be performed.

Pregnancy

One of the important sites where extrathymic T cells exist, is the uterus, especially the decidua of the uterus in pregnant mice. In recent studies, we proposed that these extrathymic T cells as well as NK cells in the decidua might be very important for inhibiting the invasion of fetal tissues (e.g., placental trophoblasts) into the mother (96). As is well established, the trophoblasts of the fetus lack the expression of polymorphic MHC antigens on the surface (97–99). Accordingly, these fetal tissues are not rejected by the maternal immune system. Instead, a danger of the invasion of fetal tissues into the mother arises.

The accumulation of NK cells and extrathymic T cells into the decidua becomes prominent at the late stage of pregnancy (96). The next question is how this activation of primordial lymphocytes is regulated in pregnant animals. Two major factors are pointed out: (i) estrogen and (ii) sympathetic nerve stress. At the late stage of pregnancy, a large amount of estrogen is released from the placenta for the maturation of the uterus in the mother. This estrogen is found to stimulate the differentiation of extrathymic T cells both in the uterus and the liver. This effect of estrogen was confirmed in nonpregnant mice injected with estrogen (80).

Another important factor inducting the differentiation of extrathymic T cells is sympathetic nerve stress. As already mentioned in the section on stress, both NK cells and extrathymic T cells carry adrenergic receptors on the surface. Therefore, sympathetic nerve stress at a late stage of pregnancy induces the activation of these primordial T cells. Granulocytes are also known to carry adrenergic receptors (86–89), and the levels of granulocytes in the blood and other immune organs, including the uterus, increased prominently at the late stage of pregnancy. These granulocytes are beneficial for the protection of the mother from infection and from the invasion of fetal tissues. Under normal pregnancy conditions, an appropriate sympathetic nerve dominance may be important for the maintenance of fetal growth, especially at the late stage of pregnancy. However, the overactivation of granulocytes and primordial lymphocytes carrying adrenergic receptors on the surface sometimes induce tachycardia, hypertension (i.e., severe sympathetic stress) and renal failure, and result in pregnant toxicosis or preeclampsia.

It is known that HLA-G is expressed on the surface of fetal trophoblasts (68,69). There is a possibility that some self-antigens are recognized by uterine extrathymic T cells in the context of this monomorphic MHC antigen. In any case, TCR^{int} cells are intimately responsible for the physiology and pathology of immunological responses during pregnancy.

Malignancy

When we observed tumor-bearing mice, a large proportion of tumor-infiltrating lymphocytes (TILs) were estimated to be TCR^{int} cells as well as NK cells (100,101). We speculated that extrathymic T cells may play an important role for the immunological surveillance of malignant cells. This speculation was also occasioned by the fact that TCR^{int} cells mediate cytotoxicity against established tumor cell lines, even if they are of syngeneic origin (36). Generally, TCR^{int} cells have lesser cytotoxic activity against NK-sensitive targets than do NK cells. However, TCR^{int} cells could mediate the cytotoxicity against NK-resistant tumor targets. In this case, the cytotoxicity was found to be augmented in the presence of antibody against TCR$\alpha\beta$, TCR$\gamma\delta$, or CD3. There is a possibility that the cytotoxicity is mediated by TCR^{int} cells through their TCR-CD3 complex. This seems to be quite different from the mechanisms involved in NK cytotoxicity.

How are NK cells, extrathymic T cells, and conventional cytotoxic lymphocytes (CTLs) associated with tumor immunity? To answer this question, further investigation is required.

In recent studies, Seki et al. (102,103) and Arase et al. (104) have demonstrated that TCR^{int} cells or NKT cells are intimately associated with the inhibition of tumor metastasis into the liver and lung in tumor-bearing mice. Since these TCR^{int} cells or NKT cells are abundantly present in these organs, they may act as an important surveillance system for circulating tumor cells.

We have also demonstrated that there is massive infiltration of TCR^{int} cells into the tumor sites in mice that show a spontaneous onset of melanoma due to *ret* transgene (101). At least under some specific conditions or against specific tumor targets, TCR^{int} cells or NKT cells are important effectors *in vivo* against malignant cells.

Chronic Graft-Versus-Host Diseases (GVHD)

In contrast to acute GVHD, chronic GVHD often shows autoimmune-like symptoms after allogeneic bone marrow transplantation (BMT). Usually chronic GVHD is induced after allogeneic BMT into mice and humans in immunosuppressive states. When bone marrow cells contain a considerable proportion of TCR^{high} cells, severe GVHD (i.e., acute GVHD) tends to be evoked. This is true when mice are injected with allogeneic splenocytes (i.e., TCR^{high} cells). However, when bone marrow cells depleted of TCR^{high} cells are injected into mice in immunosuppressive states, chronic GVHD is induced. It is found that almost all of the recovering cells are TCR^{int} cells of donor origin in these mice (58). In other words, TCR^{int} cells are associated with the onset of chronic GVHD and, therefore, chronic GVHD resembles autoimmune diseases. The reactivity and cytotoxicity of TCR^{int} cells are usually lesser than those of TCR^{high} cells. Due to this situation, the symptoms induced by the association of TCR^{int} cells tend to be mild, and such TCR^{int} cells induce chronic GVHD rather than acute GVHD.

It is known that chronic GVHD is induced even when syngeneic BMT is performed with mice in immunosuppressive states (58). Since TCR^{int} cells mediate self-reactivity as well as alloreactivity, there is a possibility that such syngeneic GVHD is induced by their own TCR^{int} cells, and we may conclude that the liver is always a major target organ where TCR^{int} cells are primarily present.

Chronic GVHD is induced under conditions of MHC class II disparity (e.g., B6 mice vs. *bm12* mice). In this situation, the expanding T cells, which induce chronic GVHD are also found to be TCR^{int} cells (manuscript submitted for publication). This result also suggests that TCR^{int} cells recognize some antigens in the context not only of monomorphic MHC class I antigen (e.g., CD1 and TL) but also of polymorphic class II antigens. As mentioned above, TCR^{int} cells could recognize even allogeneic polymorphic MHC class I (and II) disparity.

EXTRATHYMIC T CELLS IN HUMANS

Human Counterparts of Extrathymic T Cells

Small populations of T cells carrying NK markers are found in the peripheral blood of humans. Such T cells include CD56^{+}T cells and CD57^{+}T cells (105–107). As with murine NK-T cells, all properties of CD56^{+}T cells and CD57^{+}T cells are unique.

They have the morphology of granular lymphocytes. The cell size of these NK-T cells is smaller than those of CD56$^+$NK cells and CD57$^+$NK cells, and NK-T cells have fewer numbers of cytoplasmic granules than do NK cells. Human CD56$^+$T cells and CD57$^+$T cells include DN CD4$^-$8$^-$ cells, as well as single-positive cells, and always contain a significant proportion of γδ T cells (up to 25%). However, CD56$^+$T cells and CD57$^+$T cells have some properties that differ from those of murine NK-T cells. Human NK-T cells do not constitutively express IL-2Rβ and acquire a high density of TCR-CD3 complex comparable to that of conventional T cells. During phylogenetic development, NK-T cells may somewhat change their phenotype or function.

Although CD56$^+$T cells and CD57$^+$T cells are minor populations in the peripheral blood, CD56$^+$T cells are abundant in the liver, while CD57$^+$T cells are abundant in the bone marrow (107) (see Fig. 4.10). CD56$^+$T cells have higher NK-like cytotoxicity than do CD57$^+$T cells (108). Considering these tissue distributions and functions, CD56$^+$T cells resemble the NK1.1$^+$ subset of TCR^{int} cells in mice, and CD57$^+$T cells resemble the NK1.1$^-$ subset of TCR^{int} cells. Possibly reflecting this situation, the levels of CD56$^+$T cells increase in patient with viral hepatitis and the levels of CD57$^+$T cells increase in patients subjected to bone marrow transplantation.

Physiological and Pathological Roles of Human Extrathymic T Cells

In the cord blood of neonates, there are no CD56$^+$T cells and CD57$^+$T cells (i.e., 0%). A significant proportion of CD56$^+$NK cells, but not CD57$^+$ NK cells, is already pres-

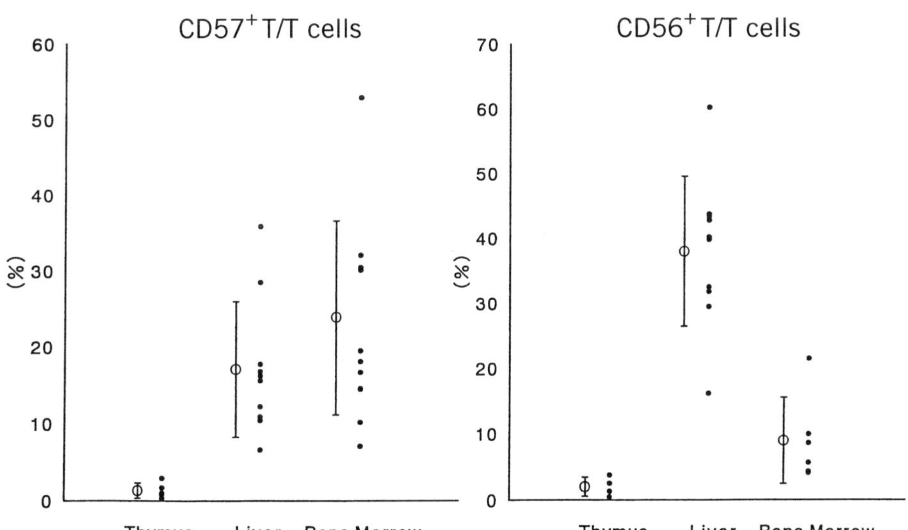

Figure 4.10. Extrathymic T cells or NK-T cells in humans. CD57$^+$T cells and CD56$^+$T cells in humans may correspond to NK-T cells in mice. CD57$^+$T cells are abundant in the bone marrow (and the liver), whereas CD56$^+$T cells are abundant in the liver. Considering their tissue distribution and function, CD56$^+$T cells correspond to NK1.1$^+$ subset of TCR^{int} cells, while CD57$^+$T cells correspond to the NK1.1$^-$ subset of TCR^{int} cells in mice.

ent at this age. Both CD56$^+$T cells and CD57$^+$T cells appear in the peripheral blood in childhood, and the proportions increase as a function of age. In a recent study (108), we have examined the levels of CD56$^+$T cells and CD57$^+$T cells in the peripheral blood of 51 centenarians. Surprisingly, the proportions of CD56$^+$T cells and CD57$^+$T cells overcome those of conventional CD56$^-$T and CD57$^-$T cells. It is conceivable that abnormal cells generated with aging might be eliminated by NK-T cells in aged persons. Similar to the case of Vα14$^+$ cells on NK-T cells in mice, there was a report that the Vα24$^+$ cells exist in human (109). However, Vα24$^+$ cells are a relatively minor population among CD56$^+$T cells and CD57$^+$T cells. In sharp contrast, almost all of NK-T cells are Vα14$^+$ in mice.

As in mice, the proportions of CD56$^+$T cells or CD57$^+$T cells tend to increase in patients with autoimmune diseases such as rheumatoid arthritis and systemic lupus erythematosus (manuscript submitted for publication). It remains obscure whether these CD56$^+$T cells or CD57$^+$T cells are simply associated with the onset of autoimmune diseases or have a regulatory role.

It has been reported that CD56$^+$NK cells and CD56$^+$T cells are abundant in the decidua of pregnant women (110,111). In a recent study, the levels of CD56$^+$T cells and/or CD57$^+$T cells are elevated in patients with pregnant toxicosis (or pregnancy-associated hypertension) (manuscript submitted for publication). Primarily, NK-T cells are very important for surveillance of the invasion of fetal tissue into the mother. However, the overactivation of such NK-T cells is very dangerous and results in tissue damage (e.g., to the kidney and liver). Indeed, many NK cells and NK-T, cells as well as granulocytes, appear in the urine of patients with proteinuria due to toxicosis of pregnancy. Since NK cells, NK-T cells, and granulocytes carry adrenergic receptors on the surface, the sympathetic nerve strain at the late stage of pregnancy may be associated with the mechanisms involved in the onset of toxicosis of pregnancy.

CONCLUSION

Extrathymic T cells have been demonstrated both in mice and humans. Concerning their morphology, phenotype, and function, extrathymic T cells are at an intermediate position between NK cells and conventional T cells in phylogenic development. Conventional T cells are very important for the surveillance of the foreign antigens. On the other hand, extrathymic T cells are important for the surveillance of abnormal self cells, including rapidly dividing cells, cells infected with intracellular pathogens, and malignant cells. However, the overactivation of extrathymic T cells also contains the potential to induce autoimmune diseases. In some cases, extrathymic T cells play a role for regulating autoreactive lymphocytes. This situation reminds us of the importance of extrathymic T cells in our immune systems. Since the liver develops phylogenetically from the intestinal diverticulum, both liver and intestine contain extrathymic T cells. The recent evidence for the existence of c-kit$^+$ stem cells in the liver and intestine is also noteworthy. Almost all of extrathymic T cells existing in the digestive tract arise from these c-kit$^+$ stem cells in the bone marrow.

REFERENCES

1. Ohteki, T., Seki, S., Abo, T., and Kumagai, K. 1990. Liver is a possible site for the proliferation of abnormal $CD3^+4^-8^-$ double-negative lymphocytes in autoimmune MRL-*lpr/lpr* mice. *J. Exp. Med.* 172:7–12.
2. Abo, T., Ohteki, T., Seki, S., Koyamada, N., Yoshikai, Y., Masuda, T., Rikiishi, H., and Kumagai, K. 1991. The appearance of T cells bearing self-reactive T cell receptor in the livers of mice injected with bacteria. *J. Exp. Med.* 174:417–424.
3. Seki, S., Abo, T., Ohteki, T., Sugiura, K., and Kumagai, K. 1991. Unusual αβ-T cells expanded in autoimmune lpr mice are probably a counterpart of normal T cell in the liver. *J. Immunol.* 147:1214–1221.
4. Sato, K., Ohtsuka, K., Hsegawa, K., Yamagiwa, S., Watanabe, H., Iwanaga, T., Takahashi-Iwanaga, H., Asakura, H., and Abo, T. 1995. Evidence for extrathymic generation of intermediate TCR cells in the liver revealed in thymectomized, irradiated mice subjected to bone marrow transplantation. *J. Exp. Med.* 182:759–767.
5. Watanabe, H., Miyaji, C., Kawachi, Y., Iiai, T., Ohtsuka, K., Iwanaga, T., Takahashi-Iwanaga, H., and Abo, T. 1995. Relationships between intermediate TCR cells and $NK1.1^+T$ cells in various immune organs. $NK1.1^+T$ cells are present within a population of intermediate TCR cells. *J. Immunol.* 155:2972–2983.
6. Watanabe, H., Miyaji, C., Seki, S., and Abo, T. 1996. c-kit^+ stem cells and thymocyte precursors in the livers of adult mice. *J. Exp. Med.* 184:687–693.
7. Kanamori, Y., Ishimaru, K., Nanno, M., Maki, K., Ikuta, K., Nariuchi, H., and Ishikawa, H. 1996. Identification of novel lymphoid tissues in murine intestinal mucosa where clusters of c-kit^+IL-$7R^+Thy1^+$ lympho-hemopoietic progenitors develop. *J. Exp. Med.* 184:1449–1459.
8. Abo, T., Watanabe, H., Iiai, T., Kimura, M., Ohtsuka, K., Sato, K., Ogawa, M., Hirahara, H., Hashimoto, S., Sekikawa, H., and Seki, S. 1994. Extrathymic pathways of T-cell differentiation in the liver and other organs. *Int. Rev. Immunol.* 11:61–102.
9. Kawachi, Y., Watanabe, H., Moroda, T., Haga, M., Iiai, T., Hatakeyama, K., and Abo, T. 1995. Self-reactive T cell clones in a restricted population of IL-2 receptor β^+ cells expressing intermediate levels of the T cell receptor in the liver and other immune organs. *Eur. J. Immunol.* 25:2272–2278.
10. Moroda, T., Kawachi, Y., Iiai, T., Tsukahara, A., Suzuki, S., Tada, T., Watanabe, H., Hatakeyama, K., and Abo, T. 1997. Self-reactive forbidden clones are confined to pathways of intermediate T cell receptor cell differentiation even under immunosuppressive conditions. *Immunology* 91:88–94.
11. Watanabe, H., Ohtsuka, K., Kimura, M., Ikarashi, Y., Ohmori, K., Kusumi, A., Ohteki, T., Seki, S., and Abo, T. 1992. Details of an isolation method for hepatic lymphocytes in mice. *J. Immunol. Methods* 146:145–154.
12. Iiai, T., Watanabe, H., Seki, S., Sugiura, K., Hirokawa, K., Utsuyama, M., Takahashi-Iwanaga, H., Iwanaga, T., Ohteki, T., and Abo, T. 1992. Ontogeny and development of extrathymic T cells in mouse liver. *Immunology* 77:556–563.
13. Ohtsuka, K., Hasegawa, K., Sato, K., Arai, K., Watanabe, H., Asakura, H., and Abo, T. 1994. A similar expression pattern of adhesion molecules between intermediate TCR cells in the liver and intraepithelial lymphocytes in the intestine. *Microbiol. Immunol.* 38:677–683.

14. Ohtsuka, K., Sato, K., Watanabe, H., Kimura, M., Asakura, H., and Abo, T. 1995. Unique order of the lymphocyte subset induction in the liver and intestine of mice during *Listeria monocytogenes* infection. *Cell. Immunol.* 161:112–124.
15. Watanabe, H., Iiai, T., Kimura, M., Ohtsuka, K., Tanaka, T., Miyasaka, M., Tsuchida, M., Hanawa, H., and Abo, T. 1993. Characterization of intermediate TCR cells in the liver of mice with respect to their unique IL-2R expression. *Cell. Immunol.* 149:331–342.
16. Koyasu, S. 1994. $CD3^+CD16^+NK1.1^+B220^+$ large granular lymphocytes arise from both α-$\beta TCR^+CD4^-CD8^-$ cells and γ-δ $TCR^+CD4^-CD8^-$ cells. *J. Exp. Med.* 179:1957–1972.
17. Sato, K., Ohtsuka, K., Watanabe, H., Asakura, H., and Abo, T. 1993. Detailed characterization of $\gamma\delta$T cells within the organs of mice: classification into three groups. *Immunology* 80:380–387.
18. Sanchez, M.J., Muench, M.O., Roncarolo, M.G., Lanier, L.L., and Phillips, J.H. 1994. Identification of a common T/natural killer cell progenitor in human fetal thymus. *J. Exp. Med.* 180:569–576.
19. Arai, K., Iiai, T., Nakayama, M., Hasegawa, K., Sato, K., Ohtsuka, K., Watanabe, H., Hanyu, T., Takahashi, H.E., and Abo, T. 1995. Adhesion molecules on intermediate TCR cells. I. Unique expression of adhesion molecules, $CD44^+$L-selectin$^-$, on intermediate TCR cells in the liver and the modulation of their adhesion by hyaluronic acid. *Immunology* 84:64–71.
20. Nakayama, M., Arai, K., Hasegawa, K., Sato, K. Ohtsuka, K., Watanabe, H., Sakai, K., Rikiishi, H., and Abo, T. 1995. Adhesion molecules on intermediate TCR cells, II. Hepatoprotective effects of hyaluronic acid on acute liver injury. *Cell. Immunol.* 166:275–284.
21. Budd, R.C., Miecher, G.C., Howe, R.C., Lees, R.K., Bron, C., and MacDonald, H.R. 1987. Developmentally regulated expression of T cell receptor β chain variable domains in immature thymocytes. *J. Exp. Med.* 166:577–582.
22. Fowlkes, B.J., Kruisbeek, A.M., Ton-That, H., Weston, M.A., Coligan, J.E., Schwartz, R.H., and Pardoll, D.M. 1987. A novel population of T-cell receptor $\alpha\beta$-bearing thymocytes which predominantly expresses a single Vβ gene family. *Nature* 329:251–254.
23. Crispe, I.N., Moore, M.W., Husmann, L.A., Smith, L., Bevan, M.J., and Shimonkevitz, R.P. 1987. Differentiation potential of subsets of $CD4^-8^-$ thymocytes. *Nature* 329:336–339.
24. Takahama, Y., Kosugi, A., and Singer, A. 1991. Phenotype, ontogeny, and repertoire of $CD4^-CD8^-$ T cell receptor $\alpha\beta^+$ thymocytes. Variable influence of self-antigens of T cell receptor Vβ usage. *J. Immunol.* 146:1134–1141.
25. Egerton, M., and Scollay, R. 1990. Intrathymic selection of murine $TCR\alpha\beta^+$ $CD4^-CD8^-$ thymocytes. *Int. Immunol.* 2:157–163.
26. Huang, L., and Crispe, I.N. 1992. Distinctive selection mechanisms govern the T cell receptor repertoire of peripheral $CD4^-CD8^-$ α/β T cells. *J. Exp. Med.* 176:699–706.
27. Prud'homme, G.J., Bocarro, D.C., and Luke, E.C.H. 1991. Clonal deletion and autoreactivity in extrathymic $CD4^-CD8^-$ (double negative) T cell receptor-α/β T cells. *J. Immunol.* 147:3314–3318.
28. Dejbakhsh-jones, S., Okazaki, H., and Strober, S. 1995. Similar rates of production of T and B lymphocytes in the bone marrow. *J. Exp. Med.* 181:2201–2211.

29. Bendelac, A. 1995. Mouse NK1.1$^+$ T cells. *Curr. Opin. Immunol.* 7:367–374.

30. MacDonald, H.R. 1995. NK1.1$^+$ T cells receptor- α/β^+ cells: new clues to their origin, specificity, and function. *J. Exp. Med.* 182:633–638.

31. Bix, M., and Locksley, R.M. 1995. Natural T cells. Cells that co-express NKRP-1 and TCR. *J. Immunol.* 155:1020–1022.

32. Vicari, A.P., and Zlotnik, A. 1996. Mouse NK1.1$^+$ T cells: a new family of T cells. *Immunology Today* 17:71–76.

33. Makino, Y., Yamagata, N., Sasho, T., Adachi, Y., Kanno, R., Koseki, H., Kanno, M., and Taniguchi, M. 1993. Extrathymic development of Vα14-positive T cells. *J. Exp. Med.* 177:1399–1408.

34. Olivier, L., and Bendelac, A. 1994. An invariant T cell receptor α chain is used by a unique subset of major histocompatibility complex class I-specific CD4$^+$ and CD4$^-$CD8$^-$ T cell in mice and humans. *J. Exp. Med.* 180:1097–1106.

35. Makino, Y., Kanno, R., Koseki, H., and Taniguchi, M. 1996. Development of Vα14$^+$ NK T cells in the early stages of embryogenesis. *Proc. Natl. Acad. Sci. U.S.A.* 93:6516–6520.

36. Kawamura, T., Kawachi, Y., Moroda, T., Weerashinghe, A., Iiai, T., Seki, S., Takada, G., and Abo, T. 1996. Cytotoxic activity against tumour cells mediated by intermediate TCR cells in the liver and spleen. *Immunology* 89:68–75.

37. Moroda, T., Iiai, T., Suzuki, S., Tsukahara, A., Tada, T., Nose, M., Hatakeyama, K., Seki, S., Takeda, K., Watanabe, H., and Abo, T. 1998. Autologous killing by a population of intermediate TCR cells and its NK1.1$^+$ and NK1.1$^-$ subsets, using Fas ligand/Fas molecules. *Immunology*, 91:219–226.

38. Emoto, M., Emoto, Y., and Kaufmann, S.H.E. 1995. IL-4 producing CD4$^+$ TCR$\alpha\beta^{int}$ liver lymphocytes: influence of thymus, β_2-microglobulin and NK1.1 expression. *Int. Immunol.* 7:1729–1739.

39. Bendelac, A., Hunziker, R.D., and Lantz, O. 1996. Increased interleukin 4 and immunoglobulin E production in transgenic mice overexpressing NK1 T cells. *J. Exp. Med.* 184:1285–1293.

40. Ferguson, A., and Parrott, D.M.V. 1972. The effect of antigen deprivation on thymus-dependent and thymus-independent lymphocytes in the small intestine of the mouse. *Clin. Exp. Immunol.* 12:477–488.

41. Rocha, B. 1990. Characterization of Vβ-bearing cells in athymic (nu/nu) mice suggests an extrathymic pathway for T cell differentiation. *Eur. J. Immunol.* 20:919–925.

42. Lake, J.P., Pierce, C.W., and Kennedy, J.D. 1991. T cell receptor expression by T cells that mature extrathymically in nude mice. *Cell. Immunol.* 135:259–265.

43. Mosley, R.L., Styre, D., and Klein, J.R. 1990. Differentiation and functional maturation of bone marrow-derived intestinal epethelial T cells expressing membrane T cell receptor in athymic radiation chimeras. *J. Immunol.* 145:1369–1375.

44. Ebert, E.C. 1990. Intra-epithelial lymphocytes: interferon-gamma production and suppressor/cytotoxic activities. *Clin. Exp. Immunol.* 82:81–85.

45. Bandeira, A., Utohara, S., Bonneville, M., Burlen-Defranoux, O., Mota-Santos, T., Coutinho, A., and Tonegawa, S. 1991. Extrathymic origin of intestinal intraepithelial lymphocytes bearing T cell antigen receptor $\gamma\delta$. *Proc. Natl. Acad. Sci. U.S.A.* 88:43–47.

46. Guy-Grand, D., Malassis-Seris, M., Briottet, C., and Vassalli, P. 1991. Cytotoxic differentiation of mouse gut thymodependent and independent intraepithelial T lymphocytes is

induced locally. Correlation between functional assays, presence of perforin and granzyme transcripts, and cytoplasmic granules. *J. Exp. Med.* 173:1549–1552.

47. Mosley, R.L., Styre, D., and Klein, J.R. 1990. Differentiation and functional maturation of bone marrow-derived intestinal epithelial T cells expressing membrane T cell receptor in athymic radiation chimeras. *J. Immunol.* 145:1369–1375.

48. Croitoru, K., Stead, R.H., Bienenstock, J., Fulop, G., Harnish, D.G., Shultz, L.D., Jeffery, P.K., and Ernst, P.B. 1990. Presence of intestinal intraepithelial lymphocytes in mice with severe combined immunodeficiency disease. *Eur. J. Immunol.* 20:645–651.

49. Guy-Grand, D., Griscelli, C., and Vassalli, P. 1978. The mouse gut T lymphocyte, a novel type of T cell. *J. Exp. Med.* 148:1664–1677.

50. Abo, T. 1992. Extrathymic differentiation of T lymphocytes and its biological function. *Biomed. Res.* 13:1–39.

51. Mabuchi, A., Komuro, T., Saizawa, T., Sakamoto, T., Watari, E., and Yokomuro, K. 1991. The liver and the hematolymphoid system, I. The regulation of nylon passed spleen cell proliferation by active factors released from syngenic nonparenchymal liver cells. *J. Leuk. Biol.* 50:402–411.

52. Matsuguchi, T., Okamura, S., Kawasaki, C., and Niho, Y. 1990. Production of interleukin 6 from human liver cell lines: production of interleukin 6 is not concurrent with the production of α-fetoprotein. *Cancer Res.* 50:7457–7459.

53. Kutteh, W.H., Rainey, W.E., and Carr, B.R. 1991. Regulation of interleukin-6 production in human fetal Kupffer cells. *Scand. J. Immunol.* 33:607–613.

54. Riches, P., Gooding, R., Millar, B.C., and Rowbottom, A.W. 1992. Influence of collection and separation of blood samples on plasma IL-1, IL-6 and TNF-α concentrations. *J. Immunol. Methods* 153:125–131.

55. Ehlers, S., Mielke, M.E.A., Blankenstein, T., and Hahan, H. 1992. Kinetic analysis of cytokine gene expression in the livers of naive and immune mice infected with *Listeria monocytogenes*. *J. Immunol.* 149:3016–3022.

56. Miyaji, C., Watanabe, H., Osman, Y., Kuwano, Y., and Abo, T. 1996. A comparison of proliferative response to IL-7 and expression of IL-7 receptors in intermediate TCR cells of the liver, spleen, and thymus. *Cell. Immunol.* 169:159–165.

57. Moroda, T., Iiai, T., Kawachi, Y., Kawamura, T., Hatakeyama, K., and Abo, T. 1996. Resteicted appearance of self-reactive clones into intermediate T cell receptor cells in neonatally thymectomized mice with autoimmune disease. *Eur. J. Immunol.* 26:3084–3091.

58. Osman, Y., Watanabe, T., Kawachi, Y., Sato, K., Ohtsuka, K., Watanabe, H., Hashimoto, S., Moriyama, Y., Shibata, A., and Abo, T. 1995. Intermediate TCR cells with self-reactive clones are effector cells which induce syngeneic graft-versus-host disease in mice. *Cell. Immunol.* 166:172–186.

59. Porcelli, S., Morita, C.T., and Brenner, M.B. 1992. CD1b restricts the response of human $CD4^-CD8^-$ T lymphocytes to a microbial antigen. *Nature* 360:593–597.

60. Bendelac, A. 1995. Positive selection of mouse $NK1^+$ T cells by CD1-expressing cortical thymocytes. *J. Exp. Med.* 182:2091–2096.

61. Porcelli, S.A., and Modlin, R.L. 1995. CD1 and the expanding universe of T cell antigens. *J. Immunol.* 155:3709–3710.

62. Watanabe, H., Ohtsuka, K., Obata, Y., Iiai, T., Kimura, M., Takahashi, T., Hirokawa, K. Utsuyama, M., and Abo, T. 1993. Generalized expansion of extrathymic T cells in various immune organs of TL-transgenic mice. *Biomed. Res.* 14:273–288.

63. Ikarashi, Y., Abo, T., Kawai, K. Iiai, T., Watanabe, H., Suzuki, K., Matsumoto, Y., Omata, S., and Fujiwara, M. 1994. Expansion of intermediate TCR cells of mice with autoimmune-like graft-versus-host disease. *Immunology* 83:205–212.

64. Chen, Z.W., McAdam, S.N., Hughes, A.L., Dogon, A.L., Letvin, N.L., and Watkins, D.I. 1992. Molecular cloning of orangutan and gibbon MHC class I cDNA the HLA-A and -B Loci diverged over 30 million years ago. *J. Immunol.* 148:2547–2554.

65. Ulbrecht, M., Honka, T., Person, S., Johnson, J.P., and Weiss, E.H. 1992. The HLA-E gene encodes two differentially regulated transcripts and a cell surface protein. *J. ımmunol.* 149:2945–2953.

66. Ishitani, A., and Geraghty, D.E. 1992. Alternative splicing of HLA-G transcripts yields proteins with primary structures resembling both class I and class II antigens. *Immunology* 89:3947–3951.

67. Houlihan, J.M., Biro, P.A., Fergar-Payne, A., Simpson, K.L., and Holmes, C.H. 1992. Evidence for the expression of non-HLA-A, -B, -C class I genes in the human fetal liver. *J. Immunol.* 149:668–675.

68. Kirszenbaum, M., Moreau, P., Gluckman, E., and Dausset, J. 1994. An alternatively spliced form of *HLA-G* mRNA in human trophoblasts and evidence for the presence of *HLA-G* transcript in adult lymphocytes. *Proc. Natl. Acad. Sci. U.S.A.* 91:4209-4213.

69. Yelavarthi, K.K., Schmidt, C.M., Ehlenfeldt, R.G., Orr, H.T., and Hunt, J.S. 1993. Cellular distribution of HLA-G mRNA in transgenic mouse placents. *J. Immunol.* 151:3638–3645.

70. Lanier, L.L., Ruitenberg, J.J., and Phillips, J.H. 1988. Functional and biochemical analysis of CD16 antigen on natural killer cells and granulocytes. *J. Immunol.* 141:3478–3485.

71. Edberg, J.C., Barinsky, M., Redecha, P.B., Salmon, J.E., and Kimberly, R.P. 1990. FcγRIII expressed on cultured monocytes is a N-glycosylated transmembrane protein distinct from FcγRIII expressed on natural killer cells. *J. Immunol.* 144:4729–4734.

72. Hardy, R.R., Hayakawa, K., Shimizu, M., Yamasaki, K., and Kishimoto, T. 1987. Rheumatoid factor secretion from human Leu-1$^+$ B cells. *Science* 236:81–83.

73. Hayakawa, K., Hardy, R.R., Parks, D.R., and Herzenberg, L.A. 1983. The "Ly-1B" cell subpopulation in normal, immunodefective, and autoimmune mice. *J. Exp. Med.* 157:202–218.

74. Herzenberg, L.A., Stall, A.M., Lalor, P.A., Sidman, C., Moore, W.A., Parks, D.R., and Herzenberg, L.A. 1986. The Ly-1B cell lineage. *Immunol. Rev.* 93:81–102.

75. Ohteki, T., Abo, T., Kusumi, A., Sasaki, T., Shibata, S., Seki, S., and Kumagai, K. 1993. Age-associated increase of CD5$^+$ B cells in the liver of autoimmune (NZB x NZW) F_1 mice. *Microbiol. Immunol.* 37:221–228.

76. Tsuchida, M., Hashimoto, S., Abo, T., Miyamura, H., Hirono, T., and Eguchi, S. 1993. CD5$^+$ B cells in the thymus of patients with myasthenia gravis. *Biomed. Res.* 14:19–25.

77. Datta, S.K., Patel, H., and Berry, D. 1987. Induction of a cationic shift in IgG anti-DNA autoantibodies. Role of T helper cells with classical and novel phenotypes in three murine modes of lupus nephritis. *J. Exp. Med.* 165:1252–1268.

78. Sainis, K., and Datta, S.K. 1988. CD4+ T cell lines with selective patterns of autoreactivity as well as CD4$^-$ CD8$^-$ T helper cell lines augment the production of idiotypes shared by pathogenic anti-DNA autoantibodies in the NZB x SWR model of lupus nephritis. *J. Immunol.* 140:2215–2224.

79. Kusumi, A., Abo, T., Masuda, T., Sugiura, K., Seki, S., Ohteki, T., Okuyama, R., and Abo, T. 1992. Lymphotoxin activates hepatic T cells and simultaneously induces profound thymic atrophy. *Immunology* 77:177–184.

80. Okuyama, R., Abo, T., Seki, S., Ohteki, T., Sugiura, K., Kusumi, A., and Kumagai, K. 1992. Estrogen administration activates extrathymic T cell differentiation in the liver. *J. Exp. Med.* 175:661–669.

81. Hirahara, H., Ogawa, M., Kimura, M., Iiai, T., Tsuchida, M., Hanawa, H., Watanabe, H., and Abo, T. 1994. Glucocorticoid independence of acute thymic involution induced by lymphotoxin and estrogen. *Cell. Immunol.* 153:401–411.

82. Nakayama, M., Ohtsuka, K., Sato, K., Hsegawa, K., Osuman, Y., and Abo, T. 1996. Activation by estrogen of the number and function of self-reactive forbidden T cell clones in intermediate T-cell receptor cells. *Cell. Immunol.* 172:163–171.

83. Masuda, T., Ohteki, T., Abo, T., Seki, S., Nose, M., Nagura, H., and Kumagai, K. 1991. Expansion of the population of double negative $CD4^-8^-$ T$\alpha\beta$-cells in the liver is a common feature of autoimmune mice. *J. Immunol.* 147:2907–2912.

84. Iiai, T., Kimura, M., Kawachi, Y., Hirokawa, K., Watanabe, H., Hatakeyama, K., and Abo, T. 1995. Characterization of intermediate TCR cells expanding in the liver, thymus and other organs in autoimmune *lpr* mice: parallel analysis with their normal counterparts. *Immunology* 84:601–608.

85. Yamagiwa, S., Kuwano, Y., Hsegawa, K., Sato, K., Ohtsuka, K., Iiai, T., Tomiyama, K., Watanabe, H., Sugahara, S., Seki, S., Asakura, H., and Abo, T. 1996. Existence of a small population of IL-2Rβ^{hi} T cell receptor^{int} cells in SCG and MRL-*lpr/lpr* mice which produce normal Fas mRNA and Fas molecules from the *lpr* gene. *Eur. J. Immunol.* 26:1409–1416.

86. Fukuda, M., Moroda, T., Toyabe, S., Iiai, T., Kawachi, Y., Takahashi-Iwanaga, H., Iwanaga, T., Okada, M., and Abo, T. 1996. Granulocytes induced by increasing sympathetic nerve activity contributes to the incidence of acute appendicitis. *Biomed. Res.* 17:171–181.

87. Yamamura, S., Arai, K., Toyabe, S., Takahashi, E.H., and Abo, T. 1996. Simultaneous activation of granulocytes and extrathymic T cells in number and function by excessive administration of nonsteroidal anti-inflammatory drugs. *Cell. Immunol.* 173:303–311.

88. Yamamura, S., Miyaji, C., Watanabe, H., Kawamura, T., Fukuda, M., and Abo, T. 1996. Paradoxical effects of glycyrrhizin on the induction of granulocytes and extrathymic T cells between normal mice and mice with preexisting granulocytosis. *Acta Medica Biol.* 44:177–185.

89. Tsukahara, A., Tada, T., Suzuki, S., Iiai, T., Moroda, T., Maruyama, S., Minagawa, M., Musha, M., Shimizu, T., Hatakeyama, K., and Abo, T. 1998. Adrenergic stimulation simultaneously induces the expansion of granulocytes and extrathymic T cells in mice. *Biomed. Res.*, 18:237–247.

90. Toyabe, S., Iiai, T., Fukuda, M., Kawamura, T., Suzuki, S., Uchiyama, M., and Abo, T. 1998. Identification of nicotinic acetylcholine receptors on lymphocytes in periphery as well as thymus in mice. *Immunology*, 92:201–205.

91. Abo, T., Kawate, T., Itoh, K., and Kumagai, K. 1981. Studies on the bioperiodicity of the immune response, I. Circadian rhythms of human T, B, and K cell traffic in the peripheral blood. *J. Immunol.* 126:1360–1363.

92. Kawate, T., Abo, T., Hinuma, S., and Kumagai, K. 1981. Studies on the bioperiodicity of the immune response, II. Co-variations of murine T and B cells and a role of corticosteroid. *J. Immunol.* 126:1364–1367.

93. Takeda, Y., Watanabe, H., Yonehara, S., Yamashita, T., Saito, S., and Sendo, F. 1993. Rapid acceleration of neutrophil apoptosis by tumor necrosis factor-α. *Int. Immunol.* 5:691–695.

94. Yuo, A., Kitagawa, S., Suzuki, I., Urabe, A., Okada, T., Saito, M., and Takaku, F. 1989. Tumor necrosis factor as an activator of human granulocytes. Potentiation of the metabolisms triggered by the Ca^{2+}-mobilizing agonists. *J. Immunol.* 142:1678–1684.

95. Hasegawa, K., Ohtsuka, K., Shimizu, F., Kawachi, Y., Nakayama, M., Sato, K., Yamagiwa, S., Asakura, H., and Abo, T. 1996. Induction of NK cells and intermediate TCR cells with protective ability form viral infectious death, at the early phase of herpes virus infection. *Biomed. Res.* 17:67–79.

96. Kimura, M., Hanawa, H., Watanabe, H., Ogawa, M., and Abo, T. 1995. Synchronous expansion of intermediate TCR cells in the liver and uterus during pregnancy. *Cell. Immunol.* 162:16–25.

97. Faulk, W.P., and Temple, A. 1976. Distribution of β_2 microglobulin and HLA in chorionic villi of human placentae. *Nature* 262:799–802.

98. Goodfellow, P.N., Barnstable, C.J., Bodmer, W.F., Snary, D.E., and Crumpton, M.J. 1976. Expression of HLA system antigens on placenta. *Transplantation* 22:595–603.

99. Galbraith, R.M., Kantor, R.R.S., Ferrar, G.B., Ades, E.W., and Galbraith, G.M.P. 1981. Differential anatomical expression of transplantation antigens within the normal human placental chorionic villus. *Am. J. Reprod. Immunol.* 1:331–335.

100. Ohmori, K., Iiai, T., Watanabe, H., Tanaka, T., Miyasaka, M., and Abo, T. 1993. Activation of extrathymic T cells in the liver of mice bearing syngeneic tumors. *Biomed. Res.* 14:65–79.

101. Iiai, T., Watanabe, H., Iwamoto, T., Nakashima, I., and Abo, T. 1994. Predominant activation of extrathymic T cells during melanoma development of metallothionein/*ret* transgenic mice. *Cell. Immunol.* 153:412–427.

102. Hashimoto, W., Takeda, K., Anzai, R., Ogasawara, K., Sakihara, H., Sugiura, K., Seki, S., and Kumagai, K. 1995. Cytotoxic NK1.1Ag$^+$ $\alpha\beta$T cells with intermediate TCR induced in the liver of mice by IL-12. *J. Immunol.* 154:4333–4340.

103. Takeda, K., Seki, S., Ogasawara, K., Anzai, R., Hashimoto, W., Sugiura, K., Takahashi, M., Satoh, M., and Kumagai, K. 1996. Liver NK1.1$^+$ CD4$^+$ $\alpha\beta$T cells activated by IL-12 as a major effector in inhibition of experimental tumor metastasis. *J. Immunol.* 156:3366–3373.

104. Arase, H., Arase, N., Kobayashi, Y., Nishimura, Y., Yonehara, S., and Onoé, K. 1994. Cytotoxicity of fresh NK1.1$^+$ T cell receptor α/β^+ thymocyte population associated with intact FAS antigen expression on the target. *J. Exp. Med.* 180:423–432.

105. Takii, Y., Hashimoto, S., Iiai, T., Watanabe, H., Hatakeyama, K., and Abo, T. 1994. Increase in the proportion of granulated CD56$^+$ Tcells in patients with malignancy. *Clin. Exp. Immunol.* 97:522–527.

106. Hashimoto, S., Takii, Y., Iiai, T., Tsuchida, M., Watanabe, H., Shinada, S., Shibata, A., and Abo, T. 1995. CD56$^+$ Tcells in humans: their abundance in the liver and similarity to extrathymic T cells in mice. *Biomed. Res.* 16:1–9.

107. Okada, Y., Iiai, T., Kawachi, Y., Moroda, T., Takii, Y., Hatakeyama, K., and Abo, T. 1995. Origin of CD57$^+$ T cells which increase at tumour sites in patients with colorectal cancer. *Clin. Exp. Immunol.* 102:159–166.

108. Miyaji, C., Watanabe, H., Minagawa, M., Toma, H., Nohara, Y., Nozaki, H., Sato, Y., and Abo, T. 1998. Numerical and functional characteristics of lymphocyte subsets in centenarians. *J. Clin. Immunol.*, 17:420–429.

109. Dellsbona, P., Padovan, E., Casorati, G., Brochhaus, M., and Lanzavecchia, A. 1994. An invariant Vα24-JαQ/ Vβ11 T cell receptor is expressed in all individuals by clonally expanded $CD4^{-}8^{-}$ T cells. *J. Exp. Med.* 180:1171–1176.

110. Deniz, G., Christmas, S.E., Brew, R., and Johnson, P.M. 1994. Phenotypic and functional cellular differences between human $CD3^{-}$ decidual and peripheral blood leukocytes. *J. Immunol.* 152:4255–4261.

111. Hayakawa, S., Saito, S., Nemoto, N., Chishima, F., Akiyama, K., Shiraishi, H., Hayakawa, J., Karasaki-Suzuki, M., Fujii, K.T., Ichijo, M., et al. 1994. Expression of recombinase-activating genes (RAG-1 and 2) in human decidual mononuclear cells. *J. Immunol.* 153:4934–4939.

CHAPTER 5

LIVER TOLERANCE

ROY CALNE
Addenbrooke's Hospital, Cambridge, United Kingdom

Garnier (1) in Paris was the first to describe prolonged survival of a porcine liver allograft, and Terblanche et al. in Bristol reported similar findings (2). At that time, working with Binns in Cambridge, I had developed a repeatable model of porcine renal allografting and had observed rejection in most cases similar in timing and histology to that occurring in other species. We therefore felt that the porcine liver allograft should be interesting to study in an attempt to learn more about allograft rejection. We published our first studies in 1967 (3,4). Following a further paper in 1969 (Nature) (5), a Lancet editorial headed "Strange English Pigs" (6) reviewed the subject with some scepticism, although they concluded that the pig liver allografts had revealed an important phenomenon.

In the intervening years we have studied the subject in many different experimental and clinical settings. We still do not have all the answers, but some of the picture is now reasonably clear. I will begin by stating the facts and then attempt an analysis of the findings. I will conclude with some speculations on how the liver tolerance effect might be harnessed to tolerance protocols in the clinic.

THE FACTS

1.

Liver allografted across both class I and II major histocompatability complex (MHC) disparities, in immunologically competent pigs, rats, and mice can survive indefinitely without any immunosuppression manipulations (7–12). An immune reaction occurs between 7 and 14 days after the procedure, with the histological changes and biochemical disturbances typical of cellular rejection. The immune reaction resolves

T Lymphocytes in the Liver: Immunobiology, Pathology, and Host Defense, Edited by I. Nicholas Crispe
ISBN 0-471-19218-X

spontaneously, leaving the liver functioning normally, and restored to normal histological appearance.

This phenomenon is not universal and, in rats and mice, liver allograft acceptance depends on the strains selected. In general, low-responder recipients are more likely to accept MHC disparate livers. High-responder animals can reject livers completely, with the death of the animal occurring in 7–14 days.

2.

Other organs transplanted together with the liver may be protected from rejection (13). In the pig, donor skin grafts have prolonged survival but were slowly rejected without the loss of the liver (4). In rats, donor skin grafting after the initial unstable rejection phase have prolonged and sometimes indefinite survival (14). Of all tissues grafted, skin is the most difficult to maintain by any immunological or immunosuppressive stratagem; thus skin graft survival is generally accepted as a rigorous demonstration of tolerance.

3.

In a series of retransplantation experiments, Sriwatanawongsa (15) worked with a chimeric rat liver graft model. Liver allografts from the DA to the PVG strain are accepted, and in the course of 30 days there are dynamic changes in donor bone-marrow-derived cells, which leave the liver and are widely distributed in the recipient. Concurrently, recipient bone-marrow-derived cells repopulate the liver with lymphocytes, Kupffer cells, dendritic, and stem cells. These chimeric livers have now donor MHC hepatocytes, bile duct cells, and vascular endothelial cells, but recipient MHC bone-marrow-derived cells. Chimeric livers were retransplanted into naive DA or PVG rats. All the livers were accepted, but the crucial test of skin grafting revealed prolongation of graft survival; however full tolerance was not achieved when the skin graft was from a chimeric liver of donor hepatocyte MHC. When the skin came from a donor of bone-marrow-derived MHC there was no prolongation or shortening of survival time—full tolerance required both components, namely hepatocytes and bone-marrow-derived cells to be present in the liver allograft. Tu et al. (16) have shown that donor irradiation will prevent liver allograft acceptance in rats.

4.

In man and animals, soluble MHC class I antigens can be detected in the serum (17). Van Rood, Davies, and Pollard (18) showed that approximately 50% of the circulating class I antigens are derived from the liver when it is functioning normally. Zavazava (19) reported that human leukocyte antigen (HLA) class I molecules induce apoptosis in primary alloreactive CD8 and T cells. Quian et al. (20) showed that, in murine liver allografts that were accepted, infiltrating lymphocytes became apoptotic, peaking at day 7.

5.

Patients with long-surviving liver allografts may be able to stop immunosuppression without rejection occurring (21,22). The longest survivor, who was operated on 25 years ago, has taken no immunosuppressive agents for the past 15 years. Cautious weaning from immunosuppression of long-term liver allograft recipients would suggest that some 30% can come off all immunosuppression without penalty after 5 years of good function of the allograft. Stopping immunosuppression in recipients of other organ allografts usually results in their rejection. In man, the liver also protects other organs from the same donor source from rejection (23–25).

DISCUSSION

The phenomenon of liver tolerance has been substantiated by independent laboratories. It is unique in immunologically mature animals: No other single organ allograft succeeds across an MHC disparity without immunosuppressive induction regimens, although in rats multiple nonhepatic vascularized organ grafts can produce a similar result (26). In man, liver allograft rejection is common despite standard immunosuppression, and protocol biopsies at a week frequently show mononuclear cell infiltration of the portal triads typical of rejection in patients with normal allograft function (27). The nature and role of these "bystander" cells is not known, but they could be participating in an immunological engagement that may lead to graft acceptance and the eventual cessation of the need for continued immunosuppression. Opelz (28) has reported that one steroid-responsive acute rejection reaction does not prejudice the long-term survival of organ allografts. Liver allograft rejection that does not respond to a short course of steroids and recurrent rejection are bad prognostic signs, chronic untreatable rejection being a likely sequel.

It is unlikely that liver allograft tolerance is a simple all or none phenomenon. Every long-term organ allograft has a precarious existence that may be upset towards acute rejection or an insidious chronic rejection by infections or inflammatory allergic episodes. Experimentally, a donor skin graft can in some cases upset the immunological balance and lead to rejection of an apparently stable well-functioning organ graft. I would argue that the liver produces and maintains its tolerance effect by the following collaborative mechanisms:

1. A continuous and plentiful source of soluble class I antigens exported into the circulation.
2. A large pool of passenger bone-marrow-derived cells, including stem cells and Kupffer cells unique to the liver, which can lead to a protective immunological engagement with recipient bone-marrow-derived cells. Establishment of some of the cells in the recipient as microchemic donor cell rests, at least temporarily, may contribute to the beneficial effects of the liver (29).
3. The liver has rapid and extensive regeneration properties and can repair damage of a self-limiting rejection reaction.

CONCLUSIONS

The clinician is now "embarrassed with riches" in terms of numerous powerful immunosuppressive agents. It is possible to cause profound inhibition of T cell activity but this carries dangers: first, excessive immunosuppression carries an increased risk of infection by bacteria, fungi, and viruses; secondly, there is increased susceptibility to all type of malignancy, particularly those associated with viruses and especially the Epstein Barr virus. It would appear that the B cell proliferative effect is normally under inhibitory control by T cells; if T cell function is lost, B cells are likely to proliferate in response to the Epstein-Barr virus in a polyclonal manner. This progresses to a monoclonal malignancy. Lymphomas are common in immunosuppressed patients and their occurence is proportional to the degree of lymphocyte inhibition.

Excessive immunosuppression probably impairs normal control of the immune system. The protective response to an antigenic challenge is a rapid clonal proliferation of lymphoid cells specifically dedicated to produce cellular and humoral immunity against the antigens in question. This proliferative response is controlled by poorly understood mechanisms that probably involve both cellular and humoral "switch-off" actions. If these are inhibited by "blunderbuss" immunosuppression, an allograft may be established but the recipient will not become tolerant and the patient will need substantial doses of maintenance immunosuppressive drugs indefinitely. The next goal of transplantation that ought to be soluble is the production of "tolerance" or "almost tolerance." At present most patients with good functioning organ allografts require immunosuppression indefinitely.

In most laboratory models of tolerance an unstable period of immunological engagement between donor and recipient occurs before tolerance is established. During this period there is a danger of graft rejection and, in the case of bone marrow transplants, graft-versus-host disease is a hazard due to aggressive donor T cell action. This risk is directly related to the degree of MHC compatibility of donor and recipient. Thus, when there is a reasonable match, graft acceptance is easier to achieve. In the clinic, strategies of tolerance will probably require initial use of powerful immunosuppressive agents and "almost tolerance" may be the first stage in moving toward complete operational tolerance (30). Woodruff (31) reported the case of a patient with a kidney graft from his father who was maintained on 10 mg per day of azathioprine; yet when the azathioprine was stopped there was an acute violet rejection reaction. How such a minute dose of azathioprine prevented rejection is not understood. It has also been possible in some patients to stop azathioprine and maintain the graft with very low doses of corticosteroids (32). These cases are examples of "almost tolerance." An important well-recognised hazard of any tolerance protocol is the commonly observed rejection crisis that can follow any acute infection. Careful long-term surveillance will be necessary with any transplant, and any signs of rejection will require rapid treatment with immunosuppressive agents.

In the new strategies that are being conceived to induce tolerance to organ grafts, immunosuppressive drug treatment will probably be necessary initially to prevent aggressive T cell reaction between the recipient's immune system and that of the donor. In order to confer specificity for graft acceptance, bone-marrow-derived cells of donor origin may be required to supplement those already present in the graft. There may, therefore, be a window of opportunity for immunological engagement (WOFIE) between donor and recipient which is required in order to achieve "tolerance" or "almost tolerance." Excessive immunosuppression during this unstable period could irreversibly prevent the emergence of tolerance, although the graft might be maintained with good function by continuous standard immunosuppression. Clinical "operational" tolerance would now seem to be a realistic goal for the current decade. The fulfillment of this transplanters' dream would be a great boon to our patients.

In all varieties of graft acceptance that do not required full-dose maintenance immunosuppression, immunological engagement of donor and recipient and an early unstable period have been observed. On the basis of the hypothesis that elimination of aggressive T cell function should tip the balance in favor of a tolerant state, experiments have been performed using donor bone-marrow-derived cells in renal allografted, MHC mismatched pigs. An interrupted course of seven 25 mg/kg intravenous doses of cyclosporin was given and a period of 2–3 days without immunosuppression. In using this dose schedule following kidney transplants between mismatched pigs, prolonged survival was observed in more than half the animals without any evidence of chronic rejection (33). This protocol with a hypothetical "WOFIE" could be suitable for clinical application. Excessive immunosuppression might prevent this engagement and the emergence of a tolerant state.

Knechtle and his colleagues (34) have produced tolerance in a very difficult rhesus monkey model using a powerful anti-CD3 monoclonal antibody linked to a modified diphtheria immunotoxin. Three doses of the immunotoxin were given intravenously, on three successive days, starting 7 days prior to renal transplantation. The total dose of 2 mg/kg given over the 3 days produced little toxicity, and tolerance was produced in most animals receiving mismatched kidneys. Donor skin grafts were usually accepted long-term, but in one case the skin graft was slowly rejected and the kidney was also rejected. The immunotoxin produced profound lymphocyte depletion, which was slow to recover, and it was postulated that depletion of T lymphocytes throughout the body was necessary in addition to purging the blood. The mechanism could be similar to the effect of high-dose cyclosporine in the porcine experiments, summarized above.

In clinical organ grafting there is a spectrum of immunological engagement from tolerance to hyperacute rejection. Most patients with organ grafts require continuous dosage with immunosuppressive drugs. The objective would be to shift the curve to the left so that the majority of patients are "operationally tolerant" or "almost tolerant" and require only minimal immunosuppression (Fig. 5.1).

The preceding discussion would suggest that although, in man, liver allografts in the absence of immunosuppression are unlikely to result in tolerance and destructive rejection would be expected, nevertheless the human liver possesses the same "tolerагenic" properties found in the pig and rodents; however, these are not sufficient to overcome the complex and very effective human rejection apparatus.

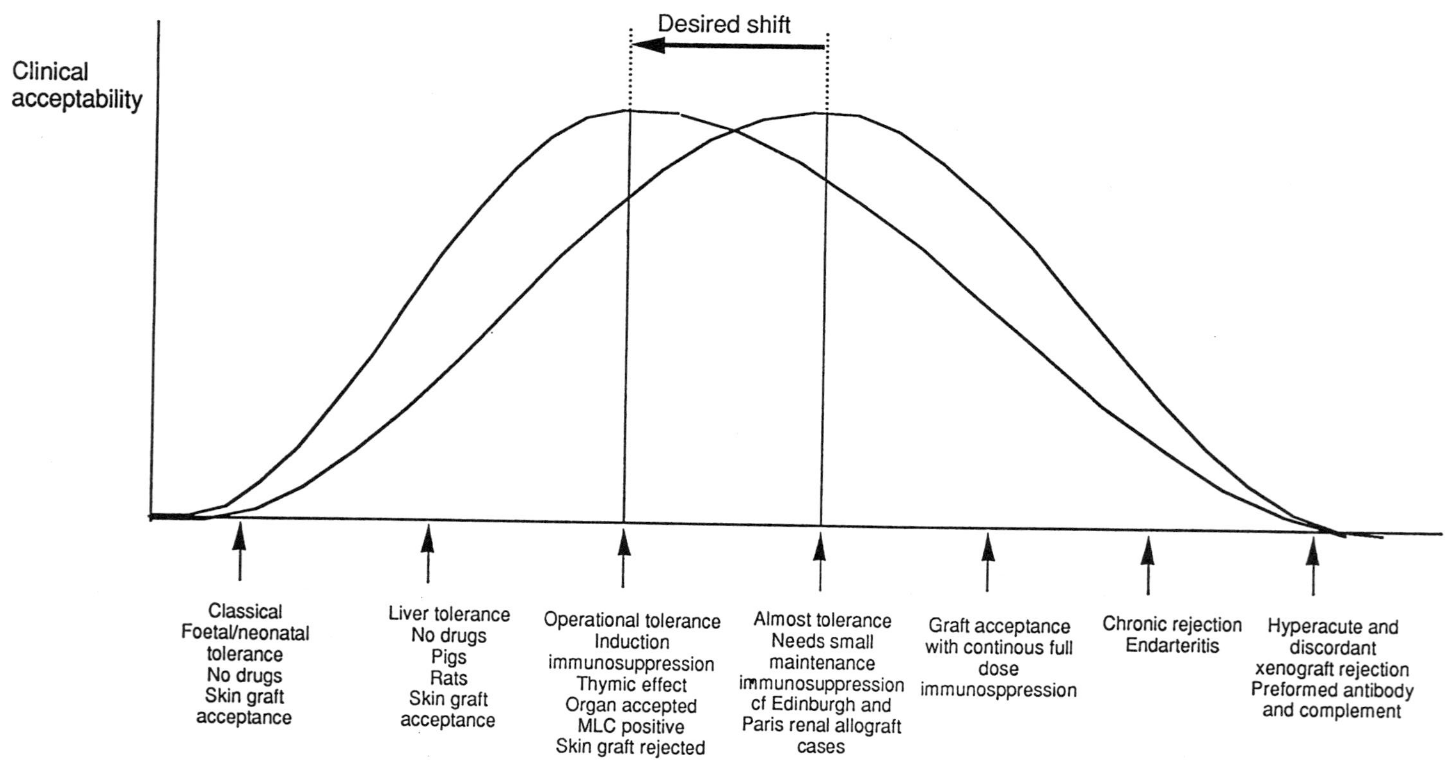

Figure 5.1. Spectrum of immunity and tolerance in liver allografts. Right-hand curve is current experience. Left-hand curve indicates the goal of immunosuppressive therapy.

CADAVERIC RENAL ALLOGRAFTS IN AN "ALMOST" TOLERANCE PROTOCOL

The monoclonal antibody CAMPATH 1H (35) is a potent lymphocyte depleting agent with some properties that resemble the CD3-diptheria immunotoxin used by Knechtle (34) in his impressive experiments. Treatment produces a profound lymphopenia, which typically lasts for 4–6 weeks. This is immunosuppressive, and patients may be at risk of infection, particularly reactivation of viral infections. Monocytes and B cells regenerate rapidly within the first few weeks; T cells regenerate more slowly. As is typical following lymphocyte depletion, the regenerating T cells are biased toward the CD8 population and CD4+ cells are relatively reduced in number, possibly for years following the treatment. So far, this does not appear to be associated with obvious side effects (e.g., opportunistic infections), but the clonality and immunophenotype of the repopulating lymphocytes as naive or memory cells has not been characterized in detail.

We have embarked on a trial of this agent given in two doses, one just before and the second the day after liver allografting. A period of 48 hours without immunosuppression is left for the postulated "WOFIE" engagement to take place. The only candidates available for the engagement would be hematopoietic stem cells that are resistant to CAMPATH 1H. Monotreatment of cyclosporin is given to maintain a blood level of approximately 100 mg/ml. 31 recipients have functioning renal allografts 3–15 months after operation. There have been no serious infections nor malignancies and only 3 acute rejection episodes all of which responded to steroids.

REFERENCES

1. Garnier, H., Clot, J.-P., Bertrand, M., et al. 1965. Biologie Experimentale - Greffe de foie chez le Porc: approche chirurgicale. *C. R. Acad. Sci.* 260:5621–5626.
2. Terblanche, J., Peacock, J.H., Bowes, J., et al. 1967. The use of the pig as an experimental animal for orthotopic liver homotransplantation. Paper presented at the meeting of the Surgical Research Society, Institute of Child Health, Gt Ormond Street, London on 18 and 10 November 1966. *Br. J. Surg.* 54:231.
3. Calne, R.Y., White, H.J., Yoffa, D.E., et al. 1967. Observations of orthotopic liver transplantation in the pig. *BMJ* 2:478–480.
4. Calne, R.Y., White, H.J., Yoffa, D.E., et al. 1967. Prolonged survival of liver transplants in the pig. *BMJ* 4:645–648.
5. Calne, R.Y., Sells, R.A., Pena, J.R., et al. 1969. Induction of immunological tolerance by porcine liver allografts. *Nature* 223:472–476.
6. Editorial. 1969. "Strange English Pigs." *Lancet* 2:940–941.
7. Calne, R.Y., White, H.J., Binns, R.M., et al. 1969. Immunosuppressive effects of the orthotopically transplanted porcine liver. *Transplant. Proc.* 1:321–324.
8. Zimmermann, F.A., Butcher, G.W., Davies, H.S., et al. 1979. Techniques for orthotopic liver transplantation in the rat and some studies of the immunologic responses to fully allogeneic liver grafts. *Transplant. Proc.* 11:571–577.

9. Zimmermann, F.A., Knoll, P.P., Davies, H.ff.S., et al. 1983. The fate of orthotopic liver allografts in different rat strain combinations. *Transplant. Proc.* 25:1272–1275.
10. Kamada, N. 1985. The immunology of experimental liver transplantation in the rat. *Immunology* 55:369–389.
11. Kamada, N. 1996. The liver as an immunosuppressive organ. In *Transplantation Biology: Cellular and Molecular Aspects*, Tilney, N.L., Strom, T.B., and Paul, L.C., eds. Philadelphia: Lippincott-Raven Publishers, pp 531–539.
12. Qian, S., Demetris, A.J., Murase, N., et al. 1994. Murine liver allograft transplantation: tolerance and donor cell chimerism. *Hepatology* 19:916–924.
13. Calne, R.Y., Sells, R.A., Marshall, V.C., et al. 1972. Multiple organ grafts in the pig. Techniques and results of pancreatic, hepatic, cardiac and renal allografts. *Br. J. Surg.* 59:969–977.
14. Kamada, N., Brons, G., and Davies, H.S. 1980. Fully allogeneic liver grafting in rats induces a state of systemic nonreactivity to donor transplantation antigens. *Transplantation* 29:429–431.
15. Sriwatanawongsa, V., Davies, H.ff.S., Calne, R.Y. 1995. The essential roles of parenchymal tissues and passenger leukocytes in the tolerance induced by liver grafting in rats. *Nature Medicine* 1:428–432.
16. Tu, Y., Arima, T., and Flye, M.W. 1997. Rejection of spontaneously accepted rat liver allografts with recipient interleukin-2 treatment or donor radiation. *Transplantation* 63:177–181.
17. Van Rood, A., van Leeuwen, A., and van Santen, M. 1970. Anti HL-A2 inhibitor in normal human serum. *Nature* 226:366–367.
18. Davies, H.ff.S., Pollard, S.G., and Calne, R.Y. 1989. Soluble HLA antigens in the circulation of liver graft recipients. *Transplantation* 47:524–527.
19. Zavazava, N., and Krönke, M. 1996. Soluble HLA class 1 molecules induce apoptosis in alloreactive cytotoxic T lymphocytes. *Nature Medicine* 2:1005–1010.
20. Qian, S., Lu, L., Li, Y., et al. 1997. Apoptosis of graft-infiltrating cytotoxic T cells: A mechanism underlying “split tolerance” in mouse liver transplantation. *Transplant. Proc.* 29:1168–1169.
21. Ramos, H.C., Reyes, J., Abu-Elmagd, K., et al. 1995. Weaning of immunosuppression in long-term liver transplant recipients. *Transplantation* 59:212–217.
22. Mazariegos, G.V., Reyes, J., Marino, I.R., et al. 1997. Weaning of immunosuppression in liver transplant recipients. *Transplantation* 63:243–249.
23. Rasmussen, A., Davies, H.F., Jamieson, N.V., et al. 1995. Combined transplantation of liver and kidney from the same donor protects the kidney from rejection and improves kidney graft survival. *Transplantation* 59:919–921.
24. Margreiter, R., Kornberger, R., Koller, J., et al. 1988. Can a liver graft from the same donor protect a kidney from rejection? *Transplant. Proc.* 1:522–523.
25. Gnowa, T.A., Nery, J.R., Husberg, B.S., et al. 1988. Simultaneous liver and renal transplantation in man. *Transplantation* 46:690–693.
26. Sun, J., Sheil, A.G., Wang, C., et al. 1996. Tolerance to rat liver allografts. *Transplantation* 62:1725–1730.
27. European FK506 Multicentre Liver Study Group. 1994. Randomised trial comparing tacrolimus (FK506) and cyclosporin in prevention of liver allograft rejection. *Lancet* 344:423–428.

28. Opelz, G. 1996. *Collaborative Transplant Study (CTS) Newsletter*. 4 December.
29. Starzl, T.E., Demetris, A.J., Murase, N., et al. 1992. Cell migration, chimerism and graft acceptance. *Lancet* 339:1579–1582.
30. Calne, R.Y. 1995. An opportunity in organ transplantation. *Nature Medicine* 1:20–22.
31. Woodruff, M.F.A., Nolan, B., Anderton, J.L., et al. 1976. Long survival after renal transplantation in man. *Br. J. Surg.* 63:85–101.
32. Compos, H., Kreis, H., Rious, P., et al. 1994. Azathioprine withdrawal in renal transplant recipients. *Transplantation* 38:29–31.
33. Calne, R.Y., Watson, C.J., Brons, I.G., et al. 1994. Tolerance of porcine renal allografts induced by donor spleen cells and seven days' treatment with cyclosporine. *Transplantation* 57:1433–1435.
34. Knechtle, S.J., Vargo, D., Fechner, J., et al. 1997. FN18-CRM9 immunotoxin promotes tolerance in primate renal allografts. *Transplantation* 63:1–6.
35. Hale, G., Dyer, M.J., Clark, M.R., et al. 1988. Remission induction in non-Hodgkin lymphoma with reshaped human monoclonal antibody CAMPATH-1H. *Lancet* 2:1394–1399.
36. Calne, R., Friend, P., Moffatt, S., et al. 1998. Prope Tolerance: perioperative campath 1H, and low-dose cyclosporin monotherapy in renal allograft recipients. *Lancet* 351:1701–1702.

CHAPTER 6

INDUCTION OF PERIPHERAL TOLERANCE BY PORTAL VEIN ADMINISTRATION OF ANTIGEN

ALLAN McI MOWAT
University of Glasgow, Glasgow, Scotland

INTRODUCTION

Several routes and procedures can be used to induce peripheral tolerance of T cells, including the intravenous or mucosal administration of antigen. One model that has analogies to both is the phenomenon by which tolerance can be induced via the portal vein. This has been recognized for several years and has received attention as a potential means of inhibiting allospecific immunity in transplantation medicine. In addition, it is possible that the physiological drainage of intestinal material to the portal vein may account in part for the tolerogenic properties of orally administered soluble antigens. In this review, we will discuss the nature of the peripheral tolerance induced via the portal vein and outline the potential mechanisms and applications.

ORAL TOLERANCE

Of all the phenomena of peripheral tolerance, that induced by the oral route is most similar to portal vein tolerance. Oral tolerance has been studied in great depth in recent years and the resulting information offers important insights into the mechanisms that may operate after injection of antigen into the portal vein.

T Lymphocytes in the Liver: Immunobiology, Pathology, and Host Defense, Edited by I. Nicholas Crispe
ISBN 0-471-19218-X

Induction of Tolerance and Immunity by the Oral Route

Primary immune responses are rarely found after oral administration of inert antigens such as a soluble protein, and the animal becomes refractory to subsequent systemic challenge with the antigen in an immunogenic form. This state of oral tolerance can be induced by a wide range of antigens and has been described in most laboratory and domestic species as well as in man (1,2,3).

Tolerance of all aspects of CD4 T cell–mediated systemic immunity can be induced by prior feeding of antigen. However, oral tolerance of T helper cell type 1 (Th1)-dependent cell-mediated immune responses, such as delayed-type hypersensitivity (DTH), contact sensitivity, IgG2a antibodies and γ interferon-γ (IFNγ) production, can generally be induced with low doses of antigen and is long-lasting. In comparison, it is more difficult to elicit tolerance to Th2-dependent humoral immune responses and the production of interleukin-4 (IL-4), IL-5, and IL-10 and these return to normal more quickly (3–12). One exception to this general rule is that IgE antibody responses are readily suppressed by feeding antigen, despite the clear dependence of this response on IL-4 *in vivo* (13–16). Tolerance of CD8-dependent cytotoxic T cell and contact sensitivity responses can both be induced by this route (6,17,18). Oral tolerance may be very long-lasting, as studies in mice indicate that tolerance of systemic cell-mediated immunity may be preserved almost lifelong after a single feed of protein antigen (19).

Mechanisms of Oral Tolerance

Several regulatory mechanisms have been implicated in oral tolerance. Initial work suggested that fed antigens preferentially induced a population of $CD8^+$ "suppressor" T cells, which inhibited the function of other effector T cells (1). Although the idea of these cells subsequently fell into disrepute, more recent studies have suggested that although classical $CD8^+$ cytotoxic T lymphocytes (CTL) may be suppressed by feeding antigen, a regulatory population of $CD8^+$ T cells may be activated under these circumstances (6). This dichotomy could reflect the existence of distinct functional subsets of $CD8^+$ T cells, as found with Th1 and Th2 $CD4^+$ cells (20), or the presence of regulatory $CD8^+$ T cells expressing γδ T cell receptors (TCR) (see below).

Oral tolerance occurs normally in mice depleted of $CD8^+$ T cells by genetic knockout or monoclonal antibodies, and most current evidence indicates a critical role for $CD4^+$ T cells in the induction of unresponsiveness (2,3). This has been associated with preferential upregulation of Th2 cells, accompanied by enhanced production of the Th2-dependent cytokines, IL-4 and IL-10 and concomitant suppression of Th1-dependent production of IL-2 and γIFN (3, 7–9,21–24). Nevertheless, it should be noted that Th2-dependent IgE production is highly susceptible to oral tolerance, and oral tolerance develops normally in the absence of Th2 cells in IL-4 knockout mice (25) and in mice treated with neutralizing anti-IL-4 antibodies (26). One explanation for these apparently discrepant findings comes from the suggestion that tolerance may be mediated by a unique subset of regulatory $CD4^+$ T cells, the Th3 cells (3,21,22,27,28). Although these cells may make Th2 products such as IL-4 and IL-10, they are characterized by a unique ability to produce transforming growth factor β (TGFβ). There is preferential retention of TGFβ production in T cell receptor (TCR) transgenic mice fed high doses of ovalbumin (OVA) or OVA peptide (28,29), and TGFβ-secreting T cells can be cloned from normal mice made tolerant by the oral route (22,23,30,31). $CD8^+$ T cells have also been reported to produce TGFβ in oral tolerance (32).

Not all studies support a role for active suppressor mechanisms in oral tolerance, and there is also evidence for direct inactivation of antigen-specific $CD4^+$ T cells via clonal anergy or deletion (2,3). Clonal deletion has been identified only in TCR transgenic mice fed very high doses of antigen (29,33) and in wild-type mice fed the superantigen SEB (34). It cannot be observed under more physiological conditions when adoptive recipients of TCR transgenic T cells are fed doses of OVA equivalent to those that induce tolerance in normal animals (35). It is more likely that when induction of oral tolerance leads to direct inactivation of T cells in the absence of active regulatory mechanisms, this is due to anergy of specific T cells. There is considerable indirect evidence for this in normal animals fed antigen (3,7,36–40) and it has been confirmed directly using the TCR transgenic adoptive transfer model (28,35). As in other models of peripheral tolerance, the development of clonal anergy is preceded by rapid, but transient expansion of $CD4^+$ T cells in systemic lymphoid tissues. These findings support the idea that fed antigens are presented inappropriately to T cells, probably because they associate with antigen presenting cells (APCs) that lack costimulatory activity. The nature and source of these cells is unknown, but they may include class II MHC expressing enterocytes, or conventional, but non-costimulatory APCs, such as resting B cells and dendritic cells, either in the intestine or in systemic lymphoid organs. As we shall discuss, it is also possible that selective presentation within the liver may play an important role.

At present, the consensus is that whether feeding antigen induces active regulatory mechanisms or clonal inactivation is determined by the regime of feeding. Thus, single high doses of antigen are considered to cause clonal anergy (or deletion), whereas multiple low doses appear to stimulate bystander suppression, mediated by Th3 etc. (3).

γδ T Cells and Oral Tolerance

Recent studies have suggested that mucosal tolerance may be mediated by T cells expressing the γδ TCR. Aerosol-induced tolerance in rats is transferable by $CD8^+$ γδ T cells, which suppress IgE production selectively and produce IFNγ (41–43). Diabetes in non-obese diabetic (NOD) mice can also be prevented by $CD8^+$ γδ T cells induced by aerosol administration of insulin (44), and subsequent studies have shown that γδ T cells can transfer orally induced tolerance (45). Oral tolerance to proteins can be prevented or even abrogated by depleting γδ T cells with antibody *in vivo* (46,47) and cannot be induced in δ TCR knockout mice that lack γδ T cells (47). Although the molecular basis for these effects remains to be established, they are consistent with other recent evidence that γδ T cells may play an important immunoregulatory role under other conditions, as well as with findings in tolerance induced via the portal vein.

PORTAL VEIN TOLERANCE

Introduction

Studies performed 25–30 years ago first indicated that administration of antigen into the portal vein was not as effective as other venous routes in priming immune responses and, in fact, induced immunological unresponsiveness (48–50). Subsequent work confirmed the unusual ability of this protocol to induce systemic tolerance (51–55) and, stimulated by the realization that liver allografts were not rejected as efficiently as other organs, several studies have explored the possibility of exploiting the route for inhibiting allogeneic responses *in vivo*.

Scope of Portal Vein Tolerance

In contrast to the wide range of species and antigens that have been examined in studies of oral tolerance, the equivalent portal vein phenomenon has been investigated predominantly in laboratory rodents. However, it was first described in pigs (48), and has also been identified in dogs (56). Similarly, although heterologous red blood cells, proteins, purified allogeneic class I MHC proteins, haptens (48–50,57–59) and Schistosome eggs (60) have been used, the vast majority of work has concentrated on infusion of allogeneic or xenogeneic lymphoid or hematopoietic cells. In this way, it has been possible to enhance the survival of a variety of allografts or xenografts, including skin, heart, kidney, pancreatic islets, and small intestine (61–69). Furthermore, delayed rejection of highly immunogenic tissues such as small intestine can be achieved by establishing venous drainage via the portal, rather than systemic venous route (70,71). Xenografts of pancreatic islets are also rejected at reduced rates if transplanted intrahepatically (69). The focus on allogeneic leukocytes as antigens for portal administration probably reflects the interest in using this route as a means of suppressing clinical allograft rejection. However, it is also interesting to note that one study has reported that the ability of allogeneic cells to induce the phenomenon reflects preferential uptake of hemopoietic stem cells in the liver via specific lectin-binding receptors (72). Whether this process is essential for the induction of portal vein tolerance, or merely enhances it, remains an open question, and more studies of other kinds of antigen are required. Interestingly, one recent report indicates that collagen arthritis can be inhibited by portal vein inoculation of collagen type II in mice, but this has not yet been confirmed (73).

Most aspects of systemic T cell–mediated immunity have been reported to be suppressed after portal vein infusion of antigen, including DTH (51–54), proliferative T cell activity (55), and specific cytotoxic T cell responses (53,55). Conversely, serum antibody responses may be primed by the procedure (52,54), a finding that may correlate with the relative sensitivity of individual cytokine-producing subsets of $CD4^+$ T cells.

Due to the technical difficulties of the procedure, little is known about host factors such as age, genetic background, or microbial colonization, which might influence the induction of portal vein tolerance. Similarly, the effects of different antigen doses have not been characterized, although those studies in which soluble antigen has been used have reported effective tolerance induction with remarkably small amounts of material (e.g., 10 μg) (57–59,73). In view of the influence all these factors have on orally induced tolerance and their possible influence on clinical applicability in man, it would be important to establish their role in portal vein tolerance.

Mechanisms of Portal Vein Tolerance

Immunoregulatory Mechanisms Studies of specific regulatory mechanisms have been limited by the technical difficulties of the procedure and by the fact that few well-defined nominal antigens have been employed. Most work has concentrated on the idea that active suppressor mechanisms are responsible for portal vein tolerance. The tolerant state can be transferred with spleen or hepatic lymphocytes (74,75), although the nature of these cells remains contentious. In one study, it was suggested that $CD4^-8^-$ αβ TCR-expressing T cells were responsible (74), but more recent work by Gorczynski and colleagues (66,67,75) has identified a potential role for γδ TCR-expressing T cells. Portal vein tolerance of skin graft rejection in mice can be transferred by enriched hepatic γδ TCR^+ T cells or by γδ TCR-expressing hybridomas derived from the Peyer's patches (PP) of tolerant animals (75,76). Activation of γδ TCR^+ T cells has also been reported in the PP, mesenteric lymph node, and intraepithelial compartments of tolerant mice and rats (66,67) and, in rats, γδ TCR^+ T cells enriched from PP can transfer the tolerant state (67). Although these latter studies do not prove that γδ TCR^+ T cells are essential for the induction of portal vein tolerance, this is suggested by the fact that tolerance is compromised by depletion of γδ TCR^+ T cells using antibody *in vivo* and in γδ knockout mice (66,76). Much remains to be learned about the nature of these regulatory γδ TCR^+ T cells. Although their activity is antigen specific, the antigens recognized and the restriction elements used, if any, are unknown. Recent studies suggesting that the γδ TCR^+ T cells activated in tolerant mice are oligoclonal in nature are interesting, but do not shed much light on this question (66). Clearly a role for unusual T cells such as γδ TCR^+ T cells or $CD4^-8^-$ αβ TCR^+ T cells is of particular interest, given the evidence discussed elsewhere in this volume for the predilection such populations may have for the liver. However, in view of the evidence from other models of peripheral tolerance, including oral tolerance, it would also seem premature to exclude completely a role for conventional αβ TCR^+ T cells.

The weight of available evidence supports the view that regulatory lymphocytes may act in portal vein tolerance by production of the cytokines which have also been implicated in orally induced tolerance, including IL-4, IL-10, and TGFβ. Initial work suggested that IL-4 production was relatively unaffected by induction of portal vein tolerance (77) and, subsequently, it has been shown that T cells and hybridomas derived from tolerant animals may produce increased levels of IL-4 and IL-10 (64,66,67,76,78). In parallel, the production of the Th1-derived cytokines IL-2 and γIFN is markedly suppressed, and the tolerant state can be reduced by regimes which favor Th1 activity, such as administration of IL-12 or anti-IL-10 antibody (64,76,78). However, anti-IL-4 antibody has no effect (78), although administration of exogenous IL-13 and anti-IL-12 enhances tolerance (79). Enhanced production of TGFβ has also been reported (67,76) and, in combination with anti-IL-10, anti-TGFβ antibody prevents the induction of portal vein tolerance (80). In many cases, the source of these regulatory cytokines is believed to be the activated γδ TCR$^+$ T cells discussed above (64,66,67,76,80). As would be predicted from this evidence, recent studies indicate that induction of portal vein tolerance to minor histocompatibility antigens can allow "bystander suppression" of the response to third party allografts given at the same time as challenge with grafts expressing the original antigen (80). This is analogous to what occurs in certain models of oral tolerance and was mediated by antigen-specific γδ TCR$^+$ T cells of limited receptor heterogeneity that produce IL-10 and TGFβ.

In contrast to these findings supporting a role for regulatory T cells, others have reported that antibody-containing serum, but not lymphocytes, can transfer tolerance from mice injected via the portal vein (51,54,81). This activity correlates with the ability of portal vein inoculation to selectively prime antibody responses *in vivo* and with the apparent presence of antibodies directed at the effector T cells that would normally cause DTH (52). Although the postulated role of anti-idiotypic antibody is consistent with the apparent upregulation of IL-4, these studies have never been followed up in detail and their significance remains unclear.

There are no direct studies of T cell anergy or deletion in portal vein tolerance. However, early studies found that tolerised lymphocytes maintained their unresponsive state *in vivo* when transferred into naive recipients in the absence of active suppression (51). In addition, exogenous IL-2 reverses T cell unresponsiveness *in vitro* and *in vivo* (65,75), findings that would support a role for T cell anergy induced by portal vein administration of antigen. This idea needs to be examined directly using appropriate TCR transgenic models when available.

Antigen Processing and Presentation in the Liver No direct studies have been performed to address the possibility that the peripheral T cell tolerance induced via the portal vein is due to inappropriate presentation of antigen. However, APC isolated from the liver can induce tolerance when given by systemic intravenous injection and preferentially stimulate the production of Th2 cytokines *in vitro* (82). A number of experiments indicate that one particular population of potential hepatic APCs is important for the tolerant state. Ablation of Kupffer cells (KCs) *in vivo* with the rare earth metal gadolinium prevents the induction of portal vein tolerance (60,83–87), an observation that supports the view that these cells play a central role in the phenomenon. The basis for this remains uncertain, although there is considerable evidence to suggest that KCs may act as APCs. Thus, purified KCs are normally capable of presenting antigen to class II MHC-restricted T cells (86,88–91) and this can be prevented by gadolinium treatment (86,89,90). Gadolinium has no effect on class II MHC expression by KCs (89), but gadolinium-treated KCs cause lymphocyte suppression, which appears to be mediated by enhanced production of nitric oxide (NO) (89,86,92). That endogenous NO may normally prevent portal vein tolerance is supported by other findings that inhibition of inducible NO synthase *in vivo* enhances the induction of portal vein tolerance (93). Together, these findings suggest that induction of portal vein tolerance normally requires activation of specific T cells by KC-associated antigen and that inhibition of this effect results in abrogation of tolerance. It would be of interest now to examine directly whether *in vivo* antigen-pulsed KCs can indeed induce a state of partial T cell activation, as is found in other states of peripheral tolerance, including oral tolerance. However, KCs appear to express costimulatory molecules such as B7.2, suggesting that they should be able to prime T cells fully (91), an idea supported by those studies which have examined presentation of antigen to T cells directly (86, 88–91). Thus it would be important to determine if KCs preferentially present antigen to the subpopulations of regulatory T cells implicated in portal vein tolerance. The other nonprofessional class II MHC-expressing APCs that have been implicated in portal vein tolerance are sinusoidal endothelial cells but, like KCs, these have been found to prime T cells normally and to express B7.2 (91).

An alternative explanation for the involvement of KCs in portal vein tolerance is that, after engulfing antigen, KCs release immunosuppressive mediators such as arachidonic acid metabolites, NO, or reactive oxygen intermediaries. This has been shown with KCs isolated from animals injected with allogeneic cells by the portal vein, and the associated induction of tolerance can be prevented by administration of the cyclooxygenase inhibitor indomethacin (94). This idea is attractive, particularly as it might explain why portal vein tolerance can be induced most readily with intact cells. However, the resulting state of tolerance would not be antigen specific, unless the immunosuppression was localized to those antigen-specific T cells in the immediate vicinity.

Relationship of Portal Vein Tolerance to Other Models of Peripheral Tolerance

Intravenous administration of antigen is often associated with induction of tolerance, and the question must therefore arise as to the uniqueness of the portal route. It was reported originally that injection into the systemic venous system does not reproduce the effects of portal vein injection (51,55) and regulatory $\gamma\delta$ T cells cannot be activated by systemic intravenous injection (67). Nevertheless, some similarities have been identified, including the fact that intravenous tolerance can also be partly prevented by gadolinium (87), while KCs from intravenously injected mice also produce increased amounts of prostaglandin E_2 (PGE2) (94). These findings may simply indicate that both routes induce equivalent regulatory mechanisms in different sites. Alternatively, access to a specialized population of tolerogenic APCs in the liver may account for the immunodulatory effects of systemic intravenous injection. The ability of portal vein inoculation to induce allograft tolerance in association with upregulated Th2 cytokines can be reproduced by intravenous administration of antigen in combination with antibodies to adhesion molecules such as LFA-1, ICAM-1, or VCAM-1 (78,95). Anti-ICAM-1 also enhances the phenomenon of portal vein tolerance (96). One explanation for these findings is that blockade of adhesion molecules alters the localization of the cells used to induce tolerance, such that they now are no longer able to enter organized lymphoid organs and accumulate in the liver, where they are accessible to "tolerogenic" APCs such as KCs. An alternative possibility is that, by interfering with the costimulatory interaction between T cells and APCs, inhibition of adhesion molecule function alters the nature of the resultant immune response. This is supported by findings that presentation of antigen by splenic APCs in presence of anti-LFA-1 preferentially induces Th2 cytokine production *in vitro*, allowing them to behave more like APCs isolated from the liver (82). Resolution of these issues would both contribute to understanding hepatic tolerance and provide important information on the anatomical basis of immune responses in general.

Practical Implications of Portal Vein Tolerance

A Role for the Liver in Oral Tolerance? Most of the blood draining from the intestine goes directly to the liver via the portal venous system, and large amounts of antigen are therefore likely to enter the liver rapidly after oral administration. As we have discussed, the states of systemic unresponsiveness induced via the oral and portal routes appear to have many features in common, including the preferential suppression of DTH and γIFN responses, with concomitant upregulation of IL-4 and IL-10 production and possible roles for TGFβ and/or γδ TCR^+ T cells. Furthermore, the potentially unusual properties of KCs as APCs might help explain the apparent involvement of ineffective antigen presentation in oral tolerance. Nevertheless, it is still unclear how much the liver contributes to the phenomenon of oral tolerance. Although one early study reported that bypass of the liver by porto-caval shunt had no effect on the induction of oral tolerance by feeding rats bovine serum albumin (97), exactly opposite findings were made in more recent experiments using OVA (98). The reasons for this discrepancy are unknown, but the interpretation of these studies is complicated by the many side effects of this surgical maneuver. Currently, other methods of interfering with liver function in oral tolerance have not been published and it would, for instance, be interesting to examine the effects of KC blockade using gadolinium. It would also be important to explore more fully the immunological consequences of portal administration of protein antigens, so that studies of the two routes could be compared more directly. One topic of particular interest would be to examine if portal administration of protein results in the appearance of tolerogenic antigen in serum within a few minutes, as has been described in oral tolerance (99–104). Elucidation of where this material is generated would be an important advance in our understanding of how the immune system handles potentially antigenic food proteins.

Use of the Portal Route to Induce Tolerance Therapeutically Induction of antigen-specific tolerance would be desirable for the prevention or treatment of allograft rejection, chronic inflammatory disease, and autoimmune disease. Clearly, the need for surgical intervention may limit the potential scope of the portal route for these purposes. However, as we have noted, most studies of portal tolerance have used allogeneic cells or tissues, with the aim of preventing allograft rejection. In this case, the practical difficulties of administering antigen can be obviated by transplanting the graft itself with portal vein drainage. In addition, oral tolerance is currently being investigated as a therapy for a number of clinical and experimental autoimmune diseases (105). Thus if the portal route could be shown to be more effective and/or long-lasting, surgical intervention might be justified.

REFERENCES

1. Mowat, A.M. 1987. The regulation of immune responses to dietary protein antigens. *Immunol. Today* 8:93–98.
2. Mowat, A.M., and Weiner, H.L. 1998. Oral tolerance: basic mechanisms and clinical implications. In *Handbook of Mucosal Immunology, 2nd ed.*, Ogra, P.L., Mestecky, J., Lamm, M.E., Strober, W. McGhee, J.R., Bienenstock, J., eds. San Diego: Academic Press, in press.
3. Weiner, H.L., Friedman, A., Miller, A., Khoury, S.J., Al-Sabbagh, A., Santos, L., Sayegh, M., Nussenblatt, R.B., Trentham, D.E., and Hafler, D.A. 1994. Oral tolerance: Immunologic mechanisms and treatment of animal and human organ-specific autoimmune diseases by oral administration of autoantigens. *Ann. Rev. Immunol.* 12:809–838.
4. Mowat, A.M., Stobel, S., Drummond, H.E., and Ferguson, A. 1982. Immunological responses to fed protein antigens in mice, I. Reversal of oral tolerance to ovalbumin by cyclophosphamide. *Immunology* 45:104–113.
5. Mowat, A.M., Thomas, M.J., Mackenzie, S., and Parrott, D.M.V. 1986. Divergent effects of bacterial lipopolysaccharide on immunity to orally administered protein and particulate antigens in mice. *Immunology* 58:677–684.
6. Ke, Y., and Kapp, J.A. 1996. Oral antigen inhibits priming of $CD8^+$ CTL, $CD4^+$ T cells and antibody responses while activating $CD8^+$ suppressor T cells. *J. Immunol.* 156:916–921.
7. Melamed, D., and Friedman, A. 1994. In vivo tolerization of Th1 lymphocytes following a single feed with ovalbumin: Anergy in the absence of suppression. *Eur. J. Immunol.* 24:1974–1981.
8. Fishman-Lobell, J., Friedman, A., and Weiner, H.L. 1994. Different kinetic patterns of cytokine gene expression in vivo in orally tolerant mice. *Eur. J. Immunol.* 24:2720–2724.
9. Melamed, D., Fischmann-Lobell, J., Uni, Z., Weiner, H.L., and Friedman, A. 1996. Peripheral tolerance of Th2 lymphocytes induced by continuous feeding of ovalbumin. *Int. Immunol.* 8:717–724.
10. von Herrath, M.G., Dyrberg, T., and Oldstone, M.B.A. 1996. Oral insulin treatment suppresses virus-induced antigen-specific destruction of β cells and prevents autoimmune diabetes in transgenic mice. *J. Clin. Invest.* 98:1324–1331.
11. Claessen, A.M.E., Von Blomberg, B.M.E., De Groot, J., Wolvers, D.A.E., Kraal, G., and Scheper, R.J. 1996. Reversal of mucosal tolerance by subcutaneous administration of interleukin-12 at the site of attempted sensitization. *Immunology* 88:363–367.
12. Husby, S., Mestecky, J., Moldoveanu, Z., Holland, S., and Elson, C.O. 1994. Oral tolerance in humans: T cell but not B cell tolerance after antigen feeding. *J. Immunol.* 152:4663–4670.
13. Vaz, N.M., Maia, L.C.S., Hanson, D.G., and Lynch, J.M. 1977. Inhibition of homocytotropic antibody responses in adult inbred mice by previous feeding of the specific antigen. *J. Allergy Clin. Immunol.* 60:110–115.
14. Ngan, J., and Kind, L.S. 1978. Suppressor T cells for IgE and IgG in Peyer's patches of mice made tolerant by the oral administration of ovalbumin. *J. Immunol.* 120:861–865.
15. Jarrett, E.E., and Hall, E. 1984. The development of IgE-suppressive immunocompetence in young animals: Influence of exposure to antigen in the presence or absence of maternal immunity. *Immunology* 53:365–373.

16. Saklayen, M.G., Pesce, A.J., Pollak, V.E., and Michael, J.G. 1984. Kinetics of oral tolerance: Study of variables affecting tolerance induced by oral administration of antigen. *Int. Arch. Allergy Appl. Immunol.* 73:75–79.

17. Garside, P., Steel, M., Liew, F.Y., and Mowat, A.M. 1995. $CD4^+$ but not $CD8^+$ T cells are required for the induction of oral tolerance. *Int. Immunol.* 7:501–504.

18. Desvignes, C., Bour, H., Nicholas, J.F., and Kaiserlian, D. 1996. Lack of oral tolerance but oral priming for contact sensitivity to dinitrofluorobenzene in major histocompatibility antigen deficient mice and in $CD4^+$ T cell-depleted mice. *Eur. J. Immunol.* 26:1756–1761.

19. Strobel, S., and Ferguson, A. 1987. Persistence of oral tolerance in mice fed ovalbumin is different for humoral and cell mediated immune responses. *Immunology* 60:317–318.

20. Mosmann, T.R., and Sad, S. 1996. The expanding universe of T-cell subsets: Th1, Th2, and more. *Immunol. Today* 17:138–146.

21. Khoury, S.J., Hancock, W.W., and Weiner, H.L. 1992. Oral tolerance to myelin basic protein and natural recovery from experimental autoimmune encephalomyelitis are associated with downregulation of inflammatory cytokines and differential upregulation of transforming growth factor β, interleukin 4, and prostaglandin E expression in the brain. *J. Exp. Med.* 176:1355–1364.

22. Chen, Y., Kuchroo, V.K., Inobe, J.-I., Hafler, D.A., and Weiner, H.L. 1994. Regulatory T cell clones induced by oral tolerance: Suppression of autoimmune encephalomyelitis. *Science* 265:1237–1240.

23. Chen, Y., Inobe, J.-I., Kuchroo, V.K., Baron, J.L., Janeway, C.A., and Weiner, H.L. 1996. Oral tolerance in myelin basic protein T-cell receptor transgenic mice: Suppression of autoimmune encephalomyelitis and dose-dependent induction of regulatory cells. *Proc. Natl. Acad. Sci. U.S.A.* 93:388–391.

24. Neurath, M.F., Fuss, I., Kelsall, B.L., Presky, D.H., Waegell, W., and Strober, W. 1996. Experimental granulomatous colitis in mice is abrogated by induction of TGF-b-mediated oral tolerance. *J. Exp. Med.* 183:2605–2616.

25. Garside, P., Steel, M., Worthey, E.A., Satoskar, A., Alexander, J., Bluethmann, H., Liew, F.Y., and Mowat, A.M. 1995. Th2 cells are subject to high dose oral tolerance and are not essential for its induction. *J. Immunol.* 15:5649–5655.

26. Wolvers, D.A.W., van der Cammen, M.J.F., and Kraal, G. 1997. Mucosal tolerance is associated with, but independent of, upregulation of Th2 responses. *Immunology* 92:328–333.

27. Fukaura, H., Kent, S.C., Pietrusewicz, M.L., Khoury, S.J., Weiner, H.L., and Hafler, D.A. 1996. Induction of circulating myelin basic protein and proteolipid protein-specific transforming growth factor-β1-secreting Th3 cells by oral administration of myelin in multiple sclerosis. *J. Clin. Invest.* 98:70–77.

28. Chen, Y., Hancock, W., Marks, R., Gonnella, P.A., and Weiner, H.L. 1997. Mechanisms of recovery from cell-mediated autoimmune disease: T cell deletion and immune deviation following encephalomyelitis in myelin basic protein T cell receptor transgenic mice. *Cell. Immunol.*, in press.

29. Chen, Y., Inobe, J.-I., Marks, R., Gonnella, P., Kuchroo, V.K., and Weiner, H.L. 1995. Peripheral deletion of antigen-reactive T cells in oral tolerance. *Nature* 376:177–180.

30. Santos, L.M.B., Al-Sabbagh, A., Londono, A.A., and Weiner, H.L. 1994. Oral tolerance to myelin basic protein induces regulatory TGR-β secreting cells in Peyer's patches of SJL mice. *Cell. Immunol.* 157:439–447.

31. Wang, Z.Y., Link, H., Ljungdahl, A., Hojeberg, B., Link, J., He, B., Qiao, J., Melms, A., and Olsson, T. 1994. Induction of interferon-γ, interleukin-4 and transforming growth factor-β in rats orally tolerized against autoimmune myaesthenia gravis. *Cell. Immunol.* 157:353–368.

32. Miller, A., Lider, O., Roberts, A.B., Sporn, M.B., and Weiner, H.L. 1992. Suppressor T cells generated by oral tolerization to myelin basic protein suppress both in vitro and in vivo immune responses by the release of transforming growth factor β after antigen-specific triggering. *Proc. Natl. Acad. Sci. U.S.A.* 89:421–425.

33. Marth, T., Strober, W., and Kelsall, B.L. 1996. High dose oral tolerance in ovalbumin TcR-transgenic mice: Systemic neutralisation of interleukin 12 augments TGFβ secretion and T cell apoptosis. *J. Immunol.* 157:2348–2357.

34. Migita, K., and Ochi, A. 1994. Induction of clonal anergy by oral administration of staphylococcal enterotoxin B. *Eur. J. Immunol.* 24:2081–2086.

35. Van Houten, N., and Blake, S.F. 1996. Direct measurement of anergy of antigen-specific T cells following oral tolerance induction. *J. Immunol.* 157:1337–1341.

36. Whitacre, C.C., Gienapp, I.E., Orosz, C.G.A., and Bitar, D.M. 1991. Oral tolerance in experimental autoimmune encephalitis, III. Evidence for clonal anergy. *J. Immunol.* 147:2155–2163.

37. Melamed, D., and Friedman, A. 1993. Direct evidence for anergy in T lymphocytes tolerized by oral administration of ovalbumin. *Eur. J. Immunol.* 23:935–942.

38. Friedman, A., and Weiner, H.L. 1994. Induction of anergy or active suppression following oral tolerance is determined by antigen doseage. *Proc. Natl. Acad. Sci. U.S.A.* 91:6688–6692.

39. Hirahara, K., Hisatune, T., Nishijima, K.-I., Kato, H., Shiho, O., and Kaminogowa, S. 1995. $CD4^+$ T cells anergized by high dose feeding establish oral tolerance to antibody responses when transferred in SCID and nude mice. *J. Immuno.* 154:6238–6245.

40. Inada, S., Yoshino, S., Haque, M.A., Ogata, Y., and Kohashi, O. 1996. Clonal anergy is a potent mechanism of oral tolerance in the suppression of acute antigen-induced arthritis in rats by oral administration of the inducing antigen. *Cell. Immunology* 175:67–75.

41. McMenamin, C., Pimm, C., McKersey, M., and Holt, P.G. 1994. Regulation of IgE responses to inhaled antigen in mice by antigen-specific γδ T cells. *Science* 265:1869–1871.

42. McMenamin, C., McKersey, M., Kuhnlein, P., Hunig, T., and Holt, P.G. 1995. γδ T cells down-regulate primary IgE responses in rats to inhaled soluble protein antigens. *J. Immunol.* 154:4390–4394.

43. McMenamin, C., Oliver, J., Girn, B.J., Kees, U.R., Thomas, W.R., and Holt, P.G. 1991. Regulation of T-cell sensitization at epithelial surfaces in the respiratory tract: Suppression of IgE responses to inhaled antigens by $CD3^+TcR\alpha^-/\beta^-$ lymphocytes (putative γ/δ T cells). *Immunology* 74:234–239.

44. Harrison, L.C., Dempsey-Collier, M., Kramer, D.R., and Takahashi, K. 1996. Aerosol insulin induces regulatory CD8 γδ T cells that prevent murine insulin-dependent diabetes. *J. Exp. Med.* 184:2167–2174.

45. Wildner, G., Hünig, T., and Thurau, S.R. 1996. Orally induced, peptide-specific γ/δ TcR+ cells suppress experimental autoimmune uveitis. *Eur. J. Immunol.* 26:2140–2148.

46. Mengel, J., Cardillo, F., Aroeira, L.S., Williams, O., Russo, M., and Vaz, N.M. 1995. Anti-gammadelta T cell antibody blocks the induction and maintenance of oral tolerance to ovalbumin in mice. *Immunol. Lett.* 48:97–102.

47. Ke, Y., Pearce, K., Lake, J.P., Ziegler, H.K., and Kapp, J.A. 1997. γδ T lymphocytes regulate the induction of oral tolerance. *J. Immunol.* 158:3610–3618.

48. Battisto, J.R., and Miller, J. 1962. Immunologic unresponsiveness produced in adult pigs by parenteral introduction of minute quantities of hapten or protein antigen. *Proc. Soc. Exp. Biol. Med.* 111:111–113.

49. Cantor, H.M., and Dumont, A.E. 1967. Hepatic suppression of sensitization to antigen absorbed into the portal vein. *Nature* 215:744–745.

50. Triger, D.R., Cynamon, M.H., and Wright, R. 1973. Studies on the hepatic uptake of antigen, I. Comparison of inferior vena cava and portal vein routes of immunisation. *Immunology* 25:941–946.

51. Qian, J.-H., Hashimoto, T., Fujiwara, H., and Hamaoka, T. 1985. Studies on the induction of tolerance to alloantigens, I. The abrogation of potentials for delayed-type hypersensitivity responses to alloantigens by portal venous inoculation with allogeneic cells. *J. Immunol.* 134:3656–3661.

52. Sato, S., Qian, J.-H., Kokudo, S., Ikegami, R., Suda, T., Hamaoka, T., and Fujiwara, H. 1988. Studies on the induction of tolerance to alloantigens, III. Induction of antibodies directed against alloantigen-specific delayed-type hypersensitivity T cells by a single injection of allogeneic lymphocytes via portal venous route. *J. Immunol.* 140:717–722.

53. Kokudo, S., Sato, S., Qian, J.-H., Wada, K., Ikegami, R., Hamaoka, T., and Fujiwora, H. 1988. Tolerance induction of alloreactivity by portal venous inoculation with allogeneic cells followed by the injection of cyclophosphamide, II. Cellular and molecular mechanisms underlying tolerance. *Microbiol. Immunol.* 32:283–292.

54. Fujiwara, H., Qian, J.-H., Satoh, S., Kokudo, S., Ikegama, R., and Hamacka, T. 1986. Studies on the induction of tolerance to alloantigens, II. The generation of serum factor(s) able to transfer alloantigen-specific tolerance for delayed-type hypersensitivity by portal venous inoculation with allogeneic cells. *J. Immunol.* 136:2763–2768.

55. Gorczynski, R.M., and Holmes, W. 1991. Specific manipulation in vivo of immunity to skin grafts bearing multiple minor histocompatibility differences. *Immunol. Lett.* 27:163–171.

56. Hirakawa, K., Yoshimura, N., Lee, C., Yasui, H., Ohsaka, Y., Hamashima, T., and Oka, T. 1993. Impact of perioperative portal venous administration of donor lymphocytes on survival of rat cardiac allografts and renal grafts of the mongrel dog. *Transplant. Proc.* 25:346–347.

57. Ghobrial, R.R., Hamashima, T., Wang, M.E., Wang, M., Stepkowski, S.M., and Kahan, B.D. 1996. Induction of transplantation tolerance by chimeric donor/recipient class I RT1.Aa molecules. *Transplantation* 62:1002–1010.

58. Wang, M., Stepkowski, S.M., Wang, M.E., Tian, L., Qu, X., Tu, Y., He, G., and Kahan, B.D. 1996. Induction of specific allograft immunity by soluble class I MHC heavy chain protein produced in a baculovirus expression system. *Transplantation* 61:448–457.

59. Wang, M., Stepkowski, S.M., Yu, J., Wang, M., and Kahan, B.D. 1997. Localization of cryptic tolerogenic epitopes in the α1-helical region of the RT1.Au alloantigen. *Transplantation* 63:1373–1379.

60. Cuison, A., Tasaka, K., Chuang, C.K., Minai, M., Yoshikawa, H., and Nakajima, Y. 1995. Schistosome eggs in the portal vein can induce tolerance. *Int. J. Parasitol.* 25:993–998.

61. Nakafusa, Y., Goss, J.A., Roland, C.R., and Flye, M.W. 1993. The effect of portal venous tolerance on the survival of small bowel allografts in the rat. *Transplantation* 56:1279–1282.
62. Fecteau, A., Tchervenkov, J., Guttman, F., Takara, T., and Rosenmann, E. 1994. Small bowel transplantation: The effect of intraportal donor-specific transfusion 24 hours pretransplant and low-dose cyclosporine. *Transplantation* 58:399–402.
63. Gorczynski, R.M., Fu, X.M., Chung, S., Sullivan, B., and Chen, Z. 1995. Manipulation of xenogeneic skin and/or renal graft survival in the rat-mouse concordant combination by portal vein pretransplant transfusion. *Transpl. Immunol.* 3:321–329.
64. Gorczynski, R.M. 1995. Regulation of IFN-γ and IL-10 synthesis *in vivo*, as well as continuous antigen exposure, is associated with tolerance to murine skin allografts. *Cell. Immunol.* 160:224–231.
65. Yu, S., Nakafusa, Y., and Flye, M.W. 1994. Portal vein administration of donor cells promotes peripheral allospecific hyporesponsiveness and graft tolerance. *Surgery* 116:229–234.
66. Gorczynski, R.M., Chen, Z., Hoang, Y., and Rossi-Bergman, B. 1996. A subset of γδ T-cell receptor positive cells produce T-helper type 2 cytokines and regulate mouse skin graft rejection following portal venous pretransplant preimmunization. *Immunology* 87:381–389.
67. Gorczynski, R.M., Cohen, Z., Levy, G., and Fu, X.M. 1996. A role for gamma(delta)TCR+ cells in regulation of rejection of small intestinal allografts in rats. *Transplantation* 62:844–851.
68. Bolling, S.F., Lin, H., Wei, R.-Q., and Turka, L.A. 1996. Preventing allograft rejection with CTLA4Ig: Effect of donor-specific transfusion route or timing. *J. Heart Lung Transplant.* 15:928–935.
69. Goss, J.A., Flye, M.W., and Lacy, P.E. 1996. Induction of allogeneic islet survival by intrahepatic islet preimmunization and transient immunosuppression. *Diabetes* 45:144–147.
70. Gorczynski, R.M., Cohen, Z., Plapler, H., Levy, G., Wojcik, D., and Koh, I. 1993. Functional activity in host and graft lymphoid tissue of rats receiving syngeneic heterotopic small bowel transplants with portal or systemic drainage. *Immunol. Lett.* 38:189–194.
71. Gorczynski, R.M., Chan, Z., Chung, S., Cohen, Z., Levy, G., Sullivan, B., and Fu, X.M. 1994. Prolongation of rat small bowel or renal allograft survival by pretransplant transfusion and/or by varying the route of allograft venous drainage. *Transplantation* 58:816–820.
72. Zhang, Y., Yasumizu, R., Sugiura, K., Hashimoto, F., Amoh, Y., Lian, Z., Cherry, A., Nishio, N., and Ikehara, S. 1994. Fate of allogeneic or syngeneic cells in intravenous or portal vein injection: Possible explanation for the mechanism of tolerance induction by portal vein injection. *Eur. J. Immunol.* 24:1558–1565.
73. Ogasawara, H., Watari, E., Shirai, Y., and Yokomuro, K. 1997. Inhibitory effects of portal venous injection of type II collagen in collagen-induced arthritis. *Nippon Ika Daigaku Zasshi* 64:220–224.
74. Koyamada, N., Ohteki, T., Abo, T., Fukimori, T., Ohkouchi, N., Satomi, S., Taguchi, Y., Kusumi, A., Mori, S., and Kumagai, K. 1993. Induction of specific tolerance by hepatic double negative CD4-8- αβ T cells of mice immunized with allogeneic cells via the portal vein *in vivo*. *Cell. Immunol.* 149:107–116.
75. Gorczynski, R.M. 1994. Adoptive transfer of unresponsiveness to allogeneic skin grafts with hepatic γδ + T cells. *Immunology* 81:27–35.

76. Gorczynski, R.M., Cohen, Z., Leung, Y., and Chen, Z. 1996. $\gamma\delta$ TcR+ hybridomas derived from mice preimmunized via the portal vein adoptively transfer increased skin allograft survival *in vivo*. *J. Immunol.* 157:574–581.

77. Gorczynski, R.M. 1992. Immunosuppression induced by hepatic portal venous immunization spares reactivity in IL-4 producing T lymphocytes. *Immunol. Lett.* 33:67–77.

78. Gorczynski, R.M., and Wojcik, D. 1994. A role for nonspecific (cyclosporin A) or specific (monoclonal antibodies to ICAM-1, LFA-1, and IL-10) immunomodulation in the prolongation of skin allografts after antigen-specific pretransplant immunization or transfusion. *J. Immunol.* 152:2011–2019.

79. Gorczynski, R.M., Cohen, Z., Fu, X.M., Hua, Z., Sun, Y., and Chen, Z. 1996. Interleukin-13, in combination with anti-interleukin-12, increases graft prolongation after portal venous immunization with cultured allogeneic bone marrow-derived dendritic cells. *Transplantation* 62:1592–1600.

80. Gorczynski, R.M., Chen, Z., Zeng, H., and Fu, X.M. 1997. Specificity for in vivo graft prolongation in $\gamma\delta$ T cell receptor+ hybridomas derived from mice given portal vein donor-specific preimmunization and skin allografts. *J. Immunol.* 159:3698–3706.

81. Yoshimura, N., Matsui, S., Hamashima, T., Lee, C., Ohsaka, Y., and Oka, T. 1990. The effects of perioperative portal venous inoculation with donor lymphocytes on renal allograft survival in the rat, I. Specific prolongation of donor grafts and suppressor factor in the serum. *Transplantation* 49:167–171.

82. Gorczynski, R.M., and Wojcik, D. 1992. Antigen presentation by murine splenic, but not hepatic, antigen-presenting cells to induce IL-2/IL-4 production from immune T cells is regulated by interactions between LFA-1/ICAM-1. *Immunol. Lett.* 34:177–181.

83. Callery, M., Kamei, T., and Flye, M. 1989. Kupffer cell blockade inhibits induction of tolerance by the portal venous route. *Transplantation* 47:1092–1094.

84. Kamei, T., Callery, M.P., and Flye, M.W. 1990. Kupffer cell blockade prevents induction of portal venous tolerance in rat cardiac allograft transplantation. *J. Surg. Res.* 48:393–396.

85. Squiers, E., Salomon, D., Pickard, L., Howard, R., and Pfaff, W. 1990. Abrogation of the induction of portal venous tolerance in cardiac transplant model resulting from Kupffer cell inhibition by gadolinium. *Transplantation* 50:171–173.

86. Roland, C.R., Walp, L., Stack, R.M., and Flye, M.W. 1994. Outcome of Kupffer cell antigen presentation to a cloned murine Th1 lymphocyte depends on the inducibility of nitric oxide synthase by IFN-γ. *J. Immunol.* 153:5453–5464.

87. Sato, K., Yabuki, K., Haba, T., and Maekawa, T. 1996. Role of Kupffer cells in the induction of tolerance after liver transplantation. *J. Surg. Res.* 63:433–438.

88. Nadler, P.I., Klingenstein, R.J., Richman, L.K., and Ahmann, G.B. 1980. The murine Kupffer cell, II. Accessory cell function in in vitro primary antibody responses, mitogen-induced proliferation, and stimulation of mixed lymphocyte responses. *J. Immunol.* 125:2521–2525.

89. Roland, C.R., Mangino, M.J., Duffy, B.F., and Flye, M.W. 1993. Lymphocyte suppression by Kupffer cells prevents portal venous tolerance induction: A study of macrophage function after intravenous gadolinium. *Transplantation* 55:1151–1158.

90. Squiers, E.C., Brunson, M.E., and Salomon, D.R., 1993. Kupffer cells can present alloantigen in vitro: An effect abrogated by gadolinium. *J. Surg. Res.* 55:551–554.

91. Lohse, A.W., Knolle, P.A., Bilo, K., Uhrig, A., Waldmann, C., Ibe, M., Schmitt, E., Gerken, G., and Meyer Zum Buschenfelde, K.H. 1996. Antigen-presenting function and

B7 expression of murine sinusoidal endothelial cells and Kupffer cells. *Gastroenterology* 110:1175–1181.

92. Roland, C.R., Mangino, M.J., and Flye, M.W. 1993. Lanthanide "blockade" of antigen-presenting cells suppresses lymphocyte proliferation by inducing nitric oxide synthesis. *J. Surg. Res.* 45:401–410.
93. Gorczynski, R.M., Rossi-Bergman, B., Sullivan, B., and Chen, Z. 1995. Role of reactive nitrogen intermediates in the regulation of allogeneic skin graft survival in mice after portal vein pretransplant transfusion. *Transplantation* 60:707–713.
94. Perez, R.V., Swanson, C., Morgan, M., Erickson, K., Hubbard, N.E., and German, J.B. 1997. Portal venous transfusion up-regulates Kupffer cell cyclooxygenase activity: A mechanism of immunosuppression in organ transplantation. *Transplantation* 64:135–139.
95. Gorczynski, R.M., Chung, S., Hoang, Y., Sullivan, B., and Chen, Z. 1996. Altered patterns of migration of cytokine-producing T lymphocytes in skin-grafted naive or immune mice following in vivo administration of anti-VCAM-1 or -ICAM-1. *Immunology* 87:573–580.
96. Chung, S.W., Gorczynski, R.M., Dziadkowiec, I., and Levy, G.A. 1995. Induction of T-cell hyporesponsiveness by intrahepatic modulation of donor antigen-presenting cells. *Immunology* 85:582–590.
97. Thomas, H.C., Ryan, C.J., Benjamin, I.S., Blumgart, L.H., and MacSween, R.N.M. 1976. The immune system response in cirrhotic rats. The induction of tolerance to orally administered protein antigens. *Gastroenterology* 71:114–117.
98. Yang, R., Liu, Q., Grosfeld, J.L., and Pescovitz, M.D. 1994. Intestinal drainage through liver is a pre-requisite for oral tolerance induction. *J. Pediatr. Surg.* 29:1145–1148.
99. Strobel, S., Mowat, A.M., Drummond, H.E., Pickering, M.G., and Ferguson, A. 1983. Immunological responses to fed protein antigens in mice, II. Oral tolerance for CMI is due to activation of cyclophosphamide sensitive cells by gut processed antigen. *Immunology* 49:451–456.
100. Peng, H.-J., Turner, M.W., and Strobel, S. 1990. The generation of a "tolerogen" after the ingestion of ovalbumin is time-dependent and unrelated to serum levels of immunoreactive antigen. *Clin. Exp. Immunol.* 81:510–515.
101. Furrie, E., Turner, M.W., and Strobel, S. 1995. Partial characterization of a circulating tolerogenic moiety which, after a feed of ovalbumin, suppresses delayed-type hypersensitivity in recipient mice. *Immunology* 86:480–486.
102. Furrie, E., Turner, M.W., and Strobel, S. 1994. Failure of scid mice to generate an oral tolerogen after a feed of ovalbumin: A role for a functioning gut-associated lymphoid system. *Immunology* 83:562–567.
103. Bruce, M.G., and Ferguson, A. 1986. Oral tolerance to ovalbumin in mice: Studies of chemically modified and of "biologically filtered" antigen. *Immunology* 57:627–630.
104. Bruce, M.G., and Ferguson, A. 1986. The influence of intestinal processing on the immunogenicity and molecular size of absorbed, circulating ovalbumin in mice. *Immunology* 59:295–300.
105. Weiner, H.L. 1997. Oral tolerance: Immune mechanisms and treatment of autoimmune diseases. *Immunol. Today* 18:335–343.

CHAPTER 7

THE IMMUNOBIOLOGY OF VIRAL HEPATITIS

FRANCIS V. CHISARI
The Scripps Research Institute, La Jolla, CA

OVERVIEW

The immune response to viral antigens is thought to be responsible for viral clearance and disease pathogenesis during hepatitis B and C virus infections. It is generally acknowledged that the humoral antibody response contributes to the clearance of circulating virus particles and the prevention of viral spread within the host, while the cellular immune response eliminates infected cells. The T cell response to the hepatitis B virus (HBV) is vigorous, polyclonal, and multispecific in acutely infected patients who successfully clear the virus, and relatively weak and narrowly focussed in chronically infected patients, suggesting that clearance of HBV is T cell dependent. In contrast, the T cell response to the hepatitis C virus (HCV) is relatively strong, polyclonal, and multispecific in chronically infected patients. This very interesting observation suggests that HCV may be more immunogenic than HBV but less responsive to control by the T cell response. The molecular and immunological basis for this seeming paradox is not understood.

The pathogenetic and antiviral potential of the cytotoxic T lymphocyte (CTL) response to HBV has been proven by the induction of a severe necroinflammatory liver disease following the adoptive transfer of hepatitis B surface antigen (HBsAg) specific CTL into HBV transgenic mice. The sheer number of potentially infectible hepatocytes in infected patients is so large, however, relative to the number of virus-specific T cells, that it may not be possible for the immune system to reach, recognize, and destroy all of the infected cells. Viral clearance from the liver, therefore, may require more than simply the killing of virus-infected cells. According to this hypothesis, clearance may only be achievable if the infecting viruses are responsive to

T Lymphocytes in the Liver: Immunobiology, Pathology, and Host Defense, Edited by I. Nicholas Crispe
ISBN 0-471-19218-X

antiviral signals induced in the infected cells by cytokines released from virus-specific T cells following antigen recognition. In keeping with this hypothesis, HBV replication is abolished, noncytopathically, by type 1 inflammatory cytokines secreted by antigen-specific CTL in HBV transgenic mice.

The dominant cause of viral persistence during HBV infection is the development of a weak antiviral immune response to the viral antigens, with corresponding inability to kill or to cure all of the infected cells. Alternatively, chronic hepatitis may be caused by the development of an inappropriate T cell response that can kill but cannot cure infected hepatocytes because it fails to produce sufficient quantities of the appropriate cytokines to clear the infection noncytopathically. Other factors that could contribute to viral persistence are immunological tolerance, mutational epitope inactivation or T cell receptor antagonism, incomplete downregulation of viral replication, and infection of immunologically privileged tissues. None of these pathways is likely to be the primary determinant of viral persistence, however, since they become apparent only in the setting of an ineffective immune response, which is, therefore, more fundamental. The basis for viral persistence during HCV infection is not as well understood, primarily because satisfactory experimental systems to study this question do not yet exist.

INTRODUCTION

Viral hepatitis is a necroinflammatory liver disease of variable severity. Persistent infection by HBV and HCV is often associated with chronic liver disease that can lead to the development of cirrhosis and hepatocellular carcinoma (HCC). An important feature of these viruses is their high mutation rate. This creates the opportunity for selection to occur during persistent infections if a mutation confers a growth advantage to a mutant viral genome or deletes a recognition site for the host immune response. The existence of substantial nucleotide and amino acid sequence heterogeneity in different isolates of HBV and HCV, and the emergence of specific mutations in the HBV genome in individual patients are well-established events that may contribute to the pathogenesis and natural history of the associated diseases.

Most studies suggest that the hepatitis viruses are not directly cytopathic, or at least not highly cytopathic, for the infected hepatocyte (1–3). Because the disease spectrum associated with these viruses is extraordinarily variable, it has been a longstanding prediction that the host response to these viruses must play a critical role in the pathogenesis of the associated diseases. Indeed, based on fairly extensive studies of HBV pathogenesis in man and animal models, there is considerable evidence that viral hepatitis is initiated by an antigen-specific antiviral intrahepatic cellular immune response that sets in motion a cascade of antigen-nonspecific cellular and molecular effector systems that actually cause most of the damage to the liver. For the hepatitis B virus, there is a great deal of evidence that both the cellular and humoral limbs of the immune response are required for viral clearance to occur. While clearance of most virus infections is widely thought to reflect the

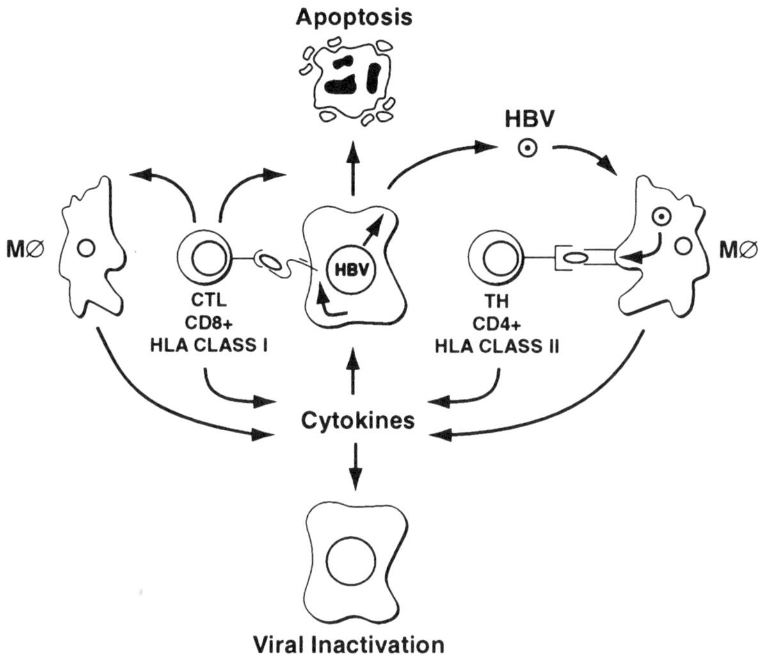

Figure 7.1. Noncytolytic clearance of HBV from the hepatocyte by T cell–derived cytokines. Upon antigen activation, $CD8^+$ CTLs deliver two signals to their target cells. One signal kills the target by apoptosis, while the other cures the infection by secreted antiviral cytokines including IFNγ and TNFα. The curative effect of the CTL response is orders of magnitude more efficient than its destructive effect. Antigen-activated $CD4^+$ T cells secrete the same cytokines when they recognize antigen presented by intrahepatic macrophages. Like CTLs, they induce an inflammatory liver disease and inhibit HBV replication, although less efficiently. The outcome of an infection may depend on the relative balance of these two effects, with a predominantly curative response leading to viral clearance, and a predominantly destructive response leading to viral persistence and chronic liver disease. Importantly, if the curative process abolishes viral gene expression and replication but does not eliminate the viral cccDNA from the hepatocyte, it could paradoxically lead to viral persistence by rendering the virus immunologically invisible without removing its transcriptional template.

killing of infected cells by virus-specific T cells, recent data also suggest that noncytolytic intracellular viral inactivation by certain inflammatory cytokines released by activated lymphomononuclear cells may play an important role in the clearance of at least some of these viruses from the infected cell (see Fig. 7.1).

THE T CELL RESPONSE TO HBV

Antiviral T cells are believed to play a major role in control of HBV infection by virtue of their capacity to identify and kill virus-infected cells and to secrete antiviral cytokines that can inhibit viral gene expression in infected cells without killing them (4). The peripheral blood and intrahepatic T cell response to HBV is vigorous, polyclonal, and multispecific in patients with acute hepatitis who ultimately clear the virus (Table 7.1), and it is relatively weak and more restricted in patients with chronic hepatitis (Table 7.2), except during acute exacerbations of chronic disease (5). Many class I and class II restricted T cell epitopes have been defined in the various HBV proteins with the class II restricted, $CD4^+$ helper T cell response being focused principally on the nucleocapsid antigens of HBV, while the envelope and polymerase antigens are more often targeted by the class I restricted $CD8^+$ CTL response in acutely infected patients (4).

Despite the vigor of the T cell response to HBV during acute viral hepatitis, however, it is now known that very low levels of HBV DNA, detectable only by nested polymerase chain reaction, are present in the serum and peripheral blood mononuclear cells (PBMC) for several decades following complete clinical and serological resolution of disease (6). Interestingly, recent studies indicate that long-term persistence of trace amounts of viral DNA is associated with equally long-term persistence of HBV-specific CTL in these individuals (7), suggesting that the viral DNA is transcriptionally active and able to produce viral antigens that actively maintain the CTL response, perhaps for life. This implies that traces of virus, not only viral DNA, persist in the face of the CTL response after recovery from acute viral hepatitis. It also implies that acute and chronic HBV infection may simply be points on a quantitative spectrum rather than being qualitatively different from each other. The fascinating ability of HBV to persist at low level after acute infection and to simultaneously maintain and evade the immune response is a matter of considerable interest for its own sake and for the insight it might yield into the basis for high-level persistence in "healthy" carriers and patients with chronic hepatitis. The subject of viral persistence will be considered in further detail later in this review.

TABLE 7.1 HBV-Specific CTL Response in Acute Viral Hepatitis

Readily detectable early during acute infection
Strong, polyclonal, multispecific for HBV envelope, capsid, and polymerase antigens
Major determinant of viral clearance and liver disease
Persists indefinitely after recovery
Maintained by traces of virus that also persist

TABLE 7.2 HBV-Specific CTL Response in Chronic Viral Hepatitis

Weak and narrowly focused in most patients
Not sufficient to terminate infection
Sufficient to cause liver disease
Strong and multispecific following remission
Inducible by epitope-specific immunotherapy
CTL escape mutants occur in persistently infected patients, but they are rare

MECHANISMS OF HBV CLEARANCE

A large body of evidence suggests that the vigor of the CTL response to HBV is the principal determinant of viral clearance in infected patients (Table 7.1) (4). It is widely believed that the CTL response clears a viral infection by killing infected cells. While this is probably true for many viruses, it may not be possible for the CTL response to eradicate infections in which the number of infected cells outnumber the antigen-specific T cells by several orders of magnitude. This appears to be the case for at least some of the hepatitis viruses, especially HBV, which can infect virtually all of the hepatocytes in the liver.

The reasons for this are as follows. For a CTL to kill a target cell in vivo, the CTL must be induced by encountering antigen in an immunologically stimulatory microenvironment (e.g., lymphoid tissue), enter the circulation and eventually the infected tissue, stop, migrate past any tissue barriers (e.g., endothelial cells, basement membranes, etc.), reach the infected cells, recognize their cognate antigens, kill the infected cells *one at a time*, move on to find the next target cell and kill it before the CTLs are triggered to die themselves by the process of activation-induced cell death (8). Thus, viral elimination by CTL-mediated killing is not nearly as efficient in vivo as one might assume from the ease with which CTLs can kill target cells in vitro, where the only functions needed are antigen recognition and delivery of one or more death signals, and where the CTL are crowded around the target cells which have been highly selected for their exquisite sensitivity to those signals.

In addition, consider that there are approximately 10^{11} infectible hepatocytes in the human liver (Table 7.3) and that all of them can be infected by HBV (9). Consider, also, that there are approximately 10^{12} lymphocytes in the entire body and that the HBV-specific CTL precursor frequency at the height of the CTL response in a strongly reactive patient with acute hepatitis is rarely greater than 10^{-4} and usually it is much lower (10). Hence, there should be no more than 10^{8} HBV-specific CTL in the entire body at any point in time. Therefore, if every HBV specific-CTL in the entire body were to enter the liver at the same time (highly unlikely), and if most of the hepatocytes were infected (common) there would be 1 specific CTL in the liver for every 1,000 infected hepatocytes. Even considering the temporally extended dynamics of the CTL response, under these conditions it is difficult to imagine that viral clearance can be achieved simply by the destruction of infected cells. Even if only 10% of the hepatocytes were infected, the effector-to-target cell ratio in the liver

TABLE 7.3 Numerical Analysis of Viral Clearance by CTL

Can CTLs clear a viral infection if all they do is kill infected cells?
$\sim 10^{11}$ hepatocytes in the liver.
$\sim 10^{12}$ lymphocytes in the body.
$<10^{-4}$ HBV CTL precursor frequency.
$<10^{8}$ HBV specific CTLs in the body.
The CTL: infected cell ratio in situ <1:1000.

would be 1:100, well beyond the cytolytic capacity of a single T cell. Even at the 1% infection level the ratio would be 1:10, which would require every CTL to find and kill 10 infected hepatocytes that are widely separated from each other by a 100-fold excess of uninfected cells in order to clear the infection. While efficient cytolysis can sometimes be achieved in vitro at this effector-to-target cell ratio, it is very unusual; and in vitro the CTLs are surrounded by target cells, all of which express their cognate antigen, so their task is much simpler than it is in vivo. Thus, as the number of infected cells decreases, the challenge of finding them increases, further contributing to the difficulty of clearing an infection by killing alone. Furthermore, if clearance were due entirely to the destruction of infected cells one might reasonably expect the incidence of fatal acute hepatitis to be much higher than it is during HBV infection. For all of these reasons, we suggest that *although the liver disease in viral hepatitis is certainly due to the destructive potential of the CTL response, viral clearance probably requires additional CTL functions besides their ability to kill infected cells.*

CTL-INDUCED LIVER DISEASE AND VIRAL CLEARANCE IN HBV TRANSGENIC MICE

Important new insights into the pathogenetic and noncytopathic antiviral capacity of the CTL response to HBV have been forthcoming from studies in HBV transgenic mice. Proof that a major histocompatibility complex (MHC)-restricted cytolytic immune response to viral-encoded antigens expressed at the surface of the hepatocyte plays an important role in viral clearance and in the pathogenesis of HBV-induced liver disease required the development of a readily manipulable small animal model in an immunologically well-defined species. In recent years it has been shown that transgenic mice that express HBV envelope antigens in their hepatocytes (11) develop acute viral hepatitis following adoptive transfer of $CD8^{+}$, MHC class I restricted, HBsAg-specific CTL lines and clones (12,13). Furthermore, it was shown that the disease progresses through a series of clearly definable steps in an orderly fashion.

The first event occurs within 1 hour of CTL administration, with antigen recognition by the CTL and delivery of a signal that results in the death of the hepatocyte by apoptosis causing the formation of acidophilic, Councilman bodies (apoptotic hepatocytes) that are characteristic of acute viral hepatitis in man (14). Recently, we have shown that for this process to be efficient requires the simultaneous activation of death signals in the hepatocyte by both the Fas- and perforin-dependent pathways (15). This suggests that the molecular and cellular requirements for CTL-mediated killing at the level of the target cell are much more stringent in vivo than in vitro, reinforcing the concept that it is difficult to clear a virus from the liver simply by killing infected cells (Table 7.4).

The clinical significance of the direct, CTL-mediated apoptotic death of hepatocytes is minimal in this model since fewer than 5% of the hepatocytes are killed by this process. However, a second phase in the disease begins between 4 and 12 hours after CTL injection, with the recruitment of many host-derived inflammatory cells

TABLE 7.4 Cytopathic Potential of the CTL Response to HBV

HBV-specific CTLs cause a necroinflammatory liver disease in HBV transgenic mice.
Both Fas- and perforin-dependent death pathways must be activated for liver disease to occur.
Cytotoxicity is inherently inefficient, requiring direct cell–cell contact to kill HBV^+ cells.
More efficient mechanisms are probably needed to clear viruses that infect large numbers of cells.

into the immediate vicinity of the apoptotic hepatocytes. This results in the formation of necroinflammatory foci and the destruction of sufficient numbers of additional hepatocytes for jaundice to occur.

Importantly, under the conditions of the foregoing experiments, only a small fraction of the hepatocytes are killed by the CTLs and the ensuing inflammatory response (16–19). If many $HBsAg^+$ ground glass hepatocytes are present in the liver, however, the disease progresses further and, if most of the hepatocytes have ground glass features, may kill the animal due to fulminant hepatitis, because these cells are exquisitely sensitive to destruction by an antigen-nonspecific process that is triggered by interferon-γ (IFNγ) and mediated by activated hepatic macrophages (20). The striking similarities between the immunopathological and histopathological features of the current model and acute viral hepatitis in man suggest that similar events probably contribute importantly to the pathogenesis of the human disease as well.

Interestingly, the CTL clones used in the foregoing studies cannot induce a second episode of hepatitis if they are readministered to the mice less than 4 weeks after the first CTL injection (11). While studying the basis for this observation it was learned that, in addition to killing some of the hepatocytes the CTLs also downregulated the expression and replication of HBV by *all* of the hepatocytes in the liver *without killing them* (19). Using transgenic mice containing the complete viral genome as recipients of adoptively transferred CTLs it has recently been shown that all of the viral gene products, including the 3.5-kb and 2.1-kb viral RNAs, their translation products (HBcAg, HBeAg, and HBsAg) and episomal replicative DNA intermediates, are susceptible to this remarkable effect (16). This process is cytokine mediated and noncytopathic, because the regulatory effects of the CTLs can be blocked by the prior administration of antibodies to IFNγ or tumor necrosis factor alpha (TNFα) without reducing the cytopathic effects of the CTLs, and because the antiviral effect can be reproduced by perforin-deficient CTLs, which do not cause hepatitis in these animals (16). Furthermore, we have shown that the same events can be initiated by the transfer of HBsAg-specific class II restricted T cell clones into the transgenic mice when they recognize antigen presented by hepatic macrophages (Kupffer cells), not the hepatocytes (21). Recently, we have shown that interleukin-12 (IL-12) inhibits HBV replication by inducing the production of IFNγ in the liver (22). Since IFNγ is a powerful macrophage activator, it is quite possible that its antiviral effect is mediated by TNFα produced by activated macrophages. In keeping with this notion, we have shown that recombinant TNFα also inhibits HBV gene expression in these mice (23), as does IL-2, the regulatory effects of which are mediated by TNFα (24), by post-transcriptionally accelerating the degradation of HBV mRNA (24).

TABLE 7.5 Curative Potential of the CTL Response to HBV

HBV-specific CTLs activate intracellular pathways that inhibit HBV gene expression and replication.
This process is mediated by IFNγ and TNFα secreted by the CTL following antigen recognition.
Neither Fas- nor the perforin-dependent signaling pathways are involved in this process.
The curative effect of the CTLs is more effective at reducing viral burden than their cytopathic effect.
If incomplete, this process could favor viral persistence.

TABLE 7.6 Antiviral Pathways in CTL-activated Hepatocytes

IFNγ and TNFα inhibit *HBV replication* by activating the hepatocyte to destroy HBV nucleocapsid particles and their cargo of replicating viral DNA in the cytoplasm.
The same cytokines inhibit *HBV gene expression* by activating the posttranscriptional degradation of viral RNA in the nucleus of the cell.
The target elements in the virus and the signaling pathways in the cell that mediate these effects are currently unknown.

One might predict from the foregoing that coinfection or superinfection of the HBV-infected liver by other pathogens could facilitate the clearance of HBV if they induce the local production of the antiviral cytokines to which HBV is susceptible. Precisely these events have been shown to occur in the HBV transgenic mice during lymphocytic choriomeningitis virus (17), adenovirus, and cytomegalovirus (18) infection of the liver. This is reminiscent of isolated case reports suggesting that superinfection by HAV or HCV is sometimes associated with clearance of HBV in chronically infected patients (26,27). The potential of these antiviral pathways to be exploited for therapeutic purposes is self-evident.

These results suggest that a strong intrahepatic immune response to HBV can suppress viral gene expression and replication and, if the supercoiled viral genome is also eliminated by this process, perhaps even "cure" infected hepatocytes of the virus without killing them (Table 7.5). Importantly, this shows that the *infected cells can become active participants in the antiviral response* by responding to cytokine-induced signals and activating specific intracellular pathways that interrupt the viral life cycle (Table 7.6). This is a significant departure from current dogma, which views the infected cell merely as a victim of the viral infection. As a corollary of this hypothesis, the data suggest that a weak immune response or incomplete viral inactivation could contribute to viral persistence and chronic liver disease by reducing the expression of viral antigens sufficiently for the infected cells to escape immune recognition.

MECHANISMS OF HBV PERSISTENCE

For a noncytopathic virus to persist it must either not induce an effective antiviral immune response, or it must be able to overwhelm or evade it (Table 7.7). One or both

TABLE 7.7 Possible Strategies for a Virus to Escape Immune Elimination

1. Decrease its visibility to the immune system by reducing:
   a. Viral gene expression
   b. HLA gene expression
   c. Antigen processing
   d. Peptide transport
2. Decrease the effectiveness of antiviral cytokines by:
   a. Downregulating cytokine receptors and signaling pathways
   b. Producing decoy cytokines or cytokine receptors
3. Increase the resistance of infected cells to CTL-mediated killing by:
   a. Reducing Fas expression or signaling pathways
   b. Blocking perforin-/granzyme-induced signaling pathways
   c. Increasing expression of genes that block apoptosis
4. Infect immunologically privileged sites that are:
   a. Physically inaccessible
   b. Unable to process or present antigen
   c. Able to express Fas ligand and, potentially, kill CTLs
5. Induce immunological tolerance.
   a. Thymic deletion
   b. Exhaustion, suppression, anergy, etc.
6. Evasion.
   a. Epitope loss mutations
   b. Partial agonist, antagonist mutations
   c. Mutational inactivation of cytokine response elements

of the first two scenarios are probably operative in most patients chronically infected by HBV. Indeed, neonatal tolerance is probably responsible for both the lack of an antiviral immune response and for viral persistence following mother–infant transmission, which is the most common antecedent of persistent HBV infection worldwide (4). The immunological basis for viral persistence during adult onset infection is not well understood. Perhaps the simplest explanation is quantitative, based on the kinetics of infection relative to the induction of a CTL response during the early days of an infection. According to the calculations presented in Table 7.3, viral persistence would be predicted if the size of the inoculum or the replication rate of an incoming virus exceeds the kinetics of the immune response such that the effector-to-target cell ratio favors the virus even when the CTL response is fully in place.

To be consistent with the repeated observation (28–31) that the CTL response is much less vigorous in chronically infected patients than it is during acute infection, however, other factors must be involved as well. Reasonable candidates are the induction of peripheral tolerance or exhaustion of the T cell response by the high viral load that characterizes most persistently infected patients. Additionally, virus-specific CTLs that might otherwise become activated by antigen recognition in the immunostimulatory context of secondary lymphoid organs might be inactivated, if antigen is presented in the absence of costimulatory signals in the liver. Unfortunately, these attractive theories are very difficult to test in patients, since they require sequential analysis of patients at multiple time points, beginning immediately after inoculation and continuing until the infection is resolved or persistent infection is established. Examination of the earliest events in the host–virus encounter is mandatory, however, to understand the immunological basis for the poor T cell response to HBV in adult onset chronic infection. Perhaps the well-characterized animal models of hepadnavirus infection will afford this opportunity when immunological reagents to study the T cell response in chimpanzees, woodchucks, and ducks become available. In the interim, the HBV transgenic mouse model described above can serve as a surrogate model to determine if the T cell response to HBV is qualitatively or quantitatively different when antigen presentation occurs in the liver instead of the lymphoid system.

Other candidate mechanisms that could contribute to viral persistence include infection of immunologically privileged sites, viral inhibition of antigen presentation, selective immune suppression, downregulation of viral gene expression, and viral mutations that abrogate, anergize, or antagonize antigen recognition by virus-specific T cells (reviewed in reference 4). There is some evidence that privileged sites may play a role, since HBV does infect extrahepatic tissues. Also, it has been reported that, while HBV-specific CTLs can recognize viral antigens in the liver, this does not occur in the kidney or brain of HBV transgenic mice due to the limited access of these CTL to antigen-positive cells present on the other side of microvascular barriers that exist in those tissues. These barriers are not present in the liver sinusoid (12). Additionally, it has been suggested that infected cells that express Fas ligand can protect themselves against CTL-mediated injury by actively destroying them via the same Fas ligand–Fas receptor pathway that CTLs use to kill their target cells but in reverse (32). Importantly, it appears that hepatocytes can be induced to express Fas ligand during an inflammatory response (33). If this is correct, individuals whose hepatocytes can be induced to express Fas ligand most efficiently would be most likely to delete their HBV-specific CTLs and become chronically infected. An interesting correlate of this scenario is the theoretical possibility that HBV itself might be able to induce Fas ligand expression by the hepatocyte, thereby deleting the HBV-specific CTL population when it enters the liver. In either case, Fas ligand induction would have to occur without inducing hepatocyte fratricide by virtue of Fas ligand–Fas interactions between adjacent cells (33). Alternatively, HBV could theoretically downregulate Fas expression, rendering the infected hepatocyte relatively resistant to destruction by the CTL. All of this is strictly speculative at present.

Viral inhibition of antigen presentation, suppression or neutralization of antiviral cytokines, and induction of selective immune suppression are pathways that are utilized by some animal viruses in their quest for survival (reviewed in references 34 and 35). Thus far, however, there is no evidence that these processes are operative during HBV infection, or during infection by any of the other persistent hepatotropic viruses for that matter. On the other hand, as mentioned above, soluble products of a type 1 CTL response, especially IFNγ, TNFα, and IL-2, have been shown to suppress HBV gene expression and replication by the hepatocyte in vivo in HBV transgenic mice (16). Instead of leading to viral clearance, however, it could contribute to viral persistence if the viral transcriptional template (cccDNA) is resistant to suppression by these cytokines. The influence of the CTL on HBV DNA cannot be addressed in the transgenic mice because, for unknown reasons, they do not produce it in detectable amounts (36). *Therefore, the influence of CTL-derived cytokines on HBV gene expression and replication could be viewed as either a survival strategy by the virus, contributing to persistence, if it is incomplete, or as a tissue-sparing antiviral strategy by the host, contributing to viral elimination, if it is complete.* Further studies are needed to clarify this important point.

If the antiviral effect of the type 1 cytokines can fully eradicate HBV, one might expect that individuals whose immune response to this virus does not lead to type 1 cytokine production would be unable to clear it. Indeed, the cytopathic potential of the CTLs in these individuals would trigger hepatitis, while the failure of their CTLs to produce the appropriate cytokines might contribute to viral persistence. Analysis of cytokine expression in the liver of patients with chronic HBV infection should clarify this interesting hypothesis.

CTL ESCAPE MUTATIONS

The role of viral escape mutations as a cause of viral persistence has attracted considerable interest in recent years. Many conditions must be fulfilled, however, for a mutant virus to be selected by CTL-mediated immune pressure (reviewed in reference 4). Perhaps the most important condition is the occurrence of a strong CTL response that is focused on a single viral epitope. This scenario would favor the outgrowth of variant viruses because they would not be otherwise visible to the immune system. This type of CTL response is unusual, however, during HBV infection, where the CTL response is typically vigorous and multispecific during acute hepatitis and weak or undetectable during chronic hepatitis (10,29,30,37). Accordingly, mutational inactivation of CTL epitopes is extremely uncommon during chronic HBV infection (38).

Nonetheless, strong, narrowly focused CTL responses do occur occasionally in these patients (20), and in this setting viral escape mutations can occur (39). Vigorous oligoclonal expansions of T cells have been described in other persistent viral infections, especially human immunodeficiency virus (HIV) (40–43). Even in these infections, however, viral mutations that affect recognition of an epitope by some CTL clones do not automatically affect all CTL clones specific for the same epitope, since different T cell clones can bind different residues in the same epitope (44,45). While CTL escape can confer a strong survival advantage, it is important to emphasize that selection of escape variants in all of these infections occurs in the setting of a preexisting persistent infection; *that is, viral persistence probably leads to selection of escape variants, not the reverse.*

The situation may be somewhat different in early chronic HIV infection, where the CTL response is characteristically very strong yet it is unable to clear the virus (40,41). The incredibly high rate of HIV production and the exceptionally high mutation rate of this virus may cause so many different viruses to be generated each day that they exceed the capacity of the immune system to respond effectively simply on a numerical basis (45). In this regard, the ostensibly vigorous immune response to

HIV appears to be unable to compete with capacity of the virus to replicate and its ability to generate mutants. Mutational inactivation of CTL epitopes might thus play an earlier and more important role in the establishment of viral persistence for this virus than for HBV. It is important to emphasize, however, that the overwhelming rates of viral replication and spread relative to the ability of the immune system to produce enough CTLs to reach and destroy all of the infected cells, plus the immunosuppressive effects of the virus itself, are probably more important than viral mutation for the development of persistent infection.

The situation may be different again during chronic hepatitis C virus (HCV) infection, where an extensive quasispecies of viral variants can coexist with a multispecific CTL response (46–49) that is intermediate in strength between the response of patients chronically infected by HBV and HIV. Unlike HBV and HIV, where the viral load is high, the viral titer is very low during chronic HCV infection (50), so viral persistence cannot be blamed on an overwhelming infection in this instance. Therefore, escape mutants may play a greater role in the primary establishment of HCV persistence than is likely for these other viruses. Importantly, CTL escape has been observed in a chronically HCV-infected chimpanzee (51). The extent to which the mutation contributed to, or is a consequence of, persistent HCV infection in this case remains to be determined.

In view of the multispecificity of the CTL response to most persistent viruses, current data favor the notion that selection of CTL escape mutants is most likely to occur only after a persistent infection is already established. In this setting, viral mutations could solidify the chronicity of the infection and perhaps even make it irreversible. Whether such mutations can also serve as the primary cause of viral persistence in the context of a multispecific T cell response remains to be proven.

THE T CELL RESPONSE TO HCV

The mechanisms whereby HCV causes acute hepatocellular injury and initiates the sequence of events leading to chronic liver disease and ultimately hepatocellular carcinoma are not well understood. Although the immune response almost certainly plays an important, perhaps a central, role in HCV pathogenesis, chimpanzees can be repetitively infected when they are exposed to the same infectious inoculum of HCV after recovery from a previous infection and the development of what would otherwise appear to be a perfectly competent immune response (52,53). While this may be due to the well-known propensity of the virus to mutate and the presence of a diverse viral quasi-species in any given inoculum, the apparent absence of a protective neutralizing humoral or cellular response to common conserved determinants in the various viral proteins is puzzling.

Using recombinant HCV proteins to stimulate HCV-specific T cells in the peripheral blood and intrahepatic T cell infiltrate, the human leukocyte antigen (HLA) class II restricted T cell response to HCV has been studied in patients with chronic HCV infection and in subjects who have apparently recovered from acute hepatitis (54–56). As in patients with acute HBV infection, the $CD4^+$ T cell response to HCV proteins is polyclonal, multispecific, and quite strong in acutely infected patients who subsequently clear the virus. The response is especially strong to nonstructural proteins, and it can last for several years after clinical and virological remission of disease (57).

The foregoing observations suggest that the T cell response to HCV plays an important role in viral clearance during this infection. However, its true role is obscured by the fact that, in contrast to the relatively weak antiviral T cell response in patients with chronic hepatitis B, the T cell response to HCV proteins can be quite vigorous in patients with chronic hepatitis C. Indeed, the $CD4^+$ T cell response in chronically infected patients is characteristically polyclonal and multispecific, often recognizing more than one viral antigen (54,55, 58,59). This response may be compartmentalized to the liver (60). A hierarchy of T cell responsiveness to HCV proteins has been defined in these patients, with core and NS4 proteins being the most immunogenic. Furthermore, healthy carriers and individuals in remission respond more strongly than patients with ongoing liver disease. Unfortunately, however, there are no obvious clinical differences between the majority of chronically infected individuals who produce a T cell response to HCV and the substantial minority of patients who do not (59).

HLA class I restricted HCV-specific $CD8^+$ CTL are also detectable in the peripheral blood and the intrahepatic lymphocyte infiltrate in patients with chronic hepatitis C (46,57, 61–64). A similar CTL response has been demonstrated in the liver of acutely infected chimpanzees, and the response can last indefinitely, suggesting that the virus can persist in the presence of these CTLs (65). The virological and immunological basis for the survival of HCV in the face of a CTL response is unclear at the moment. The CTLs identified thus far in infected patients are able to recognize both conserved and variable regions of all of the HCV proteins in the context of several different HLA molecules (46,61–63,66). Moreover, the response is often polyclonal and multispecific in chronically infected patients.

CTL clones have been isolated from the intrahepatic compartment using only antigen-nonspecific stimuli, implying that these cells must be present at relatively high frequency within the intrahepatic infiltrate (46,47,61). In contrast, it is necessary to expand the peripheral blood CTL precursor population with HCV-derived peptides in order to demonstrate a CTL response to HCV (61–64). Nonetheless, the HCV-specific CTL response is probably stronger than the response to HBV not only because it can be relatively easily detected in the periphery during chronic infection, while the response to HBV cannot, but because virus-specific lesional T cells seem to be more highly represented in HCV-infected than in HBV-infected livers.

In sum, HCV appears to be more immunogenic than HBV in chronically infected patients, but less responsive to immunological control. This is very surprising since the expression of HLA and intercellular adhesion molecules (67) and Fas antigen (68) are upregulated in the liver during HCV infection, a development that should facilitate antigen recognition, T cell–hepatocyte binding affinity, and hepatocytolysis. Additionally, several related flaviviruses have recently been shown to upregulate MHC class I expression in infected cells (69), a finding that raises the possibility that HCV might do the same. Nonetheless, HCV is rarely eliminated despite a vigorous immune response. These observations are compatible with the notion that cell killing may not be sufficient to eradicate HCV infection even under these very favorable conditions, perhaps for the reasons summarized in Table 7.3. If HCV is also resistant to control by T-cell-derived cytokines, HCV clearance from the liver would be unlikely, so that persistent infection would occur in most patients. We favor this hypothesis for the moment, but additional studies are needed to test its premises and predictions.

THE CD4$^+$ HELPER T CELL RESPONSE TO HBV AND HCV

While we have focused primarily on the CTL response to HBV and HCV in this review, because of its presumed effector function in both infections, the importance of the class II restricted helper T cell responses to these viruses should not be underestimated. Indeed, the CD4$^+$ T cell response mirrors the CTL response to both viruses in acutely and chronically infected patients. Accordingly, it probably influences the strength, specificity, and cytokine profile of the CTL response during acute and chronic infection, as well as providing help for T-cell-dependent antibody synthesis in these patients (reviewed in reference 4). In addition to their master regulatory functions, CD4$^+$ T helper type 1 (Th1) cells can function as CTL, at least in vitro. Hence, if hepatocytes or intrahepatic macrophages can present viral antigens to virus-specific helper T cells in the liver, they might contribute to disease pathogenesis and viral clearance by killing hepatocytes and by secreting the same antiviral cytokines as CD8$^+$ CTLs (discussed in reference 30). Indeed, as mentioned above, we have recently shown that HBsAg-specific CD4$^+$ T cell clones can cause hepatitis and inhibit HBV replication in the liver of HBV transgenic mice following antigen presentation by hepatic macrophages (21).

UNIFYING CONCEPTS IN HBV AND HCV IMMUNOBIOLOGY

In light of the wealth of information regarding the immune response to HBV and HCV that has been forthcoming from many different laboratories in the past several years, a general picture is emerging that may explain the immunopathogenesis of these two infections. These concepts are summarized in Table 7.8.

First, it appears that the helper and cytotoxic T cell responses to HBV are both strong and broadly specific in acutely infected patients (4), and these T cells typically secrete type 1 cytokines such as IL-2 and IFNγ upon antigen stimulation (70,71), although type 2 cytokine profiles can also be observed (71). It is germane that type 1 cytokines have been shown to inhibit HBV gene expression and replication in the liver of transgenic mice (16–19). It is easy to envision how an immune response of this sort would be able to control a viral infection quite successfully.

Second, the T cell response to HBV is weak and, when it is detectable, narrowly focused in chronically infected patients (4), except during exacerbations of liver disease (5) or following viral clearance (10). The cytokine profile of the intrahepatic HBV-specific T cells is variable, with type 1 cytokines being produced by some clones (70–73), and type 2 cytokines or a combination of cytokines (type 0) being

TABLE 7.8 Hepatitis Virus Immunobiology

	HBV		HCV	
Parameter	Acute	Chronic	Acute	Chronic
Th Strength	Strong	Weak	Strong	Int.
Th Specificity	Broad	Narrow	Broad	Broad
CTL Strength	Strong	Weak	?	Int.
CTL Specificity	Broad	Narrow	?	Broad
Cytokine Profile	Type 1	Type 0/1/2	Type 1	Type 1
Cytokine Sensitivity	Type 1	Type 1	?	?

produced by others (73). If clearance of HBV depends on the cytokine profile of the intrahepatic T cells, the heterogeneity of the T cell response in these patients is compatible with the variable duration and severity of liver disease in chronically infected patients. It is important to realize, however, that antigen-specific T cells represent a very minor component of the intrahepatic inflammatory infiltrate in patients with chronic hepatitis (74), as has been shown in a transgenic mouse model of CTL-induced inflammatory liver disease (20). Hence, the cytokines produced by the entire intrahepatic infiltrate may be more important for viral clearance than the cytokine profile produced by the antigen-specific T cells alone. This should be examined in future studies.

Third, the helper T cell response to HCV is strong and broadly specific in patients with acute hepatitis (57), most of whom fail to clear the infection. Furthermore, the helper (54–61) and CTL responses (46,47, 61–64,66) to HCV are also quite vigorous in persistently infected patients (i.e., apparently stronger than the corresponding responses to HBV during chronic HBV infection) (75). Importantly, most of the peripheral blood and intrahepatic HCV-specific CD4 and CD8 clones that have been analyzed in acutely and chronically infected patients produce primarily type 1 cytokines (47). This is very interesting because it may not only explain the vigor of the T cell response to HCV, it may also suggest a basis for viral persistence in the face of a strong T cell response (i.e., resistance to control by inflammatory cytokines).

Consider the possibility that, as mentioned earlier, it may not be possible for the T cell response to clear a virus from the liver merely by killing infected cells, because there are too many infected cells for the T cells to reach, recognize, and kill them one at a time. If this is correct, it might not be possible to clear hepatotropic viruses that are resistant to cytokine-induced hepatocellular antiviral signaling pathways. While this is an attractive hypothesis, it is speculative because the sensitivity of HCV to T cell–derived cytokines is not known at this point. Clarification of this intriguing hypothesis will be possible when improved tissue culture and animal models are available for the propagation of HCV.

SUMMARY AND CONCLUSIONS

The diversity of clinical syndromes and disease manifestations associated with each of the hepatitis viruses strongly suggests that the clinical outcome of these infections is determined by the quality and vigor of the antiviral immune response produced by each infected individual. Antibodies to antigens expressed at the surface of virus particles can provide protection from initial infection and can prevent viral spread from cell to cell, once infection is established. Antibody-mediated immune complex formation can contribute to extrahepatic syndromes in these patients and may even play a role in liver disease if they can bind to the surface of antigen-positive hepatocytes and recruit Fc-receptor-positive killer cells, thereby mediating antibody-dependent cellular cytotoxicity. $CD4^+$ helper T cells serve a critically important regulatory function by secreting a variety of cytokines that can facilitate B cell maturation, expression, and antibody secretion (e.g., Type 2 cytokines such as IL-4, IL-5, IL-10), or that foster the development of a strong CTL response (e.g., type 1 cytokines like IL-2, IFNγ and TNFβ). $CD8^+$ CTLs can kill infected cells by direct contact, triggering them to undergo apoptosis and recruiting antigen-nonspecific inflammatory cells that amplify their cytopathic potential. They also secrete cytokines when they recognize antigen in the infected tissue, some of which have the potential to inhibit the expression and replication of at least one of the hepatitis viruses (HBV) in the hepatocyte. All limbs of the immune response must cooperate productively to terminate a viral infection. Individual differences in the efficiency of viral antigen processing by hepatocytes and professional antigen presenting cells, or at the level of antigen recognition and responsiveness by B and T lymphocytes will affect the strength of the antiviral immune response and the extent to which it contributes to viral clearance and liver disease.

While a great deal is now known about the effector limb of these responses, *clarification of the factors that determine whether a given individual will mount an effective immune response to a virus represents the greatest challenge for investigation in the future*. At the effector level, it would appear that the CTL response can activate two different pathways to eliminate a virus—namely, killing the infected cells or eliminating the virus from within the cell without killing it. These alternate scenarios can be activated simultaneously as a consequence of antigen recognition, as illustrated for HBV in Figure 7.1. According to this scenario, viral clearance depends on the development of a vigorous intrahepatic immune response, with the severity of the associated liver disease being determined by the number of infected hepatocytes and the balance between the cytopathic and antiviral regulatory effects of the intrahepatic inflammatory cells.

If the T cell response is strong and the number of infected cells is low, viral clearance should occur, rapidly and efficiently, simply by killing the infected cells, and there should be little evidence of liver disease. Even a strong T cell response may not be able to clear a massive viral infection, however, unless the curative limb of the response illustrated in Figure 7.1 is called into play. In the absence of this component, either because the virus is not susceptible to cytokine-mediated control, or because it can divert the T cell response towards production of cytokines that do not inhibit viral replication (e.g., a Th2 response), the cytopathic function of the immune response may not be able to eliminate all of the infected cells, so that the result is persistent infection and chronic liver disease. On the other hand, if for any reason the T cell response is quantitatively suboptimal, one might also expect the virus to persist, even if the appropriate antiviral cytokines are produced, since, in small amounts, they will suppress, but not abolish, viral gene expression and make the virus less visible to the immune system.

It is important to emphasize, however, that these principles need not extend to all viral infections, or even to the same virus when it infects different cells, since multiple factors must cooperate for intracellular viral inactivation by the immune response to occur. First, the appropriate cytokines must be secreted in sufficient amounts in the environment of the infected cells. Second, the infected cells must be able to respond to the cytokines by activating antiviral signaling pathways appropriate for the resident virus. Finally, the viral genome must be eradicated by this process or it will result in persistent infection.

If the foregoing is correct, strategies designed to boost the HBV-specific immune response (e.g., CTL immunotherapy) or to alter the balance between the cytopathic and the regulatory components of the response (e.g., specific cytokine immunotherapy) may be able to terminate persistent infection and ameliorate the severity and consequences of the chronic liver disease that accompanies persistent HBV infection. Whether these principles apply to the rest of the hepatitis viruses remains to be determined.

ACKNOWLEDGMENTS

I would like to thank Drs. Gerd Pape and Kyong-Mi Chang for helpful suggestions and discussions that have improved the manuscript. I am very indebted to my colleagues and collaborators, especially Drs. Barbara Rehermann, Carlo Ferrari, Luca Guidotti, Alessandra Franco, Kazuki Ando, Tetsuya Ishikawa, and Yasunari Nakamoto, and to Ms. Patricia Fowler for their contributions to the work described in this paper.

These studies were supported by grants AI20001, CA40489, CA54560 and MO1 RR00833 from the National Institutes of Health. This is manuscript number 10988-MEM from The Scripps Research Institute.

REFERENCES

1. Chisari, F.V. 1992. Hepatitis B virus biology and pathogenesis. In *Molecular Genetic Medicine,* Friedmann, T., ed. San Diego: Academic Press, pp 67–104.
2. Chisari, F.V., Ferrari, C., and Mondelli, M.U. 1989. Hepatitis B virus structure and biology. *Microb. Pathog.* 6:311–325.
3. Mondelli, M.U., Cerino, A., Boender, P., Oudshoorn, P., Middeldorp, J., Fipaldini, C., LaMonica, N., and Habets, W. 1994. Significance of the immune response to a major, conformational B cell epitope on the hepatitis C virus NS3 region defined by a human monoclonal antibody. *J. Virol.* 68:4829–4836.

4. Chisari, F.V., and Ferrari, C. 1995. Hepatitis B virus immunopathogenesis. *Annu. Rev. Immunol.* 13:29–60.
5. Tsai, S.L., Chen, P.J., Lai, M.Y., Yang, P.M., Sung, J.L., Huang, J.H., Hwang, L.H., Chang, T.H., and Chen, D.S. 1992. Acute exacerbations of chronic type B hepatitis are accompanied by increased T cell responses to hepatitis B core and e antigens. Implications for hepatitis B e antigen seroconversion. *J. Clin. Invest.* 89:87–96.
6. Michalak, T.I., Pasquinelli, C., Guilhot, S., and Chisari, F.V. 1994. Hepatitis B virus persistence after recovery from acute viral hepatitis. *J. Clin. Invest.* 93:230–239.
7. Rehermann, B., Ferrari, C., and Chisari, F.V. 1996. The hepatitis B virus and specific cytotoxic T lymphocytes persist long after recovery from acute viral hepatitis. *Nature. Med.* (submitted).
8. Razvi, E.S., Jiang, Z., Woda, B.A., and Welsh, R.M. 1995. Lymphocyte apoptosis during the silencing of the immune response to acute viral infections in normal, lpr, and Bcl-2-transgenic mice. *Am. J. Pathol.* 147:79–91.
9. Yoo, J.Y., Howard, R., Waggoner, J.G., and Hoofnagle, J.H. 1987. Peroxidase-anti-peroxidase detection of hepatitis B surface and core antigen in liver biopsy specimens from patients with chronic type B hepatitis. *J. Med. Virol.* 23:273–281.
10. Rehermann, B., Lau, D., Hoofnagle, J.H., and Chisari, F.V. 1996. Cytotoxic T lymphocyte responsiveness after resolution of chronic hepatitis B virus infection. *J. Clin. Invest.* 97:1655–1665.
11. Wirth, S., Guidotti, L.G., Ando, K., Schlicht, H.J., and Chisari, F.V. 1995. Breaking tolerance leads to autoantibody production but not autoimmune liver disease in HBV envelope transgenic mice. *J. Immunol.* 154:2504–2515.
12. Ando, K., Guidotti, L.G., Wirth, S., Ishikawa, T., Missale, G., Moriyama, T., Schreiber, R.D., Schlicht, H.J., Huang, S., and Chisari, F.V. 1994. Class I restricted cytotoxic T lymphocytes are directly cytopathic for their target cells in vivo. *J. Immunol.* 152:3245–3253.
13. Moriyama, T., Guilhot, S., Klopchin, K., Moss, B., Pinkert, C.A., Palmiter, R.D., Brinster, R.L., Kanagawa, O., and Chisari, F.V. 1990. Immunobiology and pathogenesis of hepatocellular injury in hepatitis B virus transgenic mice. *Science* 248:361–364.
14. Suzuki, Y., and Remington, J.S. 1990. The effect of anti-IFN-g antibody on the protective effect of Lyt-2^{+} immune T cells against toxoplasmosis in mice. *J. Immunol.* 144:1954–1956.
15. Nakamoto, Y., Guidotti, L.G., Pasquetto, V., Schreiber, R.D., and Chisari, F.V. 1996. Differential target cell sensitivity to cytotoxic T lymphocyte-activated death pathways in vivo. *J. Immunol.*, submitted.
16. Guidotti, L.G., Ishikawa, T., Hobbs, M.V., Matzke, B., Schreiber, R., and Chisari, F.V. 1996. Intracellular inactivation of the hepatitis B virus by cytotoxic T lymphocytes. *Immunity* 4:25–36.
17. Guidotti, L.G., Borrow, P., Hobbs, M.V., Matzke, B., Gresser, I., Oldstone, M.B.A., and Chisari, F.V. 1996. Viral cross talk: Intracellular inactivation of the hepatitis B virus during an unrelated viral infection of the liver. *Proc. Natl. Acad. Sci. U.S.A.* 93:4589–4594.
18. Cavanaugh, V.J., Guidotti, L.G., and Chisari, F.V. 1988. Inhibition of hepatitis B virus replication during adenovirus and cytomegalovirus infections in transgenic mice. *J. Virol.* 72:2630–2637.
19. Guidotti, L.G., Ando, K., Hobbs, M.V., Ishikawa, T., Runkel, R.D., Schreiber, R.D., and Chisari, F.V. 1994. Cytotoxic T lymphocytes inhibit hepatitis B virus gene expression by a noncytolytic mechanism in transgenic mice. *Proc. Natl. Acad. Sci. U.S.A.* 91:3764–3768.

20. Ando, K., Moriyama, T., Guidotti, L.G., Wirth, S., Schreiber, R.D., Schlicht, H.J., Huang, S., and Chisari, F.V. 1993. Mechanisms of class I restricted immunopathology. A transgenic mouse model of fulminant hepatitis. *J. Exp. Med.* 178:1541–1554.

21. Franco, A., Guidotti, L.G., Hobbs, M.V., Pasquetto, V., and Chisari, F.V. 1997. Pathogenetic effector function of CD4-positive T helper 1 cells in hepatitis B virus transgenic mice. *J. Immunol.*, in press.

22. Cavanaugh, V.J., Guidotti, L.G., and Chisari, F.V. 1997. Interleukin-12 inhibits hepatitis B virus replication in HBV transgenic mice. *J. Virol.* 71:3236–3243.

23. Gilles, P.N., Fey, G., and Chisari, F.V. 1992. Tumor necrosis factor-alpha negatively regulates hepatitis B virus gene expression in transgenic mice. *J. Virol.* 66:3955–3960.

24. Guidotti, L.G., Guilhot, S., and Chisari, F.V. 1994. Interleukin 2 and interferon alpha/beta downregulate hepatitis B virus gene expression in vivo by tumor necrosis factor dependent and independent pathways. *J. Virol.* 68:1265–1270.

25. Guilhot, S., Guidotti, L.G., and Chisari, F.V. 1993. Interleukin-2 downregulates hepatitis B virus gene expression in transgenic mice by a post-transcriptional mechanism. *J. Virol.* 67:7444–7449.

26. Davis, G.L., Hoofnagle, J.H., and Waggoner, J.G. 1984. Acute type A hepatitis during chronic hepatitis B virus infection: Association of depressed hepatitis B virus replication with appearance of endogenous alpha interferon. *J. Med. Virol.* 14:141–147.

27. Sheen, I.-S., Liaw, Y.-F., Lin, D.-Y., and Chu, C.-M. 1994. Role of hepatitis C and delta viruses in the termination of chronic hepatitis B surface antigen carrier state: A multivariate analysis in a longitudinal follow-up study. *J. Infect. Dis.* 170:1358–1361.

28. Penna, A., Chisari, F.V., Bertoletti, A., Missale, G., Fowler, P., Giuberti, T., Fiaccadori, F., and Ferrari, C. 1991. Cytotoxic T lymphocytes recognize an HLA-A2-restricted epitope within the hepatitis B virus nucleocapsid antigen. *J. Exp. Med.* 174:1565–1570.

29. Missale, G., Redeker, A., Person, J., Fowler, P., Guilhot, S., Schlicht, H.-J., Ferrari, C., and Chisari, F.V. 1993. HLA-A31- and HLA-Aw68 restricted cytotoxic T cell responses to a single hepatitis B virus nucleocapsid epitope during acute viral hepatitis. *J. Exp. Med.* 177:751–762.

30. Nayersina, R., Fowler, P., Guilhot, S., Missale, G., Cerny, A., Schlicht, H.-J., Vitiello, A., Chesnut, R., Person, J.L., Redeker, A.G., and Chisari, F.V. 1993. HLA A2 restricted cytotoxic T lymphocyte responses to multiple hepatitis B surface antigen epitopes during hepatitis B virus infection. *J. Immunol.* 150:4659–4671.

31. Rehermann, B., Fowler, P., Sidney, J., Person, J., Redeker, A., Brown, M., Moss, B., Sette, A., and Chisari, F.V. 1995. The cytotoxic T lymphocyte response to multiple hepatitis B virus polymerase epitopes during and after acute viral hepatitis. *J. Exp. Med.* 181:1047–1058.

32. Griffith, T.S., Brunner, T., Fletcher, S.M., Green, D.R., and Ferguson, T.A. 1995. Fas ligand-induced apoptosis as a mechanism of immune privilege. *Science* 270:1189–1192.

33. Galle, P.R., Hofmann, W.J., Walczak, H., Schaller, H., Otto, G., Stremmel, W., Krammer, P.H., and Runkell, L. 1995. Involvement of the CD95 (APO-1/Fas) receptor and ligand in liver damage. *J. Exp. Med.* 182:1223–1230.

34. Gooding, L.R. 1992. Virus proteins that counteract host immune defenses. *Cell* 71:5–7.

35. Alcami, A., and Smith, G.L. 1995. Cytokine receptors encoded by poxviruses: A lesson in cytokine biology. *Immunol. Today* 16:474–478.

36. Guidotti, L.G., Matzke, B., Schaller, H., and Chisari, F.V. 1995. High level hepatitis B virus replication in transgenic mice. *J. Virol.* 69:6158–6169.

37. Bertoletti, A., Ferrari, C., Fiaccadori, F., Penna, A., Margolskee, R., Schlicht, H.J., Fowler, P., Guilhot, S., and Chisari, F.V. 1991. HLA class I-restricted human cytotoxic T cells recognize endogenously synthesized hepatitis B virus nucleocapsid antigen. *Proc. Natl. Acad. Sci. U.S.A.* 88:10445–10449.

38. Rehermann, B., Pasquinelli, C., Mosier, S.M., and Chisari, F.V. 1995. Hepatitis B virus (HBV) sequence variation in cytotoxic T lymphocyte epitopes is not common in patients with chronic HBV infection. *J. Clin. Invest.* 96:1527–1534.

39. Bertoletti, A., Sette, A., Chisari, F.V., Penna, A., Levrero, M., DeCarli, M., Fiaccadori, F., and Ferrari, C. 1994. Natural variants of cytotoxic epitopes are T cell receptor antagonists for antiviral cytotoxic T cells. *Nature* 369:407–410.

40. Kalams, S.A., Johnson, R.P., Trocha, A.K., Dynana, M.J., Ngo, S., D'Aquila, R.T., Kurnick, J.T., and Walker, B.D. 1994. Longitudinal analysis of T cell receptor (TCR) gene usage by human immunodeficiency virus 1 envelope-specific cytotoxic T lymphocyte clones reveals a limited TCR repertoire. *J. Exp. Med.* 179:1261–1271.

41. Argaet, V.P.C., Schmidt, C.W., Burrows, S.R., Silings, S.L., Kurilla, M.G., Doolan, D.L., Suhrbier, A., Moss, D.J., Kieff, E., Sculley, T.B., and Misko, I.S. 1994. Dominant selection of an invariant T cell antigen receptor in response to persistent infection by Epstein-Barr virus. *J. Exp. Med.* 180:2335–2340.

42. Bertoletti, A., Costanzo, A., Chisari, F.V., Levrero, M., Artini, M., Sette, A., Penna, A., Giuberti, T., Fiaccadori, F., and Ferrari, C. 1994. Cytotoxic T lymphocyte response to a wild type hepatitis B virus epitope in patients chronically infected by variant viruses carrying substitutions within the epitope. *J. Exp. Med.* 180:933–943.

43. Franco, A., Southwood, S., Arrhenius, T., Kuchroo, V.K., Grey, H.M., Sette, A., and Ishioka, G. 1994. T cell receptor antagonist peptides are highly effective inhibitors of experimental allergic encephalomyelitis. *Eur. J. Immunol.* 24:940–946.

44. Kuchroo, V.K., Greer, J.M., Kaul, D., Ishioka, G., Franco, A., Sette, A., Sobel, R.A., and Less, M.B. 1994. A single TCR antagonist peptide inhibits experimental allergic encelphalomyelitis by a diverse T cell repertoire. *J. Immunol.* 153:3326–3336.

45. Ho, D.D., Newmann, A.U., Perelson, A.S., Chen, W., Leonard, J.M., and Markowitz, M. 1995. Rapid turnover of plasma virions and CD4 lymphocytes in HIV-1 infection. *Nature* 373:123–126.

46. Koziel, M.J., Dudley, D., Afdhal, N., Choo, Q.-L., Houghton, M., Ralston, R., and Walker, B.D. 1993. Hepatitis C virus (HCV)-specific cytoxic T lymphocytes recognize epitopes in the core and envelope proteins of HCV. *J. Virol.* 67:7522–7532.

47. Koziel, M.J., Dudley, D., Afdhal, N., Grakoui, A., Rice, C.M., Choo, Q.-L., Houghton, M., and Walker, B.D. 1995. HLA class I-restricted cytotoxic T lymphocytes specific for hepatitis C virus. Identification of multiple epitopes and characterization of patterns of cytokine release. *J. Clin. Invest.* 96:2311–2321.

48. Pantaleo, G., Demarest, J.F., Soudeyns, H., Graziosi, C., Denis, F., Adelsberger, J.W., Borrow, P., Saag, M.S., Shaw, G.M., Sekaly, R.P., and Fauci, A.S. 1994. Major expansion of $CD8^+$ cells with a predominant V-beta usage during the primary immune response to HIV. *Nature* 370:463–467.

49. Simmonds, P. 1995. Variability of hepatitis C virus. *Hepatology* 21:570–583.

50. Choo, Q.-L., Weiner, A.J., Overby, L.R., Kuo, G., Houghton, M., and Bradley, D.W. 1990. Hepatitis C virus: The major causative agent of viral non-A, non-B hepatitis. *Br. Med. Bull.* 46:423–441.

51. Weincr, A., Erickson, A.L., Kansopon, J., Crawford, K., Muchmore, E., Hughes, A.L.,

Houghton, M., and Walker, C.M. 1995. Persistent hepatitis C virus infection in a chimpanzee is associated with emergence of a cytotoxic T lymphocyte escape variant. *Proc. Natl. Acad. Sci. U.S.A.* 92:2755–2759.

52. Farci, P., Alter, H.J., Govindarajan, S., Wong, D.C., Engle, R., Lesniewski, R.R., Mushahwar, I.K., Desai, S.M., Miller, R.H., Ogata, N., and Purcell, R.H. 1992. Lack of protective immunity against reinfection with hepatitis C virus. *Science* 258:135–140.
53. Prince, A.M., Brotman, B., Huima, T., Pascual, D., Jaffery, M., and Inchauspe, G. 1992. Immunity in hepatitis C infection. *J. Infect. Dis.* 165:438–443.
54. Botarelli, P., Brunetto, M.R., Minutello, M.A., Calvo, P., Unutmaz, D., Weiner, A.J., Choo, Q.-L., Shuster, J.R., Kuo, G., Bonino, F., Houghton, M., and Abrignani, S. 1993. T-lymphocyte response to hepatitis C virus in different clinical courses of infection. *Gastroenterology* 104:580–587.
55. Ferrari, C., Valli, A., Galati, L., Penna, A., Scaccaglia, P., Guiberti, T., Schianchi, C., Missale, G., Marin, M.G., and Fiaccadori, F. 1994. T-cell response to structural and nonstructural hepatitis C virus antigens in persistent and self-limited hepatitis C virus infections. *Hepatology* 19:286–295.
56. Schupper, H., Hayashi, P., Scheffel, J., Aceituno, S., Paglieroni, T., Holland, P.V., and Zeldis, J.B. 1993. Peripheral blood mononuclear cell responses to recombinant hepatitis C virus antigens in patients with chronic hepatitis C. *Hepatology* 18:1055–1060.
57. Diepolder, H.M., Zachoval, R., Hoffmann, R.M., Wierenga, E.A., Santantonio, T., Jung, M.-C., Eichenlaub, D., and Pape, G.R. 1995. Possible mechanism involving T-lymphocyte response to non-structural protein 3 in viral clearance in acute hepatitis C virus infection. *Lancet* 346:1006–1007.
58. Leroux-Roels, G., Esquivel, C.A., DeLeys, R., Stuyver, L., Elewaut, A., Philippe, J., Desombere, I., Paradijs, J., and Maertens, G. 1996. Lymphoproliferative responses to hepatitis C virus core, E1, E2, and NS3 in patients with chronic hepatitis C infection treated with interferon alpha. *Hepatology* 23:8–16.
59. Hoffmann, R.M., Diepolder, H.M., Zachoval, R., Zweibel, F.-M., Jung, M.-C., Scholz, S., Nitschko, H., Riethmuller, G., and Pape, G.R. 1995. Mapping of immunodominant CD4+ T lymphocyte epitopes of hepatitis C virus and their relevance during the course of chronic infection. *Hepatology* 21:632–638.
60. Minutello, M.A., Pileri, P., Unutmaz, D., Censini, S., Kuo, G., Houghton, M., Brunetto, M.R., Bonino, F., and Abrignani, S. 1993. Compartmentalization of T-lymphocytes to the site of disease: Intrahepatic $CD4^+$ T-cells specific for the protein NS4 of hepatitis C virus in patients with chronic hepatitis C. *J. Exp. Med.* 178:17–25.
61. Koziel, M.J., Dudley, D., Wong, J.T., Dienstag, J., Houghton, M., Ralston, R., and Walker, B.D. 1992. Intrahepatic cytotoxic T lymphocyte specific for hepatitis C virus in persons with chronic hepatitis. *J. Immunol.* 149:3339–3344.
62. Cerny, A., McHutchison, J.G., Pasquinelli, C., Brown, M.E., Brothers, M.A., Grabscheid, B., Fowler, P., Houghton, M., and Chisari, F.V. 1995. Cytotoxic T lymphocyte response to hepatitis C virus-derived peptides containing the HLA A2.1 binding motif. *J. Clin. Invest.* 95:521–530.
63. Shirai, M., Akatsuka, T., Pendleton, C.D., Houghten, R., Wychowski, C., Mihalik, K., Feinstone, S., and Berzofsky, J.A. 1992. Induction of cytotoxic T cells to a cross-reactive epitope in the hepatitis C virus nonstructural RNA polymerase-like protein. *J. Virol.* 66:4098–4106.
64. Battegay, M., Fikes, J., Di Bisceglie, A.M., Wentworth, P.A., Sette, A., Celis, E., Ching,

W.-M., Grakoui, A., Rice, C.M., Kurokohchi, K., Berzofsky, J.A., Hoofnagle, J.H., Feinstone, S.M., and Akatsuka, T. 1995. Patients with chronic hepatitis C have circulating cytotoxic T cells which recognize hepatitis C virus-encoded peptides binding to HLA-A2.1 molecules. *J. Virol.* 69:2462–2470.

65. Erickson, A.L., Houghton, M., Choo, Q.L., Weiner, A.J., Ralston, R., Muchmore, E., and Walker, C.M. 1993. Hepatitis C virus-specific CTL responses in the liver of chimpanzees with acute and chronic hepatitis C. *J. Immunol.* 151:4189–4199.

66. Kita, H., Moriyama, T., Kaneko, T., et. al. 1993. HLA-B44-restricted cytotoxic T lymphocytes recognizing an epitope on hepatitis C virus nucleocapsid protein. *Hepatology* 18:1039–1044.

67. Ballardini, G., Groff, P., Pontisso, P., Giostra, F., Francesconi, R., Lenzi, M., Zauli, D., Albeti, A., and Bianchi, F.B. 1995. Hepatitis C virus (HCV) genotype, tissue HCV antigens, hepatocellular expression of HLA-A,B,C, and intercellular adhesion-1 molecules. *J. Clin. Invest.* 95:2067–2075.

68. Hiramatsu, N., Hayashi, N., Katayama, K., Mochizuki, K., Kawanishi, Y., Kasahara, A., Fusamoto, H., and Kamada, T. 1994. Immunohistochemical detection of Fas antigen in liver tissue of patients with chronic hepatitis C. *Hepatology* 19:1354–1359.

69. Mullbacher, A., and Lobigs, M. 1995. Up-regulation of MHC class I by flavivirus-induced peptide translocation into the endoplasmic reticulum. *Immunity* 3:207–214.

70. Kakumu, S., Ishikawa, T., Wakita, T., Yoshioka, K., Takayanagi, M., Tahara, H., and Kusakabe, A. 1994. Interferon-gamma production specific for hepatitis B virus antigen by intraheptic T lymphocytes in patients with acute and chronic hepatitis B. *Am. J. Gastroenterol.* 89:92–96.

71. Jung, M.-C., Diepolder, H.M., Spengler, U., Wierenga, E.A., Zachoval, R., Hoffmann, R.M., Eichelaub, D., Frosner, G., Will, H., and Pape, G.R. 1995. Activation of a heterogenous hepatitis B (HB) core and e antigen-specific $CD4^+$ T-cell population during seroconversion to anti-HBe and anti-HBs in hepatitis B virus infection. *J. Virol.* 69:3358–3368.

72. Inoue, M., Kakumu, S., Yoshioka, K., Tsutsumi, Y., Wakita, T., and Arao, M. 1989. Hepatitis B core antigen specific IFN-gamma production of peripheral blood mononuclear cells in patients with chronic hepatitis B virus infection. *J. Immunol.* 142:4006–4011.

73. Barnaba, V., Franco, A., Paroli, M., Benvenuto, R., De Petrillo, G., Burgio, V.L., Santilio, I., Balsano, C., Bonavita, M.S., Cappelli, G., Colizzi, V., Cutrona, G., and Ferrarini, M. 1994. Selective expansion of cytotoxic T lymphocytes with a $CD4^+CD56^+$ surface phenotype and a T helper type 1 profile of cytokine secretion in the liver of patients chronically infected with hepatitis B virus. *J. Immunol.* 152:3074–3087.

74. Lohr, H.F., Gerken, G., Schlicht, H.-J., Meyer zum Buschenfelde, K.-H., and Fleischer, B. 1993. Low frequency of cytotoxic liver-infiltrating T lymphocytes specific for endogenous processed surface and core proteins in chronic hepatitis B. *J. Infect. Dis.* 168:1133–1139.

75. Tsai, S.-L., Liaw, Y.-F., Yeh, C.-T., Chu, C.-M., and Kuo, G.C. 1995. Cellular immune responses in patients with dual infection of hepatitis B and C viruses: Dominant role of hepatitis C virus. *Hepatology* 21:908–912.

CHAPTER 8

IMMUNITY TO *Listeria monocytogenes* INFECTION OF THE LIVER

JOHN T. HARTY
University of Iowa, Iowa City, IA

INTRODUCTION

Listeria monocytogenes is a gram positive, facultative intracellular bacterial pathogen that causes potentially severe infections in humans and numerous other mammalian hosts (1). Human listeriosis can be particularly severe in pregnant women, infants, and the immunocompromised, and can result in abortion, septicemia, and meningitis. In general, *L. monocytogenes* infections occur after consumption of contaminated food products, particularly dairy products, since even appropriate refrigeration does not prevent the growth of the organism (1). Although the number of *L. monocytogenes* infections in the United States is not large, their impact is severe, with a 25% mortality in the susceptible population (2). The increasing number of immunocompromised individuals due to cancer chemotherapy, transplant-associated immunosuppression, and HIV disease is likely to increase the impact of *L. monocytogenes* infection in the human population (3).

Experimental infection of mice with *L. monocytogenes* provides a highly reproducible model system for in vivo analyses of bacterial pathogenesis and cell-mediated immunity to infection. *L. monocytogenes* encoded virulence factors have been identified using in vitro cell culture approaches, and the relevance of these virulence factors has been confirmed in mouse infection models. In addition, *L. monocytogenes* infection evokes a complex immunological response involving elements of innate (nonspecific) immunity and specific T cell responses. In the mouse, the primary sites of *L. monocytogenes* replication are the liver (both Kupffer cells and hepatocytes) and the spleen. Thus, *L. monocytogenes* infection of mice provides an excellent in vivo model system for bacterial infection and immunity in the liver. In this chapter we will

T Lymphocytes in the Liver: Immunobiology, Pathology, and Host Defense, Edited by I. Nicholas Crispe
ISBN 0-471-19218-X

discuss the role of specific cell types in resistance to *L. monocytogenes* infection in the liver, with particular emphasis on T-cell-mediated immunity.

Listeria Infection

L. monocytogenes is able to infect a variety of cell types in vitro, including certain nonphagocytic cell lines (4), hepatocyte-like lines (5), primary hepatocytes (6), primary macrophages, and macrophage cell lines (4). *L. monocytogenes* encoded virulence factors such as the surface molecules internalins A and B (7), and p60 (8), a secreted murein hydrolase, have been implicated in invasion of nonphagocytic eukaryotic cells. Recent experiments have revealed that the cellular receptor for one of the internalin family members, InlA, is the E-cadherin molecule (9). InlA is required for efficient invasion of some cultured epithelial cells (10). Another member of the internalin family, InlB appears to be required for invasion of some hepatocyte-like cells in vitro (10). In vivo studies with InlAB-deficient mutant *L. monocytogenes* strains by two groups provide contradictory evidence: the results of Gaillard et al. (11) support a role for InlA or InlB in hepatocyte invasion, while those of Gregory et al. (12) do not support this interpretation. These studies were performed with different InlAB-deficient mutants, and thus the issue remains to be resolved.

Shortly after experimental infection of mice, *L. monocytogenes* is cleared from the bloodstream by tissue macrophages in the spleen and liver (Kupffer cells). In vitro studies demonstrate that *L. monocytogenes* enters infected macrophages in a membrane-bound phagosome (4). Bacteria in the phagosome are exposed to an increasingly acidic and degradative environment that is the major site of antimicrobial defense mechanisms in professional phagocytes (13). Some intracellular bacteria, such as *Salmonella* species and *Mycobacterium tuberculosis*, survive in this hostile environment (14), in part due to their ability to modify the phagosome environment (15). In contrast to these organisms, *L. monocytogenes* escapes from the phagosome into the cytoplasm of the infected cell. Escape from the phagosome is mediated primarily through the actions of a pore-forming hemolysin, listeriolysin O (LLO, encoded by *hlyA*) (4,16). LLO is a member of a large family of related bacterial hemolysins (16). In contrast to the other members of this family, which are active at neutral pH, the hemolytic activity of LLO is optimal at pH 5.5 (17) which corresponds to the pH of the acidic environment of the phagosome. In macrophages, LLO^- *L. monocytogenes* strains remain vacuolar and are destroyed in the phagosome. Such LLO^- *L. monocytogenes* are completely avirulent in mouse challenge studies (18), whereas virulence is reinstated after transformation with a plasmid expressing the LLO gene (19). These results demonstrate that escape from the phagosome is a critical event in the pathogenesis of *L. monocytogenes* infection (18). This notion is supported by the finding that even virulent *L. monocytogenes* that fail to escape from the phagosome are destroyed in the vacuole (20).

Once the organism escapes from the phagosome it replicates in the relatively benign environment of the cytoplasm of the infected cell. Recent studies indicate that the presence of *L. monocytogenes* in the cytoplasm evokes a series of defined responses from host cell signaling molecules (21,22) and can affect the regulation of cytokine and cytokine receptor gene expression in macrophages (23). It is currently unclear whether *L. monocytogenes* alters specific signaling pathways in hepatocytes distinct from its effect in macrophages or epithelial cells.

Next, in a spectacular interaction between host and pathogen, *L. monocytogenes* begins to move within the cytoplasm via the polymerization of host derived F-actin, resulting in the appearance of "rocket-like" tails of polymerized actin behind the moving bacteria (24). Actin-based movement depends on the *L. monocytogenes* encoded ActA molecule (25), which is expressed at one pole of a cytoplasmic *L. monocytogenes* bacillus. Recent experiments have begun to characterize the host cell molecules involved in actin polymerization (26). ActA appears to function as the site of F-actin nucleation and is required for intercellular spread of *L. monocytogenes*, a process that occurs when the organism propels itself into cellular protrusions that are engulfed by adjacent cells (27). In this fashion, *L. monocytogenes* can spread from initially infected Kupffer cells to hepatocytes in the liver. In vitro experiments reveal ActA-dependent cell–cell spread as early as 3 hours after infection (27). Thus, *L. monocytogenes* can rapidly spread between cells without exposure to extracellular immune defenses, a finding that accounts for the inability of antibodies to mediate specific immunity against *L. monocytogenes* (28). Mutant *L. monocytogenes* strains have been generated with in frame deletion of the *actA* gene. ActA gene deletion does not prevent the organism from entering the cytoplasm of the infected cell but prevents cell–cell spread. This action results in dramatically reduced virulence for in vivo infection (25,29). Thus, cell–cell spread is also an important attribute of virulent *L. monocytogenes*.

During cell–cell spread the organism becomes encased in a double membrane vesicle in the newly infected cell. Two *L. monocytogenes* gene products with phospholipase activity, PlcA and PlcB, have been implicated in escape from this double membrane structure (30). PlcA has also been shown to facilitate escape of LLO^- *L. monocytogenes* from the phagosome of certain nonphagocytic cell lines (31). Once the organism escapes from the double membrane vesicle into the cytoplasm of the newly infected cell, the cycle of replication and cell–cell spread can resume.

A number of *L. monocytogenes* encoded virulence factors (LLO, ActA, PlcA, PlcB) are physically linked on the bacterial chromosome and are under the control of a linked positive regulatory factor, PrfA (32). PrfA mutant *L. monocytogenes* are severely attenuated for in vivo infection (33). PrfA expression is controlled in part by environmental signals that mimic the intracellular environment (34). Thus, *L. monocytogenes* encoded virulence factors are coordinately regulated for expression in the intracellular environment.

Mouse Model of *L. monocytogenes* Infection

Upon intravenous infection of mice, *L. monocytogenes* is rapidly cleared from the bloodstream by macrophages in the spleen and liver (28). It has been estimated that 60% to 70% of the organisms are taken up by the liver, while the remaining organisms are found in the spleen (35). There is an initial decrease in bacterial colony forming units (CFU) as a result of phagocyte-mediated killing. Surviving organisms then grow exponentially in the spleen and liver for the next 2–3 days (28) reaching 10^6 to 10^7 CFU/organ. During this time the organism spreads from macrophages into nonphagocytes such as hepatocytes. Experiments with hepatocytes and Kupffer cells isolated from *L. monocytogenes* infected mice reveal that *L. monocytogenes* numbers increase 200-fold in hepatocytes over the initial 3 days of infection, but do not significantly increase in the Kupffer cell population (16). Thus, hepatocytes are a major reservoir of *L. monocytogenes* during the exponential growth phase of primary infection. In an immunocompetent animal given a sublethal infection, the number of *L. monocytogenes* in the spleen and liver declines until the infection is sterilized by 2 weeks after infection (28). In contrast, a persistent infection occurs in athymic nude mice, which lack T cells, or in severe combined immunodeficiency (SCID) mice, that cannot rearrange T cell receptor or B cell receptor genes and thus lack peripheral T and B cells (36,37). Lethal doses of *L. monocytogenes* result in the death of immunocompetent animals in 4–7 days (28).

Strains of inbred mice differ in their resistance to *L. monocytogenes* infection (38). The 50% lethal dose (LD_{50}) for relatively susceptible mouse strains such as Balb/c ranges from 10^3 to 10^4 CFU after intravenous infection, while relatively resistant strains such as C57Bl/6 (B6) are 5–10 times more resistant. Sublethal infection immunizes both susceptible and resistant strains of mice and results in survival following a normally lethal secondary challenge infection. Survival from lethal challenge correlates directly with an experimentally observable 10^2–10^4-fold reduction in spleen or liver organisms at 2–3 days after infection compared to nonimmune mice.

Innate Immunity to *L. monocytogenes* Infection

Studies with SCID mice that lack mature T and B cells demonstrated a T-cell-independent mechanism for resistance to primary *L. monocytogenes* infection (39). This innate immunity to *L. monocytogenes* infection is a consequence of the recruitment and activation of neutrophils and macrophages. In vitro and in vivo studies identified a pathway where cytokines such as interleukin-12 (IL-12) and tumor necrosis factor-α (TNF)-α are produced by *L. monocytogenes* infected macrophages and stimulate interferon-γ (IFNγ) production by natural killer (NK) cells (40). These cytokines activate the microbicidal activities of macrophages and can affect the development of specific immunity to infection (41). Other studies show that neutrophils play a critical role in innate resistance to *L. monocytogenes* infection (42–44) and reveal that γδ T cells play an important role in controlling the extent of immune-mediated pathology in the livers of *L. monocytogenes* infected mice (45,46).

Experiments with gene knockout mice confirm studies with anti-cytokine antibodies and reveal the complexity of innate resistance to *L. monocytogenes* infection. The finding that IFNγ receptor and IFNγ gene (GKO-/-) knockout mice are extremely susceptible to primary *L. monocytogenes* infection (47,48) demonstrates that IFNγ is a critical mediator of innate immunity to infection. Innate immunity also depends on TNFα and perhaps lymphotoxin-α (LTα), as shown by the increased susceptibility of mice with disruption of the TNF receptor 1 (TNFR1) (49), TNFα (50) and lymphotoxin/TNFα (51) genes. TNFα may play multiple roles in the innate immune response including macrophage activation and neutrophil recruitment (52). Neutralization of IL-12 also exacerbates primary *L. monocytogenes* infection (53) likely through interference with NK cell IFNγ production (54) whereas neutralization of IL-1β may interfere with IFNγ production (54) and neutrophil recruitment (55). Similarly, disruption of the IL-6 gene (56) or nuclear factor (NF)-IL6 (57) increases susceptibility to *L. monocytogenes* infection with effects at the level of the neutrophil (56) and macrophage (57).

Acquired Immunity to *L. monocytogenes*

Early studies of acquired immunity to *L. monocytogenes* infection indicated an essential role for T cells (36,58,59) and that antibody plays little, if any, role in immunity (28). $CD4^+$ and $CD8^+$ T cells respond to *L. monocytogenes* infection in an antigen-specific fashion (60). A great deal of in vivo evidence, using antibodies to deplete T cell subsets from immune mice, as well as adoptive transfer of specific T cell subsets, suggests that $CD8^+$ T cells are very effective mediators of acquired immunity to *L. monocytogenes* infection (61–66). This finding is consistent with the cytoplasmic location of *L. monocytogenes*, which exposes the organism to the endogenous antigen presentation pathway by which peptides are displayed by surface major histocompatibility complex (MHC) class I molecules and recognized by $CD8^+$ T cells (60).

A substantial fraction of *L. monocytogenes* are unable to escape from the phagosome in macrophages and are destroyed in this compartment (20). Thus, *L. monocytogenes* antigens are also presented by the exogenous pathway by which peptides are bound to MHC class II molecules for recognition by $CD4^+$ T cells. In contrast to the experiments demonstrating effective $CD8^+$ T cell immunity to *L. monocytogenes*, the same type of experiments did not demonstrate a major role for $CD4^+$ T cells as effectors of antilisterial immunity. However, MHC class II deficient mice, which lack $CD4^+$ T cells, are slightly more susceptible to *L. monocytogenes* infection than controls, suggesting a role for $CD4^+$ T cells in resistance to primary *L. monocytogenes* infection (67). In support of these data, $CD4^+$ T cell clones and lines transfer some immunity to *L. monocytogenes* infections (68,69). However, MHC class I deficient mice exhibit more profound susceptibility to *L. monocytogenes* infection (67).

In keeping with the finding that $CD8^+$ T cells are potent effectors of acquired immunity to *L. monocytogenes*, we demonstrated that $CD8^+$ T cells with specificity only for the secreted *L. monocytogenes* proteins LLO or p60, can transfer significant immunity to naive mice (70–72). The effector mechanisms used by $CD8^+$ T cells in resistance to *L. monocytogenes* infection are an area of current research interest.

IMMUNITY TO *L. monocytogenes* INFECTION OF THE LIVER

Immunity to *L. monocytogenes* infection depends on the interaction of multiple cytokines and effector cells (of both the innate and acquired immune response) that provide overlapping and distinct roles in clearance of this intracellular bacterial pathogen. The prevailing notion is that the innate immune response fights off primary infection until the acquired immune response develops and eventually clears the infection. This notion is consistent with studies using gene knockout mice or antibodies that deplete cells or cytokines of the innate response. All of these studies show that the absence of an intact innate immune response dramatically lowers resistance to primary *L. monocytogenes* infection (52).

In contrast, evidence suggests that resistance to secondary *L. monocytogenes* infection can be carried out in the absence of at least some effectors, such as IFNγ, that are critical for innate resistance to primary *L. monocytogenes* infection (48). Thus, effective immunity against primary and secondary *L. monocytogenes* infection of the liver may result from different effector mechanisms and cell types.

Clear evidence from studies in the mouse model of *L. monocytogenes* infection reveal that the innate immune response can profoundly affect the nature of the developing acquired immune response (41). Recent studies also reveal that acquired immunity to *L. monocytogenes* depends on at least some elements of the innate immune response. In addition, evidence is accumulating that elements of the acquired immune response regulate the nature and extent of tissue destruction related to activation of innate immunological effector mechanisms. Although the focus of this chapter is on T cell immunity to *L. monocytogenes* infection of the liver, it is clear that many cell types interact to resist infection. For this reason the discussion of immunity to *L. monocytogenes* infection of the liver will focus on the interaction of specific cell types, particularly T cells, in primary and secondary resistance mechanisms against infection.

Resistance to Primary *L. monocytogenes* Infection in the Liver

Resistance to primary *L. monocytogenes* infection involves the interaction between the innate immune response, which provides a rapid response to infection, and the acquired immune response, which develops with time after infection. As detailed above, the innate immune response is critical for resistance to primary infection. Our discussion of resistance to primary *L. monocytogenes* infection of the liver will begin with elements of the innate immune response and finish with a discussion of elements of the acquired immune response and their ability to control the immunopathological consequences of nonspecific immune activation.

Kupffer Cells and Immigrant Macrophages As mentioned above, *L. monocytogenes* initially is taken up by Kupffer cells in the liver. Kupffer cells exhibit many characteristics of normal tissue macrophages, such as phagocytosis and MHC class II expression, but may lack some capacity to exhibit antimicrobial activities, such as H_2O_2 production, at least in vitro (73). However, these cells may elaborate other antimicrobial defenses, as evidenced by the destruction of 50% to 90% of the *L. monocytogenes* inoculum in the liver within 3 hours after injection (28). This issue is not completely clear since neutrophils also accumulate in the liver during the first 24 hours after infection and may contribute to the initial bacterial killing (35,74). However, recent experiments with transgenic mice in which an inhibitor of the IFNγ receptor was expressed only in tissue macrophages, and not immigrant macrophages or other cell types, reveal the importance of the antimicrobial activities of resident Kupffer cells in resistance to *L. monocytogenes* infection (75).

In addition, in vitro evidence suggests that cytokine-activated macrophages prevent *L. monocytogenes* from escaping the phagosome and thus destroy the bacteria in the vacuole (76). Consistent with the antimicrobial potential of macrophages is the finding that liver macrophages are not the major site of *L. monocytogenes* replication in this tissue, since analysis of Kupffer cells isolated from *L. monocytogenes* infected mice at various times after primary infection reveals little if any increase in *L. monocytogenes* numbers in these cells (6). After the initial 24 hours following infection a substantial influx of monocytes enter the liver and participate in granuloma formation and innate resistance to *L. monocytogenes* infection (73). These immigrant macrophages are essential for resistance to primary *L. monocytogenes* infection (77,78).

Neutrophils The initial influx of neutrophils into the liver following *L. monocytogenes* infection is a critical component of the innate immune response to primary infection. Treatment of mice with antibodies that inhibit neutrophil and macrophage extravasation, by blocking complement receptor type 3 interactions, greatly exacerbates *L. monocytogenes* infection by preventing accumulation of neutrophils at foci of infection (74). Histological analyses of the livers of *L. monocytogenes* infected normal mice reveal the presence of large numbers of neutrophils associated with *L. monocytogenes* infected hepatocytes that are being destroyed. These data have been interpreted to suggest that neutrophils are involved in lysis of *L. monocytogenes* infected hepatocytes as a major mechanism of innate resistance to *L. monocytogenes* infection (79). The involvement of neutrophils in the lysis of *L. monocytogenes* infected hepatocytes has been supported by similar findings in mice that have been depleted of NK cells, $CD4^+$ T cells, and $CD8^+$ T cells (80). In addition, studies with monoclonal antibodies (mAb) that specifically deplete neutrophils and eosinophils have demonstrated the importance of these cells for innate resistance to *L. monocytogenes*, since granulocyte-depleted mice are extremely susceptible to primary infection (42,44,81). Interestingly, the impact of neutrophil depletion was greatest in the livers of *L. monocytogenes* infected mice during the first 24 hours after infection (42). In these mice, *L. monocytogenes* replicated to high numbers inside hepatocytes and the focal destruction of hepatocytes, found in control mice, was absent in mice depleted of neutrophils. Currently, the mechanism by which neutrophils specifically cause the lysis of *L. monocytogenes* infected hepatocytes is unclear. One study of hepatocyte-like cells in vitro suggests that *L. monocytogenes* infection results in upregulation of intracellular adhesion molecule 1 (ICAM-1) on these cells and thus increases neutrophil adhesion to *L. monocytogenes* infected hepatocytes (81). The relevance of this result will be elucidated by analysis of mice deficient in ICAM-1 expression. An intriguing scenario that may account for the interaction of neutrophils and *L. monocytogenes* infected hepatocytes could involve upregulation of FasL (CD95L) on *L. monocytogenes* infected hepatocytes. Studies have shown that neutrophils, which are Fas^+ ($CD95^+$), will adhere to cells that express CD95L and undergo apoptosis. Dying neutrophils may release toxic granule contents that apparently mediate the rejection of CD95L-expressing tumor cells (82) and could potentially mediate lysis of *L. monocytogenes* infected hepatocytes in the vicinity. This hypothesis is also consistent with the results of recent studies of hepatitis in mouse models that suggest a role for CD95–CD95L interactions in the liver (83).

Hepatocytes It is generally accorded that activated macrophages and neutrophils provide the major route of bacterial destruction in response to *L. monocytogenes* infection of mice. However, *L. monocytogenes* also replicates in hepatocytes. Several studies of hepatocyte-like cell lines indicate that treatment of the cells with individual recombinant cytokines (e.g., IFNγ, TNFα, and IL-6) prior to infection has little or no effect on replication of virulent *L. monocytogenes* (5), but that pretreatment with combinations of these cytokines can result in partial inhibition of *L. monocytogenes* replication (84). However, these hepatocyte-like cells are unable to achieve the antimicrobial activity attained by macrophages (84). Studies with hepatocytes isolated from normal mice also suggest that these cells may elaborate some level of antimicrobial activity since IFNγ pretreatment of the cells resulted in decreased *L. monocytogenes* recovery 2 or 4 hours after infection (85). In vivo, *L. monocytogenes* numbers in hepatocytes increase significantly with time after primary infection of naive mice, and thus hepatocyte-mediated killing of *L. monocytogenes* may not play an important role in primary resistance to infection. Consistent with this view are studies where addition of cytokines to heptocyte-like cells or isolated hepatocytes at the time of *L. monocytogenes* infection resulted in no inhibition of *L. monocytogenes* replication over a 15-hour period (86). Interestingly, the latter study provided the first evidence that *L. monocytogenes* caused infected hepatocytes to undergo apoptosis, both in vivo and in vitro.

Natural Killer Cells The general consensus is that natural killer (NK) cells are the major source of IFNγ in the early stages of *L. monocytogenes* infection of mice (39,87). IFNγ is a potent activator of the microbicidal activities of macrophages, and experiments with anti-IFNγ mAb (39), IFNγ gene knockout mice (48), and IFNγ receptor gene knockout mice (47) reveal that IFNγ is a critical cytokine for resistance to primary *L. monocytogenes* infection. NK cells are thought to produce IFNγ in response to IL-12 and TNFα that are elaborated by *L. monocytogenes* infected macrophages (40). Interestingly, IFNγ neutralization appears primarily to exacerbate *L. monocytogenes* infection of the liver (85). In this regard, analysis of the influx of inflammatory cells into the liver of *L. monocytogenes* infected mice reveals a detectable increase in NK1.1 positive cells during the first 24 hours after infection.

In addition to cytokine production, activated NK cells are capable of lysing specific target cells. This type of immune response is potentially relevant for resistance to intracellular pathogens such as *L. monocytogenes*. Consistent with this notion are studies that demonstrate a small but significant increase in lysis of *L. monocytogenes* infected isolated hepatocytes, compared to uninfected hepatocytes, by lymphokine-activated NK (LAK) cells (88). The mechanism by which NK cells might recognize *L. monocytogenes* infected hepatocytes is currently unclear. NK cells express receptors that either activate or inhibit target cell killing. Inhibitory receptors, which appear to recognize MHC class I molecules, prevent killing of MHC class I expressing target cells. Interestingly, a recent report indicates that MHC class I molecules in *L. monocytogenes* infected macrophage cell lines are hyposialated (89). The consequences of this alteration for NK cell recognition of *L. monocytogenes* infected cells are currently unknown. In addition, the relevance of NK cell mediated cytolysis of *L. monocytogenes* infected cells is unclear, since perforin-deficient mice, that are deficient in NK cell mediated killing (90), show a slightly increased resistance to primary *L. monocytogenes* infection compared to wild-type mice (91). Finally, the role of CD-1 restricted NK1.1$^+$ liver T cells in resistance to primary *L. monocytogenes* infection is unknown.

γδ T Cells The function of γδ T cells in immunity to infectious disease remains enigmatic. These cells express specific antigen receptors (TCRγδ) that are derived from rearranging gene segments in a fashion similar to that of TCRαβ. In contrast, antigen recognition by γδ T cells is generally not MHC restricted as is that of αβ T cells. In fact, recent evidence suggests that γδ T cells may recognize proteins, peptides, or soluble nonpeptide antigens derived from microbes, including phosphorylated nucleotides and compounds related to prenyl pyrophospate (92).

Early studies with mAb that efficiently deplete mouse γδ T cells demonstrated that γδ T cells contribute to early resistance to *L. monocytogenes* but play little role in clearance of the primary infection (93). Other studies reveal substantial increases in γδ T cell numbers in the livers of *L. monocytogenes* infected mice early after infection (94). These results were extended by studies comparing resistance to primary *L. monocytogenes* infection in mice with targeted deletion of the TCR δ chain and the TCR α or TCR β chain that respectively lack γδ or αβ T cells. All of the TCR-deficient mice were able to control sublethal *L. monocytogenes* infection (45). However, the finding that mAb depletion of γδ T cells in the TCRαβ-deficient mice exacerbated *L. monocytogenes* infection suggests that γδ T cells are able to respond to infection in an immunologically relevant fashion. Perhaps the most interesting finding from these studies related to the differences in liver lesions in mice deficient in γδ T cells compared with mice deficient in αβ T cells. Liver lesions in the absence of γδ T cells were atypically large, with substantial tissue destruction and inflammation, whereas smaller, granulomatous lesions are found in normal mice. These results were interpreted to suggest that γδ T cells regulate the degree or nature of the inflammatory response to *L. monocytogenes* infection of the liver.

This latter result was confirmed and substantially extended with studies that used mAb-mediated depletion of γδ or αβ T cells in normal mice (46). In these studies, it was shown that γδ T cells accumulate in granulomatous lesions in normal mice after *L. monocytogenes* infection. A detailed analysis of histological changes in the livers of *L. monocytogenes* infected mice revealed that the lesions in normal mice were small, organoid structures with few neutrophils and no evidence of destruction of surrounding tissue (Fig. 8.1A). In contrast, lesions in TCRαβ-depleted mice were larger, more diffuse, and exhibited few mononuclear infiltrating cells or neutrophils (Fig. 8.1B). More strikingly, the lesions in γδ T cell–depleted mice were much larger and exhibited abscess formation, with extensive tissue destruction and large numbers of neutrophils

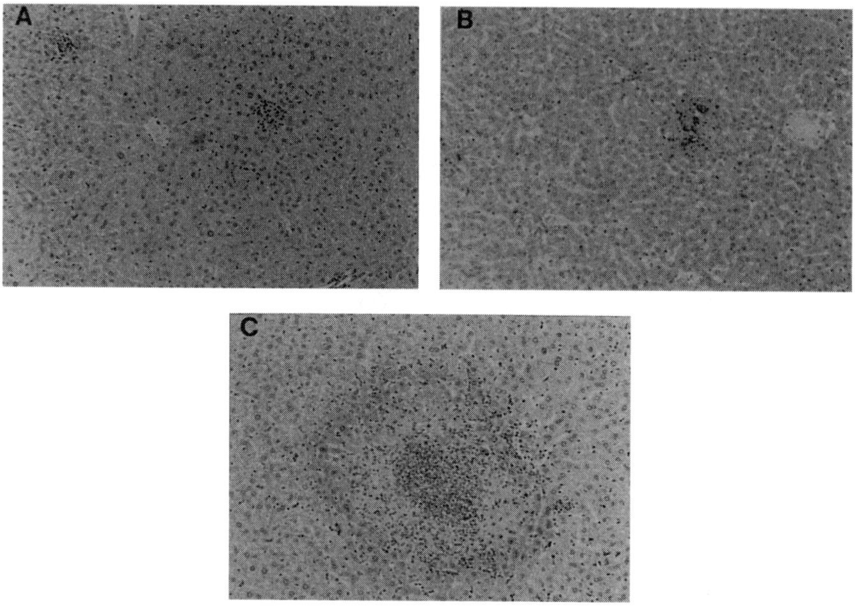

Figure 8.1. Liver lesions after primary *L. monocytogenes* infection. (**A**). Control mice. (**B**). αβ T cell deficient mice. (**C**). γδ T cell deficient mice. Figure reprinted from (Fu et al., 1994) with permission. Copyright 1994, The American Association of Immunologists.

(Fig. 8.1C). Interestingly, the early course of *L. monocytogenes* infection in SCID mice, which lack both B and T cells, was similar to that observed in γδ T cell–depleted normal mice. Transfer of enriched γδ T cells into SCID mice prior to *L. monocytogenes* infection resulted in reduced liver lesions and decreased liver destruction. Thus, it appears that one function of γδ T cells is to regulate the level of inflammation and tissue destruction that results from the influx of neutrophils into the liver in response to *L. monocytogenes* infection.

Further studies reveal that early IFNγ production in response to *L. monocytogenes* infection is impaired in TCR δ gene knockout mice (95) and that the innate immune response to infection is deficient in these animals. NK cells from TCR δ gene knockout mice are deficient in IFNγ production compared to NK cells from TCR β gene knockout mice. Thus, γδ T cells may also play a role in regulating the response of NK cells to *L. monocytogenes* infection. In this regard, it is interesting to note that γδ T cells can exhibit polarized cytokine expression profiles in response to infection. IFNγ predominates in the γδ T cell response to *L. monocytogenes* infection (96).

αβ T Cells The major classes of αβ TCR expressing T cells express either the CD4 coreceptor and recognize peptides presented by MHC class II molecules, or express the CD8 coreceptor and recognize peptides presented by MHC class I molecules. It is generally found that both $CD4^+$ and $CD8^+$ T cells are capable of responding to infection with most intracellular bacterial pathogens. However, it is less clear that both CD4$^+$ and CD8$^+$ T cells are essential for immunity against all intracellular bacteria (97). In part, this difference results from differences in the subcellular compartmentalization of intracellular bacteria. All intracellular bacteria enter eukaryotic cells in membrane-bound structures. Some intracellular bacteria such as *Mycobacterium tuberculosis* or *Salmonella typhi* remain inside vacuolar structures in the infected cell. While proteins from these organisms are readily processed and presented to CD4$^+$ T cells by the exogenous pathway of MHC class II antigen presentation, their proteins are not readily accessible to the endogenous pathway of MHC class I antigen presentation to CD8$^+$ T cells that originates in the cytoplasm of the infected cell. Presentation of antigens from vacuolar pathogens to CD8$^+$ T cells requires an exogenous MHC class I antigen presentation pathway that may not suffice for the elaboration of protective immunity (98). In contrast, *L. monocytogenes* enters the cytoplasm of the infected cell and is thus exposed to the endogenous pathway of MHC class I presentation and the attention of CD8$^+$ T cells. As mentioned above, many *L. monocytogenes* are destroyed in the phagosome prior to their escape from the vacuole and thus *L. monocytogenes* antigens are also efficiently presented by MHC class II molecules to CD4$^+$ T cells.

Recruitment of αβ T cells to the liver after primary *L. monocytogenes* infection exhibits a biphasic pattern (99). CD4$^+$ and CD8$^+$ T cell numbers increase equivalently in the liver by 1 day after infection, but return to baseline by 2 days after infection. The second phase of T cell infiltration into the liver begins at 3 days and peaks at 5–7 days after infection. CD8$^+$ T cells predominate at day 5, increasing 21-fold over baseline by day 7, while the peak of CD4$^+$ T cell accumulation (5-fold over baseline) occurs at day 7 after infection. Both CD4$^+$ and CD8$^+$ T cells then return to baseline over the next several days. Evidence that many of these liver T cells are *L. monocytogenes* specific derives from studies that reveal the capacity of T cells isolated from livers 7 days after infection to transfer antilisterial immunity to naive mice (100). Consistent with the majority of studies of specific immunity to *L. monocytogenes*, liver T cells that were depleted of the CD8$^+$ T cell subset failed to provide antilisterial immunity in transfer assays.

Depletion of either CD4$^+$ T cells or CD8$^+$ T cells prior to sublethal *L. monocytogenes* infection delays *L. monocytogenes* clearance in the liver by several weeks (101). Depletion of the CD8$^+$ T cell subset resulted in the greatest delay in bacterial clearance. Depletion of both CD4$^+$ and CD8$^+$ T cells completely prevents clearance of sublethal infection from the liver. In addition, depletion of CD4$^+$ T cells resulted in an increase of serum levels of ALT and aspartate transaminose (AST) that correlated with increases in the number and size of liver lesions compared to controls. Treatment of the CD4$^+$ T cell–depleted mice with recombinant IFNγ at the time of infection reduced the serum ALT and AST levels to those of control mice and decreased the severity of liver lesions. Another report confirms the exacerbation of *L. monocytogenes* induced liver lesions in CD4$^+$ T cell–depleted mice (102) and suggest that granuloma formation requires CD4$^+$ T cells (103). Together, these studies confirm that αβ T cells are required for sterilizing immunity against primary *L. monocytogenes* infection of the liver. In addition, these studies of primary *L. monocytogenes* infection suggest that $CD4^+$ T cells play a role in controlling liver damage, perhaps through control of the granulomatous response.

This notion is supported by studies of *L. monocytogenes* infection of MHC class I and class II deficient mutant mice that lack $CD8^+$ T cells and $CD4^+$ T cells respectively (67). Both $CD4^+$ T cell–deficient and $CD8^+$ T cell–deficient mice exhibited delayed clearance of *L. monocytogenes* infection compared to control animals. In $CD4^+$ T cell–deficient mice, liver granuloma formation at 7 days after primary *L. monocytogenes* infection was aberrant, with few defined accumulations of inflammatory cells. However, the same studies reveal that $CD8^+$ T cells may also play a role in appropriate granuloma formation in response to primary *L. monocytogenes* infection.

Secondary Resistance to *L. monocytogenes* Infection of the Liver

Resistance to secondary challenge with *L. monocytogenes* is dependent on T cells, since T-cell-deficient mice fail to develop acquired immunity and immune mice, depleted of T cells, fail to exhibit acquired immunity. In the majority of studies, $CD8^+$ T cells play a dominant role as effectors of acquired immunity to *L. monocytogenes* infection. However, $CD4^+$ T cells can contribute to acquired immunity to *L. monocytogenes* infection of the liver in the absence of $CD8^+$ T cells. Similarly, $\gamma\delta$ T cells may provide some level of acquired immunity in the absence of $\alpha\beta$ T cells, although this issue is not resolved. It is clear that at least some elements of the innate immune response, which are critical for resistance to primary infection, also contribute to the elaboration of specific resistance to secondary *L. monocytogenes* infection. In some respects, particularly the activation of macrophages, T cells control the elements of innate immunity during secondary resistance to *L. monocytogenes* infection of the liver.

Kupffer Cells and Immigrant Macrophages In mice exposed to a secondary *L. monocytogenes* infection, bacterial numbers associated with isolated Kupffer cells decrease dramatically and the organisms are eliminated after 2 days of infection (6). This result is in contrast the twofold increase in *L. monocytogenes* in the Kupffer cell population of mice after 2 days of primary infection. Thus, *L. monocytogenes* immune T cells are able to increase the microbicidal activities of Kupffer cells. In contrast to their essential role in resistance to primary *L. monocytogenes* infection, immigrant macrophages are not essential for secondary resistance to *L. monocytogenes* infection in the livers of immune mice or mice that receive immune T cells (78). Other studies reveal that secondary resistance to *L. monocytogenes* infection can occur in the absence of detectable granuloma formation (65).

Neutrophils Neutrophils are essential for resistance to primary *L. monocytogenes* infection (42–44). In contrast to the finding with immigrant macrophages, neutrophils are also required for T-cell-mediated acquired immunity to secondary *L. monocytogenes* infection of the liver (104–106). The basis for this finding is not clear. Neutrophils may be required for early control of *L. monocytogenes* infection of the liver, even in the presence of memory T cells that are specific for *L. monocytogenes* antigens. Alternatively, neutophils may be required to eliminate extracellular bacteria that are released as a consequence of $CD8^+$ T cell lysis of infected hepatocytes. A role for $CD8^+$ T-cell-mediated cytolysis, and by inference a requirement for neutrophils, is consistent with recent studies with perforin deficient mice. These mice, which lack the capacity to mediate one of the major pathways of $CD8^+$ T cell killing, are apparently deficient in secondary resistance to *L. monocytogenes* infection (91).

Hepatocytes In contrast to the dramatic increase in heptocyte-associated *L. monocytogenes* seen during the first several days of a primary infection, there is a rapid decrease in *L. monocytogenes* numbers in hepatocytes isolated from immune mice after secondary infection, and by two days after infection *L. monocytogenes* are essentially undetectable (6). It is not clear from these assays, however, whether the hepatocytes eliminated intracellular *L. monocytogenes* or if the decrease in bacterial numbers resulted from T-cell-mediated destruction of infected cells. As mentioned above, cytokine treatment of hepatocytes (78) and hepatocyte-like cell lines (84) has been found to slightly increase their resistance to *L. monocytogenes* infection. In contrast, other studies found no evidence for hepatocyte-mediated killing of *L. monocytogenes* (5,86).

Natural Killer Cells NK cells contribute to resistance against primary *L. monocytogenes* infection by production of IFNγ and the activation of macrophages. NK cell–derived IFNγ may also play a role in shifting the balance of $CD4^+$ T cell development towards a T helper type 1 (Th1) phenotype, although it is clear that IL-12 plays a dominant role in this process (41). It is not clear what role, if any, is played by NK cells in resistance to secondary *L. monocytogenes* infection. IFNγ in secondary *L. monocytogenes* infection is also produced by *L. monocytogenes* specific $CD4^+$ and $CD8^+$ T cells. Studies with neutralizing anti-IFNγ mAb either support (107) or fail to support (108) a role for IFNγ in secondary resistance to *L. monocytogenes*. In this regard, our own studies of IFNγ gene knockout mice demonstrate that $CD8^+$ T cell immunity to *L. monocytogenes* infection of the spleen and liver can develop and be expressed in the complete absence of IFNγ (48). Thus, the role of NK cells in secondary resistance to *L. monocytogenes* infection is unclear.

γδ T Cells γδ T cells play an important role in resistance to primary *L. monocytogenes* infection, apparently by controlling the nature and the degree of inflammation and tissue destruction in the liver (45,46). These cells may also contribute to the innate immune response against *L. monocytogenes* by cytokine secretion or other mechanisms (40,93). The question of whether γδ T cells develop memory responses that contribute to acquired immunity against secondary infection has not been fully answered. In studies with TCRαβ knockout mice, TCRγδ knockout mice, or mice without T cells, it was determined that vaccinated TCRαβ knockout mice exhibit more resistance than vaccinated mice that lack all T cells (45). However, these mice were less resistant than TCRγδ knockouts, which develop the same level of resistance to secondary challenge as wild-type mice. These data suggested that γδ T cells may play a role in secondary resistance to *L. monocytogenes* infection. However, the relationship described above also holds true for naive TCR-deficient and control mice.

Therefore, it is not clear that vaccination had a substantial effect on the ability of γδ T cells to resist secondary challenge with *L. monocytogenes*. Interestingly, γδ T cell depletion of mice previously immunized with *L. monocytogenes* also resulted in increased liver damage and exacerbated the level of secondary infection in the spleen, although not to the same extent as αβ T cell depletion (46). Thus, γδ T cells apparently play a role in resistance to both primary and secondary *L. monocytogenes* infection. However, the issue of whether γδ T cells develop specific memory to infection remains to be resolved.

αβ T Cells Acquired immunity to secondary *L. monocytogenes* challenge is primarily mediated by T cells. A substantial body of experiments, employing both T cell subset depletion or adoptive transfer of selected T cell subsets from immune to naive mice, reveal that $CD8^+$ T cells are the most effective mediators of acquired immunity to *L. monocytogenes* infection (63,66). However, $CD4^+$ T cells clearly respond during primary *L. monocytogenes* infection and mount a vigorous secondary response to challenge infection. This scenario is entirely consistent with the lifecycle of virulent *L. monocytogenes*, which enter the cytoplasm of infected cells and are thus exposed to the endogenous MHC class I antigen presentation pathway to $CD8^+$ T cells. However, substantial numbers of *L. monocytogenes* are also destroyed in the phagosome, and it is likely that the majority of *L. monocytogenes* antigens presented by MHC class II molecules derive from bacteria that are destroyed in the phagosome of macrophages. The dominance of $CD8^+$ T cells as effectors of secondary resistance to *L. monocytogenes* infection is also consistent with the fact that hepatocytes, which are the major cell type supporting *L. monocytogenes* replication in the infected animal, do not constitutively express MHC class II molecules, but do constitutively express MHC class I molecules. Thus, infected hepatocytes should be readily recognized by MHC class I restricted $CD8^+$ T cells and not MHC class II restricted $CD4^+$ T cells.

Recent studies have provided experimental support for $CD8^+$ T cell recognition of *L. monocytogenes* infected hepatocytes as an important aspect of secondary resistance to infection. Studies with an hepatocyte-like cell line reveal that *L. monocytogenes* antigen-specific $CD8^+$ T cells that recognize peptides from the *L. monocytogenes* encoded p60 molecule can mediate antigen-specific lysis of *L. monocytogenes* infected hepatocyte-like cells (70). Consistent with this finding are studies that describe the capacity of $CD8^+$ T cells, purified from *L. monocytogenes* immune mice, to mediate lysis of infected heptocytes (109). The latter studies also demonstrated that $CD4^+$ T cells, purified from *L. monocytogenes* immune mice, exhibit no cytolytic activity against infected hepatocytes. Thus, infected hepatocytes can be recognized and lysed by *L. monocytogenes* specific $CD8^+$ T cells in vitro.

Our laboratory has extended these observations with in vivo studies (70). We constructed radiation bone marrow chimeric mice that had been manipulated to control the MHC class I alleles expressed on bone-marrow-derived macrophages, Kupffer cells, and non-bone-marrow-derived hepatocytes. In these mice, we created situations where MHC class I molecules expressed by Kupffer cells would differ from MHC class I molecules expressed by hepatocytes. Since the $CD8^+$ T cells in immune mice are MHC restricted, and can only recognize infected cells that express appropriate

MHC class I alleles, we created an experimental situation where the $CD8^+$ T cells could recognize either *L. monocytogenes* infected macrophages and hepatocytes or only infected hepatocytes. These mice allowed us to determine if $CD8^+$ T cell recognition of *L. monocytogenes* infected hepatocytes was relevant to protective immunity. As summarized in Table 8.1, these studies revealed that $CD8^+$ T cells can provide immunity against *L. monocytogenes* by recognition of either infected macrophages or infected hepatocytes. This contention was supported by the finding that an H-$2K^b$ restricted $CD8^+$ T cell line, specific for peptides from the *L. monocytogenes* encoded LLO molecule, mediated immunity in the livers of transgenic mice that express the H-$2K^b$ MHC class I molecule only on hepatocytes. Together, these data demonstrate that $CD8^+$ T cells can provide significant immunity to *L. monocytogenes* infection through recognition of *L. monocytogenes* infected hepatocytes.

Recently, our laboratory has focused on understanding the mechanisms that $CD8^+$ T cells use to provide immunity to *L. monocytogenes* infection. $CD8^+$ T cells are capable of killing target cells that express the appropriate MHC class I–peptide complexes on their cell surface. The majority of $CD8^+$ T cell–mediated target cell lysis occurs via one of two described pathways, either perforin-dependent granule exocytosis or CD95L–CD95 interaction (110). In addition to target cell lysis, $CD8^+$ T cells elaborate significant levels of IFN–γ, TNF–α, and other cytokines that may play a role in resistance to *L. monocytogenes* infection (52). In previous studies, we determined that wild-type $CD8^+$ T cells, specific for the *L. monocytogenes* antigens LLO and p60, are able to transfer high levels of immunity against *L. monocytogenes* infection to naive mice (70–72). To address the requirement for specific $CD8^+$ T cell effector mechanisms in resistance to *L. monocytogenes*, we have made use of recently generated gene knockout mice that lack expression of potential $CD8^+$ T cell effector functions. We used these gene knockout mice to generate $CD8^+$ T cells lines that rec-

TABLE 8.1 $CD8^+$ T Cell Mediation of Immunity to *L. moncytogenes* by Recognition of Infected Hepatocytes or Kupffer Cells*

	Chimeric mice		
	Kupffer cell MHC^{bxd}	Kupffer cell MHC^b	Kupffer cell MHC^d
L. monocytogenes	Hepatocyte MHC^{bxd}	Hepatocyte MHC^{bxd}	Hepatocyte MHC^{bxd}
immune $CD8^+$ T cells	Relative immunity in the livers of T cell recipient chimeric mice		
From MHC^b mice	++++	++++	++
From MHC^d mice	++++	++	++++

*Chimeric mice were generated by reconstitution of lethally irradiated BDF1 (MHC^{bxd}) mice with bone marrow from parental B6 (MHC^b) or DBA/2 (MHC^d) mice. In the chimeric mice, bone-marrow-derived Kupffer cells express the MHC allele of the bone marrow donor (MHC^b or MHC^d) while the non-bone-marrow-derived hepatocytes express both MHC^b and MHC^d alleles. Thirteen weeks after reconstitution, the chimeric mice were used as recipients for immune $CD8^+$ T cells, recognizing *L. monocytogenes* antigens presented by either MHC^b or MHC^d class I molecules. The relative immunity to challenge infection in each group is indicated by the number of plus marks.

ognize protective *L. monocytogenes* antigens and analyzed their ability to provide immunity to infection in the absence of individual effector functions.

In the first series of studies, we examined the requirement for $CD8^+$ T cell–derived IFNγ by generating LLO- and p60-specific $CD8^+$ T cell lines from IFNγ gene knockout mice (48). IFNγ gene knockout $CD8^+$ T cells are capable of target cell lysis that is indistinguishable from that caused by wild-type $CD8^+$ T cells. In addition, IFNγ deficiency does not affect TNFα production in response to specific target cells. In transfer assays, LLO- or p60-specific $CD8^+$ T cells from IFNγ gene knockout mice provided identical levels of antilisterial immunity to naive mice as did wild-type $CD8^+$ T cells specific for the same antigens. The results of these studies demonstrated convincingly that $CD8^+$ T cell–derived IFNγ was not required for immunity to *L. monocytogenes* infection of the liver or the spleen. In other experiments with the IFNγ gene knockout mice, we were able to demonstrate that $CD8^+$ T cell immunity could develop and be expressed in the complete absence of IFNγ. These results supported earlier studies in which we found that treatment of recipient mice with a neutralizing anti-IFN–γ mAb did not inhibit the transfer of antilisterial immunity by LLO-specific $CD8^+$ T cells from wild-type mice (71). Thus, $CD8^+$ T cell–derived IFNγ is not required for immunity to *L. monocytogenes* infection.

Experiments with perforin gene knockout mice suggest that $CD8^+$ T cell immunity to *L. monocytogenes* is at least partially perforin dependent (91). We have extended these findings by generating LLO-specific $CD8^+$ T cells from perforin gene knockout mice and determining their capacity to provide antilisterial immunity (111). Somewhat to our surprise, the LLO-specific perforin-deficient $CD8^+$ T cells provide significant immunity against *L. monocytogenes* infection. Interestingly, the perforin-deficient $CD8^+$ T cells provide intermediate levels of immunity in the spleen of T cell recipients but equivalent levels of immunity in the liver, as compared to the levels of immunity provided by LLO-specific $CD8^+$ T cells from wild-type mice. These data suggest that the importance of specific $CD8^+$ T cell effector mechanisms may be different in the liver and the spleen. Since $CD8^+$ T cells are also capable of target cell lysis via CD95L–CD95 interactions, and hepatocytes express considerable levels of CD95, we also tested the requirement for CD95 expression in $CD8^+$ T cell immunity to *L. monocytogenes* infection. In these studies, we performed transfer assays with LLO-specific perforin-deficient $CD8^+$ T cells into wild-type and MRL *lpr/lpr* (CD95-deficient) hosts. These studies showed that perforin-deficient $CD8^+$ T cells could provided equivalent immunity to *L. monocytogenes* in control and CD95-deficient recipients and suggest that other effector pathways are able to function in the absence of $CD8^+$ T-cell-mediated cytolysis.

Although immune $CD8^+$ T cells appear to be the most potent effectors of secondary antilisterial immunity, immune $CD4^+$ T cells also respond to secondary challenge infection. In some experimental circumstances, *L. monocytogenes* specific $CD4^+$ T cell clones (68) and $CD4^+$ T cell lines (69) provided significant immunity when transferred into naive mice prior to *L. monocytogenes* infection. In our study (69), transfer of immunity by $CD4^+$ T cells was only observed in the livers of recipient mice and was completely abrogated by treatment of the T cell recipients with anti-IFN–γ mAb. Thus, in contrast to immunity mediated by CD8+ T cells, CD4+ T cell immunity to *L. monocytogenes* depends on IFNγ production. Recent studies have also demonstrated the capacity of *L. monocytogenes* specific $CD4^+$ T cells, purified from *L. monocytogenes* immune mice, to provide some antilisterial immunity in the livers but not spleens of recipient mice (112). Thus, cytokine production by $CD4^+$ T cells may be important in resistance to *L. monocytogenes* infection of the liver, perhaps by activating the microbicidal activities of resident Kupffer cells.

In addition to their ability to mediate cytokine production, $CD4^+$ T cells also play an important role in granuloma formation in response to secondary *L. monocytogenes* infection. Depletion of $CD4^+$ T cells from *L. monocytogenes* immune mice prior to challenge dramatically decreased the appearance of mononuclear cell foci in the livers of infected mice (65). Interestingly, depletion of $CD4^+$ T cells from the immune mice had little, if any, negative impact on the number of organisms recovered or clearance of the infection, while depletion of $CD8^+$ T cells dramatically exacerbated secondary *L. monocytogenes* infection. Thus, $CD8^+$ T-cell-mediated resistance to secondary *L. monocytogenes* infection of the liver can occur in the absence of the granulomatous response.

SUMMARY

The studies of immunity against *L. monocytogenes* infection of the liver detailed in this chapter reveal the complex interaction between cells and molecules of the innate immune response, which not only function in direct microbial killing, but also serve to shape the nature of the acquired immune response to infection. In turn, elements of the T cell immune response control the level of tissue destruction associated with the influx of neutrophils and macrophages into the liver, as well as provide the effector functions required for sterilizing immunity and acquired immunity to reinfection. The reproducibility of infection in combination with sophisticated bacterial and immunological reagents provide strong support for continued studies of murine listeriosis as an important model system for bacterial infection and immunity in the liver.

ACKNOWLEDGMENTS

The author would like to acknowledge W. Born for providing Figure 8.1, D. W. White for review of the manuscript, and the Arthritis Foundation, Roy J. Carver Charitable Trust, and the NIH for financial support.

REFERENCES

1. Farber, J.M., and Peterkin, P.I. 1991. *Listeria monocytogenes*, a food-borne pathogen. *Microbiol. Rev.* 55:476–511.
2. Rouquette, C., and Berche, P. 1996. The pathogenesis of infection by Listeria monocytogenes. *Microbiologia* 12:245–258.

3. Altekruse, S., Hyman, F., Klontz, K., Timbo, B., and Tollefson, L. 1994. Foodborne bacterial infections in individuals with the human immunodeficiency virus. *South Med. J.* 87:169–173.
4. Portnoy, D.A., Jacks, P.S., and Hinrichs, D.J. 1988. Role of hemolysin for the intracellular growth of Listeria monocytogenes. *J. Exp. Med.* 167:1459–1471.
5. Wood, S., Maroushek, N., and Czuprynski, C.J. 1993. Multiplication of Listeria monocytogenes in a murine hepatocyte cell line. *Infect. Immun.* 61:3068–3072.
6. Gregory, S.H., Barczynski, L.K., and Wing, E.J. 1992. Effector function of hepatocytes and Kupffer cells in the resolution of systemic bacterial infections. *J. Leuk. Biol.* 51:421–424.
7. Gaillard, J.L., Berche, P., Frehel, C., Gouin, E., and Cossart, P. 1991. Entry of L. monocytogenes into cells is mediated by internalin, a repeat protein reminiscent of surface antigens from gram-positive cocci. *Cell* 65:1127–1141.
8. Kuhn, M., and Goebel, W. 1989. Identification of an extracellular protein of Listeria monocytogenes possibly involved in intracellular uptake by mammalian cells. *Infect. Immun.* 57:55–61.
9. Mengaud, J., Ohayon, H., Gounon, P., Mege, R.M., and Cossart, P. 1996. E-cadherin is the receptor for internalin, a surface protein required for entry of L. monocytogenes into epithelial cells. *Cell* 84:923–932.
10. Dramsi, S., Biswas, I., Maguin, E., Braun, L., Mastroeni, P., and Cossart, P. 1995. Entry of Listeria monocytogenes into hepatocytes requires expression of inlB, a surface protein of the internalin multigene family. *Mol. Microbiol.* 16:251–261.
11. Gaillard, J.L., Jaubert, F., and Berche, P. 1996. The inlAB locus mediates the entry of Listeria monocytogenes into hepatocytes in vivo. *J. Exp. Med.* 183:359–369.
12. Gregory, S.H., Sagnimeni, A.J., and Wing, E.J. 1996. Expression of the inlAB operon by Listeria monocytogenes is not required for entry into hepatic cells in vivo. *Infect. Immun.* 64:3983–3986.
13. Harding, C.V. 1991. Pathways of antigen processing. *Curr. Opin. Immunol.* 3:3–9.
14. Hof, H. 1991. Microbial strategies for intracellular survival. *Infection* 19:s202–s205.
15. Russell, D.G. 1995. Of microbes and macrophages: Entry, survival and persistence. *Curr. Opin. Immunol.* 7:479–484.
16. Mengaud, J., Chenevert, J., Geoffroy, C., Gaillard, J.L., and Cossart, P. 1987. Identification of the structural gene encoding the SH-activated hemolysin of Listeria monocytogenes: Listeriolysin O is homologous to streptolysin O and pneumolysin. *Infect. Immun.* 55:3225–3227.
17. Geoffroy, C., Gaillard, J.L., Alouf, J.E., and Berche, P. 1987. Purification, characterization, and toxicity of the sulfhydryl-activated hemolysin listeriolysin O from Listeria monocytogenes. *Infect. Immun.* 55:1641–1646.
18. Gaillard, J.L., Berche, P., and Sansonetti, P. 1986. Transposon mutagenesis as a tool to study the role of hemolysin in the virulence of Listeria monocytogenes. *Infect. Immun.* 52:50–55.
19. Cossart, P., Vicente, M.F., Mengaud, J., Baquero, F., Perez, D.J.C., and Berche, P. 1989. Listeriolysin O is essential for virulence of Listeria monocytogenes: Direct evidence obtained by gene complementation. *Infect. Immun.* 57:3629–3636.
20. de Chastellier, C., and Berche, P. 1994. Fate of Listeria monocytogenes in murine macrophages: Evidence for simultaneous killing and survival of intracellular bacteria. *Infect. Immun.* 62:543–553.

21. Tang, P., Rosenshine, I., Cossart, P., and Finlay, B.B. 1996. Listeriolysin O activates mitogen-activated protein kinase in eucaryotic cells. *Infect. Immun.* 64:2359–2361.
22. Weiglein, I., Goebel, W., Troppmair, J., Rapp, U.R., Demuth, A., and Kuhn, M. 1997. Listeria monocytogenes infection of hela cells results in listeriolysin O-mediated transient activation of the raf-mek-map kinase pathway. *FEMS Microbiol. Lett.* 148:189–195.
23. Demuth, A., Goebel, W., Beuscher, H.U., and Kuhn, M. 1996. Differential regulation of cytokine and cytokine receptor mrna expression upon infection of bone marrow-derived macrophages with listeria monocytogenes. *Infect. Immun.* 64:3475–3483.
24. Cossart, P. 1995. Actin-based bacterial motility. *Curr. Opin. Cell Biol.* 7:94–101.
25. Kocks, C., Gouin, E., Tabouret, M., Berche, P., Ohayon, H., and Cossart, P. 1992. L. monocytogenes-induced actin assembly requires the actA gene product, a surface protein. *Cell* 68:521–531.
26. Welch, M.D., Iwamatsu, A., and Mitchison, T.J. 1997. Actin polymerization is induced by arp2/3 protein complex at the surface of Listeria monocytogenes. *Nature* 385:265–269.
27. Tilney, L.G., and Portnoy, D.A. 1989. Actin filaments and the growth, movement, and spread of the intracellular bacterial parasite, Listeria monocytogenes. *J. Cell. Biol.* 109:1597–1608.
28. Mackaness, G.B. 1962. Cellular resistance to infection. *J. Exp. Med.* 116:381–406.
29. Brundage, R.A., Smith, G.A., Camilli, A., Theriot, J.A., and Portnoy, D.A. 1993. Expression and phosphorylation of the Listeria monocytogenes ActA protein in mammalian cells. *Proc. Natl. Acad. Sci. U.S.A.* 90:11890–11894.
30. Camilli, A., Goldfine, H., and Portnoy, D.A. 1991. Listeria monocytogenes mutants lacking phosphatidylinositol-specific phospholipase C are avirulent. *J. Exp. Med.* 173:751–754.
31. Marquis, H., Doshi, V., and Portnoy, D.A. 1995. The broad-range phospholipase C and a metalloprotease mediate listeriolysin O-independent escape of Listeria monocytogenes from a primary vacuole in human epithelial cells. *Infect. Immun.* 63:4531–4534.
32. Mengaud, J., Dramsi, S., Gouin, E., Vazquez, B.J.A., Milon, G., and Cossart, P. 1991. Pleiotropic control of Listeria monocytogenes virulence factors by a gene that is autoregulated. *Mol. Microbiol.* 5:2273–2283.
33. Freitag, N.E., Rong, L., and Portnoy, D.A. 1993. Regulation of the prfA transcriptional activator of Listeria monocytogenes: Multiple promoter elements contribute to intracellular growth and cell-to-cell spread. *Infect. Immun.* 61:2537–2544.
34. Renzoni, A., Klarsfeld, A., Dramsi, S., and Cossart, P. 1997. Evidence that PrfA, the pleiotropic activator of virulence genes in Listeria monocytogenes, can be present but inactive. *Infect. Immun.* 65:1515–1518.
35. Gregory, S.H., Sagnimeni, A.J., and Wing, E.J. 1996. Bacteria in the bloodstream are trapped in the liver and killed by immigrating neutrophils. *J. Immunol.* 157:2514–2520.
36. Newborg, M.F., and North, R.J. 1980. On the mechanism of T cell-independent anti-Listeria resistance in nude mice. *J. Immunol.* 124:571–576.
37. Bancroft, G.J., Bosma, M.J., Bosma, G.C., and Unanue, E.R. 1986. Regulation of macrophage Ia expression in mice with severe combined immunodeficiency: induction of Ia expression by a T cell-independent mechanism. *J. Immunol.* 137:4–9.
38. Cheers, C., and McKenzie, I.F. 1978. Resistance and susceptibility of mice to bacterial infection: Genetics of listeriosis. *Infect. Immun.* 19:755–762.
39. Bancroft, G.J., Schreiber, R.D., and Unanue, E.R. 1991. Natural immunity: a T-cell-independent pathway of macrophage activation, defined in the scid mouse. *Immunol. Rev.* 124:5–24.

40. Tripp, C.S., Wolf, S.F., and Unanue, E.R. 1993. Interleukin 12 and tumor necrosis factor alpha are costimulators of interferon gamma production by natural killer cells in severe combined immunodeficiency mice with listeriosis, and interleukin 10 is a physiologic antagonist. *Proc. Natl. Acad. Sci. U.S.A.* 90:3725–3729.

41. Hsieh, C.S., Macatonia, S.E., Tripp, C.S., Wolf, S.F., O'Garra, A., and Murphy, K.M. 1993. Development of TH1 CD4+ T cells through IL-12 produced by Listeria-induced macrophages. *Science* 260:547–549.

42. Conlan, J.W., and North, R.J. 1994. Neutrophils are essential for early anti-Listeria defense in the liver, but not in the spleen or peritoneal cavity, as revealed by a granulocyte-depleting monoclonal antibody. *J. Exp. Med.* 179:259–268.

43. Czuprynski, C.J., Brown, J.F., Maroushek, N., Wagner, R.D., and Steinberg, H. 1994. Administration of anti-granulocyte mAb RB6-8C5 impairs the resistance of mice to Listeria monocytogenes infection. *J. Immunol.* 152:1836–1846.

44. Rogers, H.W., and Unanue, E.R. 1993. Neutrophils are involved in acute, nonspecific resistance to Listeria monocytogenes in mice. *Infect. Immun.* 61:5090–5096.

45. Mombaerts, P., Arnoldi, J., Russ, F., Tonegawa, S., and Kaufmann, S.H. 1993. Different roles of alpha beta and gamma delta T cells in immunity against an intracellular bacterial pathogen. *Nature* 365:53–56.

46. Fu, Y.X., Roark, C.E., Kelly, K., Drevets, D., Campbell, P., O'Brien, R., and Born, W. 1994. Immune protection and control of inflammatory tissue necrosis by gamma delta T cells. *J. Immunol.* 153:3101–3115.

47. Huang, S., Hendriks, W., Althage, A., Hemmi, S., Bluethmann, H., Kamijo, R., Vilcek, J., Zinkernagel, R.M., and Aguet, M. 1993. Immune response in mice that lack the interferon-gamma receptor. *Science* 259:1742–1745.

48. Harty, J.T., and Bevan, M.J. 1995. Specific immunity to Listeria monocytogenes in the absence of IFN gamma. *Immunity* 3:109–117.

49. Rothe, J., Lesslauer, W., Lotscher, H., Lang, Y., Koebel, P., Kontgen, F., Althage, A., Zinkernagel, R., Steinmetz, M., and Bluethmann, H. 1993. Mice lacking the tumour necrosis factor receptor 1 are resistant to TNF-mediated toxicity but highly susceptible to infection by Listeria monocytogenes. *Nature* 364:798–802.

50. Pasparakis, M., Alexopoulou, L., Episkopou, V., and Kollias, G. 1996. Immune and inflammatory responses in tnf-alpha-deficient mice—a critical requirement for tnf-alpha in the formation of primary b cell follicles, follicular dendritic cell networks and germinal centers, and in the maturation of the humoral immune response. *J. Exp. Med.* 184:1397–1411.

51. Eugster, H.P., Muller, M., Karrer, U., Car, B.D., Schnyder, B., Eng, V.M., Woerly, G., Lehir, M., Dipadova, F., Aguet, M., Zinkernagel, R., Bluethmann, H., and Ryffel, B. 1996. Multiple immune abnormalities in tumor necrosis factor and lymphotoxin-alpha double-deficient mice. *Int. Immunol.* 8:23–36.

52. Harty, J.T., Lenz, L.L., and Bevan, M.J. 1996. Primary and secondary immune responses to Listeria monocytogenes. *Curr. Opin. Immunol.* 8:526–530.

53. Tripp, C.S., Gately, M.K., Hakimi, J., Ling, P., and Unanue, E.R. 1994. Neutralization of IL-12 decreases resistance to Listeria in SCID and C.B-17 mice. Reversal by IFN-gamma. *J. Immunol.* 152:1883–1887.

54. Hunter, C.A., Chizzonite, R., and Remington, J.S. 1995. IL-1 beta is required for IL-12 to induce production of IFN-gamma by NK cells. A role for IL-1 beta in the T cell-independent mechanism of resistance against intracellular pathogens. *J. Immunol.* 155:4347–4354.

55. Rogers, H.W., Tripp, C.S., Schreiber, R.D., and Unanue, E.R. 1994. Endogenous IL-1 is required for neutrophil recruitment and macrophage activation during murine listeriosis. *J. Immunol.* 153:2093–2101.

56. Dalrymple, S.A., Lucian, L.A., Slattery, R., McNeil, T., Aud, D.M., Fuchino, S., Lee, F., and Murray, R. 1995. Interleukin-6-deficient mice are highly susceptible to Listeria monocytogenes infection: Correlation with inefficient neutrophilia. *Infect. Immun.* 63:2262–2268.

57. Tanaka, T., Akira, S., Yoshida, K., Umemoto, M., Yoneda, Y., Shirafuji, N., Fujiwara, H., Suematsu, S., Yoshida, N., and Kishimoto, T. 1995. Targeted disruption of the NF-IL6 gene discloses its essential role in bacteria killing and tumor cytotoxicity by macrophages. *Cell* 80:353–361.

58. North, R.J. 1973. Importance of thymus-derived lymphocytes in cell-mediated immunity to infection. *Cell. Immunol.* 7:166–176.

59. Lane, F.C., and Unanue, E.R. 1973. Immunologic events during Listeria monocytogenes infection in mice: Adjuvanticity and immunogenicity of macrophage-bound antigens. *J. Immunol.* 110:829–834.

60. Brunt, L.M., Portnoy, D.A., and Unanue, E.R. 1990. Presentation of Listeria monocytogenes to CD8+ T cells requires secretion of hemolysin and intracellular bacterial growth. *J. Immunol.* 145:3540–3546.

61. Lukacs, K., and Kurlander, R. 1989. Lyt-2+ T cell-mediated protection against listeriosis. Protection correlates with phagocyte depletion but not with IFN-gamma production. *J. Immunol.* 142:2879–2886.

62. Bishop, D.K., and Hinrichs, D.J. 1987. Adoptive transfer of immunity to Listeria monocytogenes. The influence of in vitro stimulation on lymphocyte subset requirements. *J. Immunol.* 139:2005–2009.

63. Dunn, P.L., and North, R.J. 1991. Limitations of the adoptive immunity assay for analyzing anti-Listeria immunity. *J. Infect. Dis.* 164:878–882.

64. Czuprynski, C.J., and Brown, J.F. 1990. Effects of purified anti-Lyt-2 mAb treatment on murine listeriosis: comparative roles of Lyt-2+ and L3T4+ cells in resistance to primary and secondary infection, delayed-type hypersensitivity and adoptive transfer of resistance. *Immunology* 71:107–112.

65. Mielke, M.E., Niedobitek, G., Stein, H., and Hahn, H. 1989. Acquired resistance to Listeria monocytogenes is mediated by Lyt-2+ T cells independently of the influx of monocytes into granulomatous lesions. *J. Exp. Med.* 170:589–594.

66. Mielke, M.E., Ehlers, S., and Hahn, H. 1988. T-cell subsets in delayed-type hypersensitivity, protection, and granuloma formation in primary and secondary Listeria infection in mice: Superior role of Lyt-2+ cells in acquired immunity. *Infect. Immun.* 56:1920–1925.

67. Ladel, C.H., Flesch, I.E., Arnoldi, J., and Kaufmann, S.H. 1994. Studies with MHC-deficient knock-out mice reveal impact of both MHC I- and MHC II-dependent T cell responses on Listeria monocytogenes infection. *J. Immunol.* 153:3116–3122.

68. Magee, D.M., and Wing, E.J. 1988. Cloned L3T4+ T lymphocytes protect mice against Listeria monocytogenes by secreting IFN-gamma. J. *Immunol.* 141:3203–3207.

69. Harty, J.T., Schreiber, R.D., and Bevan, M.J. 1992. CD8 T cells can protect against an intracellular bacterium in an interferon gamma-independent fashion. *Proc. Natl. Acad. Sci. U.S.A.* 89:11612–11616.

70. Harty, J.T., and Bevan, M.J. 1996. CD8 T-cell recognition of macrophages and hepatocytes results in immunity to Listeria monocytogenes. *Infect. Immun.* 64:3632–3640.

71. Harty, J.T., and Bevan, M.J. 1992. CD8+ T cells specific for a single nonamer epitope of Listeria monocytogenes are protective in vivo. *J. Exp. Med.* 175:1531–1538.
72. Harty, J.T., and Pamer, E.G. 1995. CD8 T lymphocytes specific for the secreted p60 antigen protect against Listeria monocytogenes infection. *J. Immunol.* 154:4642–4650.
73. Lepay, D.A., Steinman, R.M., Nathan, C.F., Murray, H.W., and Cohn, Z.A. 1985. Liver macrophages in murine listeriosis. Cell-mediated immunity is correlated with an influx of macrophages capable of generating reactive oxygen intermediates. *J. Exp. Med.* 161:1503–1512.
74. Rosen, H., Gordon, S., and North, R.J. 1989. Exacerbation of murine listeriosis by a monoclonal antibody specific for the type 3 complement receptor of myelomonocytic cells. Absence of monocytes at infective foci allows Listeria to multiply in nonphagocytic cells. *J. Exp. Med.* 170:27–37.
75. Dighe, A.S., Campbell, D., Hsieh, C.-S., Clarke, S., Greaves, D.R., Gordon, S., Murphy, K.M., and Schreiber, R.D. 1995. Tissue-specific targeting of cytokine unresponsiveness in transgenic mice. *Immunity* 3:657–666.
76. Portnoy, D.A., Schreiber, R.D., Connelly, P., and Tilney, L. G. 1989. Gamma interferon limits access of Listeria monocytogenes to the macrophage cytoplasm. *J. Exp. Med.* 170:2141–2146.
77. Gregory, S.H., Wing, E.J., Tweardy, D.J., Shadduck, R.K., and Lin, H.S. 1992. Primary listerial infections are exacerbated in mice administered neutralizing antibody to macrophage colony-stimulating factor. *J. Immunol.* 149:188–193.
78. Gregory, S.H., and Wing, E.J. 1993. Macrophage colony-stimulating factor and the enhanced migration of monocytes are essential in primary but not secondary host defenses to Listeria organisms. *J. Infect. Dis.* 168:934–942.
79. Conlan, J.W., and North, R.J. 1991. Neutrophil-mediated dissolution of infected host cells as a defense strategy against a facultative intracellular bacterium. *J. Exp. Med.* 174:741–744.
80. Conlan, J.W., Dunn, P.L., and North, R.J. 1993. Leukocyte-mediated lysis of infected hepatocytes during listeriosis occurs in mice depleted of NK cells or CD4+ CD8+ Thy1.2+ T cells. *Infect. Immun.* 61:2703–2707.
81. Boury, N.M., and Czuprynski, C.J. 1995. Listeria monocytogenes infection increases neutrophil adhesion and damage to a murine hepatocyte cell line in vitro. *Immunol. Lett.* 46:111–116.
82. Seino, K.I., Kayagaki, N., Okumura, K., and Yagita, H. 1997. Antitumor effect of locally produced CD95 ligand. *Nat. Med.* 3:165–170.
83. Kondo, T., Suda, T., Fukuyama, H., Adachi, M., and Nagata, S. 1997. Essential roles of the Fas ligand in the development of hepatitis. *Nat. Med.* 3:409–413.
84. Szalay, G., Hess, J., and Kaufmann, S.H. 1995. Restricted replication of Listeria monocytogenes in a gamma interferon-activated murine hepatocyte line. *Infect. Immun.* 63:3187–3195.
85. Gregory, S.H., and Wing, E.J. 1993. IFN-gamma inhibits the replication of Listeria monocytogenes in hepatocytes. *J. Immunol.* 151:1401–1409.
86. Rogers, H.W., Callery, M.P., Deck, B., and Unanue, E.R. 1996. Listeria monocytogenes induces apoptosis of infected hepatocytes. *J. Immunol.* 156:679–684.
87. Dunn, P.L., and North, R.J. 1991. Early gamma interferon production by natural killer cells is important in defense against murine listeriosis. *Infect. Immun.* 59:2892–2900.

88. Gregory, S.H., Jiang, X., and Wing, E.J. 1996. Lymphokine-activated killer cells lyse Listeria-infected hepatocytes and produce elevated quantities of interferon-gamma. *J. Infect. Dis.* 174:1073–1079.
89. Villanueva, M.S., Beckers, C., and Pamer, E.G. 1994. Infection with Listeria monocytogenes impairs sialic acid addition to host cell glycoproteins. *J. Exp. Med.* 180:2137–2145.
90. Kagi, D., Ledermann, B., Burki, K., Seiler, P., Odermatt, B., Olsen, K.J., Podack, E.R., Zinkernagel, R.M., and Hensgartner, H. 1994. Cytotoxicity mediated by T cells and natural killer cells is greatly impaired in perforin-deficient mice. *Nature* 369:31–37.
91. Kagi, D., Ledermann, B., Burki, K., Hengartner, H., and Zinkernagel, R.M. 1994. CD8+ T cell-mediated protection against an intracellular bacterium by perforin-dependent cytotoxicity. *Eur. J. Immunol.* 24:3068–3072.
92. Boismenu, R., and Havran, W. 1997. An innate view of $\gamma\delta$ T cells. *Curr. Opin. Immunol.* 9:57–63.
93. Hiromatsu, K., Yoshikai, Y., Matsuzaki, G., Ohga, S., Muramori, K., Matsumoto, K., Bluestone, J.A., and Nomoto, K. 1992. A protective role of gamma/delta T cells in primary infection with Listeria monocytogenes in mice. *J. Exp. Med.* 175:49–56.
94. Hiromatsu, K., Matsuzaki, G., Tauchi, Y., Yoshikai, Y., and Nomoto, K. 1992. Sequential analysis of T cells in the liver during murine listerial infection. *J. Immunol.* 149:568–573.
95. Ladel, C.H., Blum, C., and Kaufmann, S.H. 1996. Control of natural killer cell-mediated innate resistance against the intracellular pathogen Listeria monocytogenes by gamma/delta T lymphocytes. *Infect. Immun.* 64:1744–1749.
96. Ferrick, D.A., Schrenzel, M.D., Mulvania, T., Hsieh, B., Ferlin, W.G., and Lepper, H. 1995. Differential production of interferon-gamma and interleukin-4 in response to Th1- and Th2-stimulating pathogens by gamma-delta T cells in vivo. *Nature* 373:255–257.
97. White, D.W., Wilson, R.L., and Harty, J.T. 1996. CD8+ T cells in bacterial infections of mice. *Res. Immunol.* 147:519–524.
98. Shen, H., Miller, J.F., Fan, X., Kolwyck, D., Ahmed, R., and Harty J.T. 1998. Bacterial antigen compartmentalization: differential effects on CD8+ T cell priming and protective immunity. *Cell* 92:535–545.
99. Goossens, P.L., Jouin, H., and Milon, G. 1991. Dynamics of lymphocytes and inflammatory cells recruited in liver during murine listeriosis. A cytofluorimetric study. *J. Immunol.* 147:3514–3520.
100. Goossens, P.L., Marchal, G., and Milon, G. 1992. Transfer of both protection and delayed-type hypersensitivity against live Listeria is mediated by the CD8+ T cell subset: A study with Listeria-specific T lymphocytes recovered from murine infected liver. *Int. Immunol.* 4:591–598.
101. Sasaki, T., Mieno, M., Udono, H., Yamaguchi, K., Usui, T., Hara, K., Shiku, H., and Nakayama, E. 1990. Roles of CD4+ and CD8+ cells, and the effect of administration of recombinant murine interferon gamma in listerial infection. *J. Exp. Med.* 171:1141–1154.
102. Czuprynski, C.J., Brown, J.F., Young, K.M., and Cooley, A.J. 1989. Administration of purified anti-L3T4 monoclonal antibody impairs the resistance of mice to Listeria monocytogenes infection. *Infect. Immun.* 57:100–109.
103. Ehlers, S., Mielke, M.E.A., and Hahn, H. 1994. The mRNA-phenotype of granuloma formation: CD4+ T cell-associated cytokine gene expression during primary murine listeriosis. *Immunobiology* 191:432–440.

104. Appleberg, R., Castro, A.G., and Silva, M.T. 1994. Neutrophils as effector cells of T-cell-mediated, acquired immunity in murine listeriosis. *Immunology* 83:302–307.

105. Czuprynski, C.J., Brown, J.F., Wagner, R.D., and Steinberg, H. 1994. Administration of antigranulocyte monoclonal antibody RB6-8C5 prevents expression of acquired resistance to Listeria monocytogenes infection in previously immunized mice. *Infect. Immun.* 62:5161–5163.

106. Rakhmilevich, A.L. 1995. Neutrophils are essential for resolution of primary and secondary infection with Listeria monocytogenes. *J. Leuk. Biol.* 57:827–831.

107. Tripp, C.S., Kanagawa, O., and Unanue, E.R. 1995. Secondary response to Listeria infection requires IFN-gamma but is partially independent of IL-12. *J. Immunol.* 155:3427–3432.

108. Samsom, J.N., Langermans, J.A., Savelkoul, H.F., and Van, F.R. 1995. Tumour necrosis factor, but not interferon-gamma, is essential for acquired resistance to Listeria monocytogenes during a secondary infection in mice. *Immunology* 86:256–262.

109. Jiang, X., Gregory, S.H., and Wing, E.J. 1997. Immune CD8+ T lymphocytes lyse Listeria monocytogenes-infected hepatocytes by a classical MHC class I-restricted mechanism. *J. Immunol.* 158:287–293.

110. Kagi, D., Ledermann, B., Burki, K., Zinkernagel, R.M., and Hengartner, H. 1996. Molecular mechanisms of lymphocyte-mediated cytotoxicity and their role in imunological protection and pathogenesis. *Annu. Rev. Immunol.* 14:207–232.

111. White, D.W., and Harty, J.T. 1998. Perforin-deficient $CD8^+$ T cells provide immunity to *Listeria monocytogenes* by a mechanism which is independent of CD95 and IFNγ but requires TNFα. *J. Immunol.* 160:898–905.

112. Rakhmilevich, A.L. 1994. Evidence for a significant role of CD4+ T cells in adoptive immunity to Listeria monocytogenes in the liver. *Immunology* 82:249–254.

CHAPTER 9

MALARIA AND THE LIVER: TOLERANCE AND IMMUNITY TO ATTENUATED PLASMODIA SPOROZOITES

URSZULA KRZYCH, MIMI GUEBRE-XABIER, and ROBERT SCHWENK
Walter Reed Army Institute of Research, Washington, DC

MALARIA—AN OVERVIEW

Malaria is one of the major infectious diseases leading to morbidity and mortality of people in tropical areas of the world (1–3). Despite decades of effort devoted to unraveling mechanisms of immune responses that participate in protective immunity to Plasmodia parasites, our understanding remains incomplete. Currently, no effective vaccines are available to prevent the infection, which kills millions of people every year.

Malaria is caused by a protozoan parasite belonging to the genus *Plasmodium*. The parasites have a complex, biphasic life cycle involving an arthropod host, where the sexual stage of development occurs, and vertebrate hosts, where nonsexual development continues. In the vertebrate hosts, the parasite exhibits three distinct phases of infection—the sporozoite-stage, liver-stage, and blood-stage, which occur either extra- or intracellularly in a particular organ. At each stage, unique proteins are expressed that serve as key elements for attachment to and/or invasion of organ-specific cells that have receptors for the respective parasite ligand. The different species of Plasmodia express species-specific proteins, and despite considerable variations both at the DNA and protein level, many proteins display a high degree of structural conservation and contain areas of homology (4). These proteins, under certain conditions, also induce either cellular or antibody responses that provide protective immunity against the infection.

The short extracellular sporozoite stage comprises the release of sporozoites from the mosquito and their transport to the liver and is associated with the expression of

T Lymphocytes in the Liver: Immunobiology, Pathology, and Host Defense, Edited by I. Nicholas Crispe
ISBN 0-471-19218-X

the circumsporozoite (CS) protein, the major sporozoite stage protein that covers the entire parasite (5). Once the parasite enters the liver, it begins to develop into the exoerythrocytic form (EEF) and expresses a new set of proteins, for example, liver-stage antigens (LSA) (6). The erythrocytic stage commences upon the rupture of the infected hepatocyte and invasion of erythrocytes; the latter process defines clinical malaria. The proteins that characterize the erythrocytic stage of the plasmodia parasite include merozoite surface proteins (7) and erythrocyte-binding protein (8), and their roles in the invasion of red blood cells have been intensively studied. The vertebrate phase is completed upon a subsequent feeding by the Anopheles vector, at which point a blood stage gametocyte is taken up to initiate the next cycle, beginning with fertilization and sporogony and resulting in the production of infective sporozoites, which accumulate in the salivary glands of a mosquito and are ready for release into a vertebrate host.

The liver-stage constitutes perhaps the most important phase, since besides expressing an abundant array of new proteins, the parasite undergoes an exponential multiplication, designated schizogony, within each infected hepatocyte. Hence, in contrast to the small number of sporozoites that invade hepatocytes, the liver-stage represents a much larger parasite load and a richer pool of antigens. Moreover, in addition to liver-stage-specific proteins, liver-stage parasites produce protein antigens that belong to the erythrocytic- as well as sporozoite-stage infections. The presence of these antigens in hepatocytes singles out the liver as a major antigen depot for the plasmodial parasite. Presumably this depot is required for the induction of protective immune responses and as the target for humoral and cellular effectors of antimalarial protective immunity.

Natural infection does not lead to a full and stable protective immunity (9). Instead, immunity develops gradually, as clinical manifestations decline with increasing age. The form of immunity that develops allows intermittent episodes of parasitemia to occur, and it decays rapidly once exposure to the parasite ceases. Acquired immunity apparently is directed principally against the blood stage of the parasite and is mediated by protective antibodies, which decline rapidly in the absence of continued exposure. The reasons for this poor immunogenicity to malaria parasite are not completely understood. Whereas it may stem from inadequate immunizing doses or infrequent exposure, such as occurs in hypoendemic areas, it must be considered as a means whereby the parasite efficiently ensures its survival by evading a full engagement of the host's immune system. It perhaps is the choice of the immunologically tolerant liver as the venue for the parasite's nonsexual reproduction that allows the parasite to adapt so well to the otherwise formidable consequences of the host's immune surveillance.

In contrast to observations made during natural infection, in the model system involving exposure to attenuated sporozoites there is longer-lasting protective immunity to an infectious sporozoite challenge (10). The attenuated sporozoites fail to establish an erythrocytic stage infection, but continue to develop into liver-stage parasites. It is believed that the accumulation of aborted parasites in the liver leads to the induction of cellular and antibody responses mediating protective immunity, by mechanisms that are currently poorly understood. To maintain this form of sterile protection, however, periodic boost immunizations with attenuated sporozoites are required. The observations and hypotheses surrounding immunological responses to exoerythrocytic antigens that are induced and/or occur in the liver will be the topic of this chapter. Therefore, we shall concentrate on mechanisms of immunity in human and rodent models of radiation-attenuated plasmodial sporozoites, rather than providing an exhaustive review of the ample literature on immune responses considered to play a role in antimalarial protective immunity.

PLASMODIA COLONIZATION OF THE LIVER

Segue of Sporozoites from the Skin to the Liver

Malaria infection is initiated when sporozoites are released from the salivary glands of the plasmodia-infected anopheles mosquito to the bloodstream of the host (Fig. 9.1). Although the number of sporozoites introduced during a single blood meal has not been determined in the field, on the basis of laboratory data, it is estimated that the median number of parasites ranges from 6 to 15 (11,12). It is also known that intravenous injection of as few as two sporozoites can initiate malaria infection (13,14). The injected sporozoites quickly travel via blood from the skin to the liver, where they invade a few hepatocytes, undergo transformation into liver-stage parasites, and amplify their numbers to thousands of merozoites. It is not known if the sporozoite performs this segue solo, depending only on being swept by the bloodstream, or whether it is aided by any transport cells or proteins.

Entry of Sporozoites into the Liver

In contrast to the well-understood mechanisms surrounding invasion of erythrocytes by the parasite (15), information on sporozoite invasion of the liver is incomplete and controversial. Nevertheless, some detailing of these processes is essential for consideration of immunity to the parasite antigens that develops during this phase. Indeed, the exoerythrocytic liver phase is considered pivotal not only for survival of the parasite but also as a significant phase for the induction of the antimalarial immune response.

Electron microscopic studies in rodents showed that *Plasmodium berghei* sporozoites localize in the sinusoid or in the endocytic vacuoles of Kupffer cells (16). Because a Kupffer cell containing a parasite was observed in the space of Disse adjacent to hepatocytes, which were visualized as being invaded by the apical end of the sporozoite, it was suggested that Kupffer cells trap and then transport sporozoites from the sinusoidal lumen across the Disse space to hepatocytes. This interpretation is rather difficult to reconcile with the fact that Kupffer cells are antigen presenting cells (APC) (17), and consequently metabolically degrade the trapped parasite, which would clearly interfere with the sporozoite survival. Observations which indicate that sporozoites appear first in hepatocytes, and only later in Kupffer cells, already altered by destruction in endocytic vacuoles (18,19) seem to be a more reliable guide to the actual process.

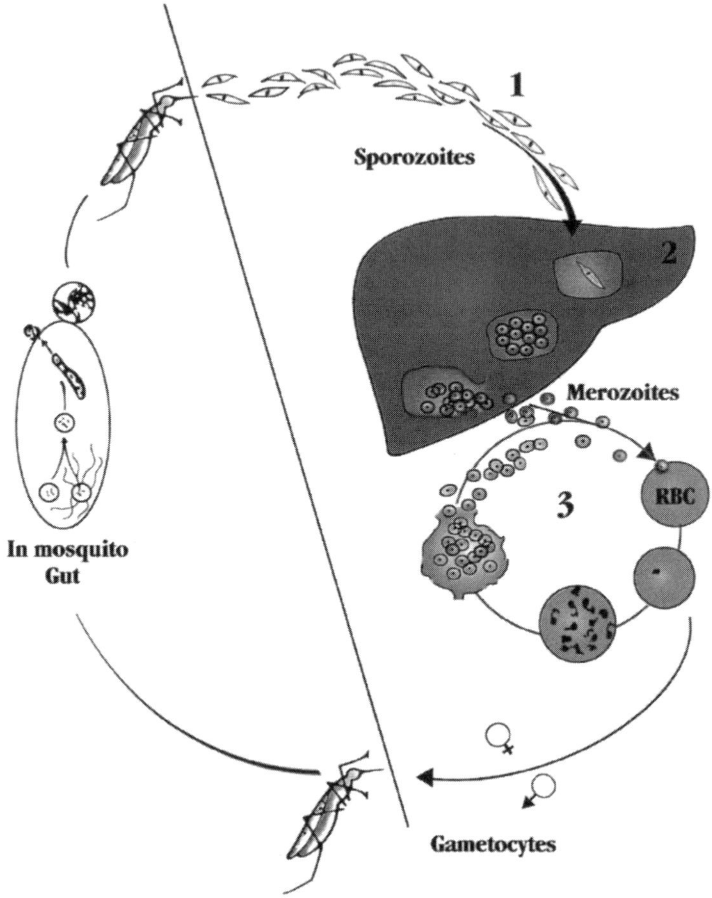

Figure 9.1. The model illustrates the life cyle of vertebrate segment of Plasmodia ssp., including (1) sporozoite-, (2) liver-, and (3) blood-stage infections. Briefly, a few sporozoites enter the bloodstream of a host during an Anopheles blood meal. The sporozoites are quickly removed by the liver and upon invasion of hepatocytes (H), initiate liver-stage infection. The formation of the exoerythrocytic forms is marked by the synthesis of proteins that belong to this and also to the blood-stage of development. In addition, sporozoites undergo amplification or schizogony. Upon completion of this developmental process, the liver merozoites are released from the ruptured hepatocytes and quickly invade red blood cells, to initiate the final stage of vertebrate infection. During the blood-stage, formation of gametocytes occurs for the initiation of the next cycle, which begins with the next mosquito blood meal.

Why would any sporozoite be found in the Kupffer cells? It is possible that only those sporozoites that fail to invade the liver end up in the Kupffer cells and that these are processed into antigenic forms for T cell activation. For example, mutation-induced changes in the surface protein, radiation-induced attenuation, or other developmental abnormalities may change the course of travel of some sporozoites and redirect them away from hepatocytes to Kupffer cells (Fig. 9.2). Another possibility is that if the invading sporozoites can, by still unknown mechanisms, paralyze Kupffer cells, they may thereby cancel or interfere with the scavenging of foreign particles and antigen processing and presentation that are properties of Kupffer cells. The parasite may then utilize the mobility of Kupffer cells, to its own advantage, for transport to hepatocytes. It has been shown that the blood-stage forms reduce phagocytic activity of circulating monocytes and possibly interfere with their function as presenting or costimulatory cells (20). The alleged paralysis of the Kupffer cells would constitute yet another mechanism by which the parasite skillfully evades the immune system of the host. Whatever the mechanism, the results from ultrastructural approaches to localize the sporozoites are difficult to interpret because very few sporozoites can be visualized ($<0.001\%$). Results of experiments examining trafficking of sporozoites through the liver of rodents during targeted destruction of Kupffer cells are equally difficult to interpret (21–23). Whereas some results point to an increased malaria infection (22), others show that Kupffer cells inhibited malaria infection (23).

Several experimental approaches have been devised to study direct interaction between macrophages or Kupffer cells and sporozoites *in vitro*. In an elegant experiment, Vandeberg and Stuart, using video microscopy, showed that although sporozoites approach macrophages, the parasites are very seldom captured by these cells. Instead, the parasite enters the macrophage and destroys it (24). In a separate study by colleagues at the Walter Reed Army Institute of Research (WRAIR), no association between sporozoites and Kupffer cells was observed (25) unless sporozoite immune serum was added, which facilitated the interaction between Kupffer cells and sporozoites and led to killing of the parasite. It is presumed that the sporozoites became opsonized and then internalized by Kupffer cells. The minimal interaction between the sporozoites and macrophages or Kupffer cells suggests that Kupffer cells do not facilitate the sporozoite invasion of hepatocytes. It seems more likely that the parasite may avoid destruction by the APC unless it has been attenuated by radiation or captured by antisporozoite antibodies, which may redirect its course from the hepatocytes to Kupffer cells.

Based on these observations, a picture emerges suggesting that sporozoite trafficking to the liver, invasion of hepatocytes, and continued development into liver merozoites are influenced by a prior immunological history involving plasmodial antigens. Because the preexisting immune milieu greatly alters the process of sporozoite infection, it also complicates data analysis and interpretation of results. Therefore, an alternative approach to studies of in vivo infection with sporozoites was devised, based on the possibility that sporozoites invade hepatocytes directly, bypassing the Kupffer cells altogether. It was also reasoned that the CS protein may contain the ligand for binding to hepatocytes, because it has been observed that sporozoites invaded hepatoma cell lines (26) and hepatocytes in primary culture (27) and that peptides representing CS protein-conserved Region I bound specifically to the hepatoma cells (28).

These studies were possible largely through the efforts of gene cloning and recombinant DNA technology, as well as production of monoclonal antibodies, which enabled identification and production of proteins associated with the various stages of the parasite life cycle. The CS protein (5), associated with the sporozoite stage, is a

35- to 45-kD glycoprotein, with a centrally located region consisting of sets of repeating octomer or quatramer amino acid motifs that define each species of Plasmodia. The central repeat region is flanked by two highly conserved regions, Region I and Region II plus. Region I is composed of the amino acids KLKQP and is located on the N-terminal boundary of the repeats. Region II plus is located in the C-terminal end of the protein and is also found in another protein of the plasmodia sporozoite stage, designated thrombospondin-related anonymous protein (TRAP) (29), or sporozoite surface protein 2 (SSP2) (30). It contains the known cell adhesion motif also found in thrombospondin and the complement components (31), F-spondin (32) and Unc-5 (33), proteins involved in the development of the nervous system, as well as Etp 100, a protein from the coccidian parasite, *Eimeria tenella* (34).

Data obtained primarily from *in vitro* experiments demonstrate that the binding of sporozoites to liver cell lines involves interaction between CS protein Region II plus and glycosaminoglycan chains of heparan sulfate proteoglycans on the surface of hepatocytes (35). This hypothesis has been supported further by observations showing specific binding of two sporozoite surface proteins, CS protein and SSP2, to the basolateral domain of hepatocytes (36,37). Furthermore, constructs containing Region II plus bound to frozen tissue sections and immunoelectron microscopy revealed that CS protein was bound exclusively on the microvilli of the basolateral region of hepatocytes in the space of Disse, a portion exposed to the circulation, but was not bound to Kupffer cells or to sections of other organs, including spleen, brain, lung, heart, and others (19). The observation that CS protein Region II plus binds to hepatocytes has been corroborated by many other studies, including experiments in vivo showing patterns of recombinant CS protein homing to the liver (38). The latter study also suggested that a certain degree of configurational preservation of the CS protein may be required for binding to hepatocytes. It has been assumed that sporozoites might bind to the liver by the same mechanism. This notion is supported by the observation that fucoidan, a branched polymer of sulfated fucose, inhibits malaria infection and also delays clearance of CS protein from circulation (19,39). In other experiments, it was found that agents that bind to heparan sulfate proteoglycans also delayed clearance of CS protein and decreased the efficiency of sporozoite infection in mice (19).

The importance of these observations needs to be interpreted in relation to liver histology. Such orientation will allow better insight into the reason why plasmodial sporozoites home to the liver to continue their development and exponential amplification in the vertebrate hosts, hence increasing the antigenic load for the host. The liver is composed of hepatocyte sheets that line vascular sinusoids and of endothelial cells lining these sinusoids. The unique feature of the endothelial cell lining in the liver is its open fenestration and lack of a basement membrane. The endothelial cells are separated from the underlying hepatocytes by a loose extracellular space called the space of Disse, where Kupffer cells migrate to clear foreign particles, including antigens like sporozoites, from the blood. Hepatocyte microvilli lie behind the fenestration of the endothelial cells in the space of Disse, which presumably allows the hepatocytes direct contact with the sporozoites (40). According to one hypothesis, the long glycosaminoglycan chains of the heparan sulfate proteoglycans protrude through the fenestrae of the endothelial cells into the sinusoid and trap the sporozoites (40).

Another possibility is that the fenestrae are quite flexible, and by increasing their diameter during sporozoite infection, they allow the sporozoite direct contact with the hepatocyte microvilli (19).

Invasion of Hepatocytes and Development of Exoerythrocytic Forms

The next phase of the liver-stage infection is the invasion of hepatocytes by sporozoites. Whether attachment and invasion constitute distinct events or a single event during liver infection has not been well established. In general, the mechanisms governing these stages of infection and the subsequent rupture of the infected hepatocytes remain poorly understood. This process must accommodate sporozoite detachment from the glycosaminoglycan chains, which is believed to require the shedding of the CS protein–heparan sulfate proteoglycans complexes (19). It has been shown *in vitro* that in the presence of anti-repeat antibodies, the CS protein is shed from sporozoites (41), and if they remain viable, a new CS protein is reexpressed (42,43). It has been speculated that this represents the situation in vivo, including resynthesis of CS protein on sporozoites internalized by hepatocytes (44). Based on studies of the plasmodial invasion of erythrocytes, micronemes and rhoptries are membranous vesicles that are involved during merozoite invasion of red cells and their contents contribute to the formation of the parasitophorous vacuole (15). Both micronemes and rhoptries are also found in sporozoites, and the TRAP/SSP2 localizes in these organelles, suggesting that, unlike CS protein, it may be involved in the invasion of hepatocytes (45). Currently, all these processes remain speculative, as mechanisms of infection of hepatocytes have not been fully elucidated; however, they are believed to occur by a chain of successive interactions involving a spate of molecules (46)

During the liver-stage, the inner membrane and subpellicular microtubules of the thin sporozoite break down shortly after invasion, creating a uninucleated trophozoite measuring 3–5 μm in diameter, which is bound by a plasma membrane and situated in a parasitophorous vacuole (47). When the trophozoite develops into a mature liver-stage schizont, it occupies most of the volume of the hepatocyte (48,49). In the case of relapsing malaria caused by *P. vivax* and *P. ovale*, the characteristic hypnozoite (the latent form of parasite persisting in the liver) is arrested as a small (5 μm in diameter) trophozoite (50), and the liver-stage can last for up to 3 years after sporozoite infection. The mechanisms responsible for the relapse remain unknown.

The duration of the liver-stage infection varies among Plasmodia species. It has been established that the liver-stage of the *P. berghei* and *P. yoelii* life cycle lasts for 2 days (51), and for the human malaria parasites (49) for a considerably longer time, 5–14 days. It is also possible that the primary liver-stage may last for 6 to 12 months. During schizogony of *P. berghei* and *P. yoelii*, the development and amplification of mature exoerythrocytic schizonts results in at least 2,000 uninucleated merozoites (51). In contrast, *P. falciparum* exoerythrocytic schizonts form around 30,000 merozoites within a schizont that is 80–100 μm in diameter (52). During schizogony, parasite antigens are found in the parasitophorous membrane, which forms deep invaginations into the infected hepatocyte (53), proximal to the hepatocyte nucleus (48). The cytoplasm of infected hepatocytes contains some parasite proteins (48), but

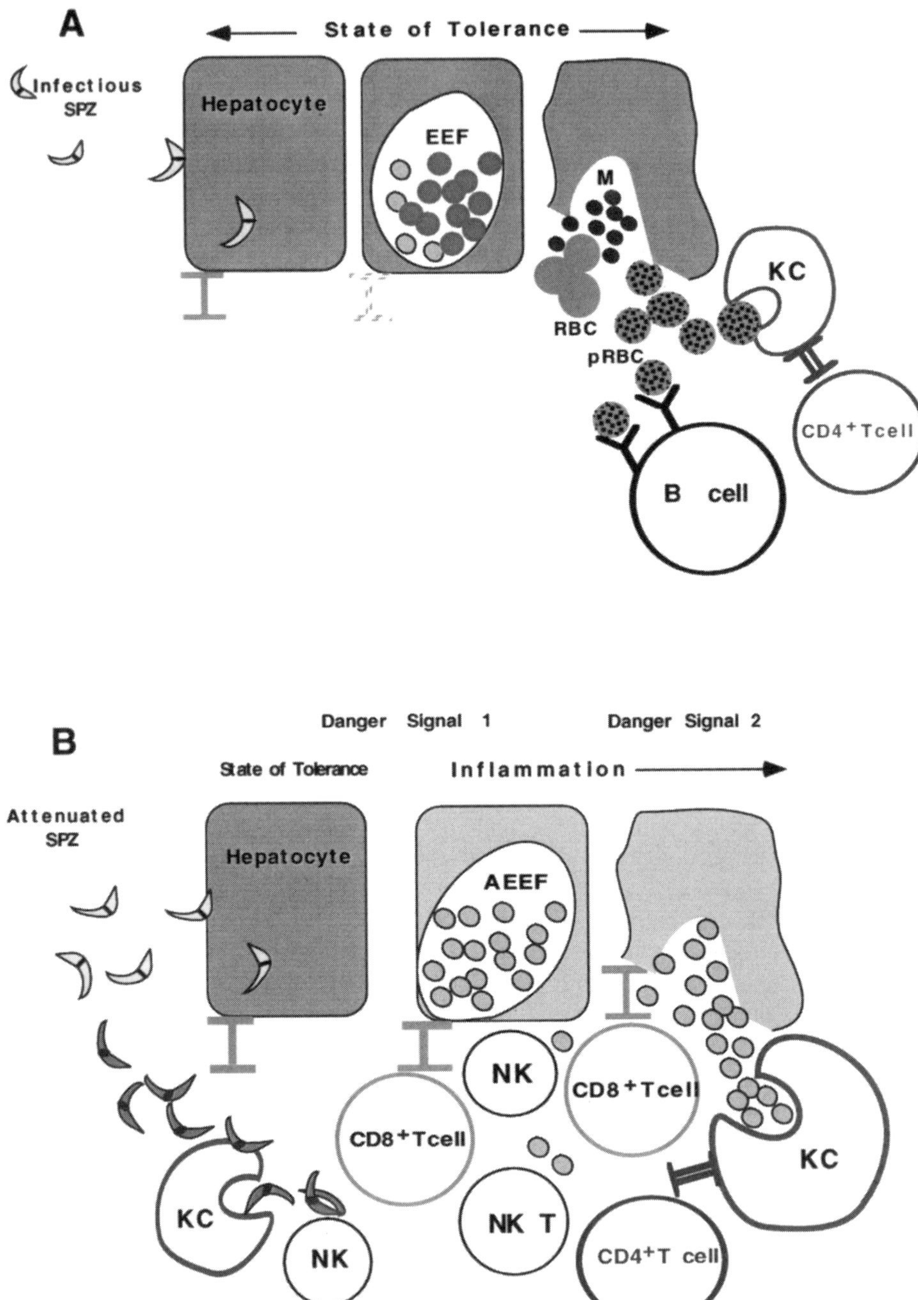
A
State of Tolerance
Infectious SPZ
Hepatocyte
EEF
M
RBC
pRBC
KC
CD4+Tcell
B cell
B
Danger Signal 1
Danger Signal 2
State of Tolerance
Inflammation
Attenuated SPZ
Hepatocyte
AEEF
NK
CD8+Tcell
CD8+Tcell
KC
NK T
CD4+T cell
KC
NK

apart from a single report (54) no parasite antigens have been detected microscopically on the hepatocyte surface. After rupture of infected hepatocytes, merozoites are released to invade erythrocytes. At this point, they may also be phagocytized by Kupffer cells (55) (Fig. 9.2).

By current immunological and/or molecular technologies, several proteins have been identified in hepatocytes infected with sporozoites. Although CS protein is thought to be carried into the hepatocytes, there is no evidence for its transcription or translation within hepatocytes (56). SSP2 is detected on the sporozoite surface and

Figure 9.2. A switch from a state of tolerance to a localized inflammation in the liver promotes development of Plasmodia antigen–specific cellular immunity. The model depicts our view of contrasting events that occur within the liver following exposure to (**A**) infectious and (**B**) attenuated sporozoites (SPZ). Liver, as an organ, prevails in a state of immunological tolerance to antigens expressed within its tissue, and this condition shields Plasmodia parasites from immune attack by the host, thus allowing development into exoerythrocytic forms (EEF). The liver-specific tolerance is mediated in part by IL-10, a cytokine produced by hepatocytes to downregulate proinflammatory responses that are constantly arising to toxins and other debris trafficking through the liver, and also by mechanisms operating to eliminate effector lymphocytes.

(**A**). Very few infectious SPZ are released into the bloodstream, whereupon they rapidly invade a small number of hepatocytes without causing malarial symptoms or a marked liver pathology, including inflammation. The hepatocytes remain intact during schizogony but they may lose MHC molecules, which prevents the induction of Plasmodia antigen–specific effector T cells. Upon the rupture of hepatocytes, liver merozoites (M) parasitize the red blood cells (pRBC). Although Kupffer cells (KC) phagocytize some pRBC, most escape phagocytic elimination and enter the circulation, where they continue their propagation as blood-stage merozoites, a manifestation of malaria infection. The unabated production of IL-10 regulates the APC activity of Kupffer cells; nonetheless these cells might still present erythrocytic antigens to T helper cells to promote T–B cell interaction for an antibody response, which constitutes a form of protective immunity against blood-stage parasites.

(**B**). Attenuation of SPZ does not inhibit, but may limit, their invasion of the liver, hence directing some SPZs to activate KCs or natural killer cells (NK). These interactions initiate a first localized "danger signal" within the liver. Attenuated SPZs that do invade hepatocytes develop into aborted exoerythrocytic forms (AEEF) unable to invade RBCs. The AEEFs accumulate within the infected hepatocyte and become metabolically degraded for presentation by intact or ruptured hepatocytes via MHC class I molecules to the respective $CD8^+$ T cells; upon hepatocyte rupture, the AEEFs also become phagocytized by Kupffer cells, a second danger signal, which enhances the inflammatory response, and also induces $CD4^+$ T cells. Activated $CD8^+$ and $CD4^+$ effector T cells secrete INF(rom), thus completing a local switch from a state of tolerance to inflammation, an uninhabitable milieu for the parasite. The inflammatory condition is, however, only temporary, and liver homeostasis is restored, presumably by IL-10 or the NK-T cells, which secrete IL-4 in response to Plasmodia antigens expressed in the liver.

throughout the liver-stage in *P. yoelii* infected hepatocytes (57). TRAP is present on the surfaces and in the micronemes of sporozoites and for a short time during the liver-stage of *P. falciparum* (58). A liver-stage characteristic protein that is detected throughout liver schizogony and increases with the maturation process is *P. falciparum* liver-stage antigen-1 (LSA-1) (59). LSA-1 is localized to flocculent material in the parasitophorous vacuole, which forms a stroma into which hepatic merozoites are released (59). The gene for LSA-1 of NF54 strain of *P. falciparum* encodes a 230-kD acidic protein containing 86 copies of the 17 amino-acid repeat sequence EQQSDLEQERLAKEKLQ (60), which is flanked by relatively invariant nonrepeat regions (59). A possible analog of LSA-1 has been found on the parasitophorous membrane of *P. berghei* and has been termed LSA-2 (53). Other proteins that have been found in association with the liver-stage infection caused by either *P. falciparum*, *P. berghei*, *P. yoelii*, *P. reichenowi*, or *P. chabaudi* include PyHEP17/PfEXP-1 (61), sporozoite threonine- and asparagine-rich protein (STARP) (62), SALSA (56), LSA-3 (63), Pbl.1 (64), PfMSP-1 (44), PfEMP2 (44).

Two main events that highlight the liver phase of the plasmodial parasite life cycle are the synthesis of newly expressed antigenic proteins, some of which belong to this phase as well as to a subsequent blood-stage infection (44), and the amplification of the parasites within a single hepatocyte. Although such events would typically engender a cascade of specific immune responses, the liver-phase infection occurs in the virtual absence of any symptoms or signs of malaria or pathology associated with the invasion of the liver. Even if some inflammatory responses do occur, they are usually transitory and do not lead to sustained immunity involving induction of effector or memory T cell responses.

CELLULAR IMMUNITY TO EXOERYTHROCYTIC FORMS OF PLASMODIA

Natural Immunity

Natural exposure to Plasmodia does not generally lead to full sterile immunity, but to responses that only partially ameliorate the illness. Protection induced by natural exposure also develops gradually, and clinical manifestations of infection decline with increasing age (3). This immunity is, however, short lived; immune individuals leaving endemic areas rapidly develop susceptibility to reinfection. It is generally believed that acquired immunity after repeated infection is principally directed against the blood-stage of the parasite antigens or toxins, and is not directed against developing liver-stage parasites (9). Although naturally induced preerythrocytic "sterile" immunity probably exists in some individuals, it has been difficult to confirm experimentally. A decline in protective antibodies following departure from endemic areas is thought to be responsible for the loss of immunity.

Based on observations describing the efficient invasion of target cells, hepatocytes, and subsequently red blood cells by the parasites, it is likely that both the sporozoites and liver-stage merozoites leave a limited opportunity for the intervention of host immune cells. The infectious sporozoites are rapidly taken up by the liver and become shielded intrahepatically from the intruding host immune cells; likewise, the numerous mature liver merozoites that are released from the ruptured hepatocytes quickly invade mature erythrocytes, which are considered to be inefficient APCs because they lack major histocompatibility complex (MHC) molecules. Consequently, neither malarial symptoms nor pathology occur during liver infection, which greatly reduces any possibility for the requisite "danger signals" (65) to initiate anti-plasmodial acquired immune responses for elimination of the parasite (Fig. 9.2A). Instead, the liver, with its persistent tolerant state, might even promote the growth and development of the parasite by controlling the emergence of any inflammatory or immune condition (66). Ample data from the transplantation literature describe the liver as an immunologically privileged site. A constant state of tolerance to any antigens expressed within the hepatocytes persists in the liver and such tolerance has far-reaching effects because it induces systemic tolerance. For example, in rodent models, allogeneic liver transplants can induce tolerance to donor MHC antigens by downregulating the expression of clonotypic T cell receptor and CD8 molecules or by T cell deletion (67). Other studies have suggested that by constitutively producing interleukin-10 (IL-10), the liver downregulates the intrahepatic lymphocytes and macrophages, including Kupffer cells (68). These mechanisms, although quite attractive, are not well understood and their relevance to malaria immunity is currently unclear.

There is, however, some evidence that natural infection induces immunity against plasmodial liver-stage antigens. LSA-specific $CD8^+$ cytolytic T cells have been detected in persons bearing the B53 HLA haplotype (69). Correlation between the appearance of these cells in the periphery and the severity of infection has been proposed (70). This observation, in particular, strengthens the notion that antigens derived from intracellular parasites activate $CD8^+$ effector T cells.

If, for the sake of argument, we accept the preerythrocytic contributions to naturally acquired immunity, tolerance-mediated elimination of $CD8^+$ T cells in the liver (71) may be one explanation for the need for constant reexposure to malaria parasites. Although cytolytic T cells specific for LSA, CS protein, and TRAP (72) have been detected in the peripheral blood of residents of endemic areas, the kinetics of these responses has not been well investigated. Whether the trafficking of these T cells might be regulated by inflammation or induction of tolerance in the liver remains unknown.

Attenuated Sporozoite Model of Protective Immunity

In contrast to naturally induced immune responses, sterile lasting protection has been achieved in human (73,74) and rodent models (75) by exposure to bites from mosquitoes infected by radiation-attenuated Plasmodia sporozoites. This form of immunity prevents the development of the erythrocytic-stage infection in response to sporozoite challenge. Although attenuated sporozoites fail to establish an erythrocytic-stage infection, they invade the liver, carrying with them the sporozoite-stage-associated antigens, CS protein, and SSP2 (10). While in the liver, sporozoites undergo aborted development into schizonts (10), expressing liver- and blood-stage antigens (76). Protection that is induced by attenuated sporozoites arises precisely because the aborted extraerythrocytic forms are either retained within hepatocytes or, unable to invade red blood cells when released from ruptured hepatocytes, are trapped by Kupffer cells (Fig. 9.2B). Although formal proof is still missing, it is thought that Kupffer cells activated by attenuated sporozoites and by aborted liver-stage parasites initiate the cascade of proinflammatory cytokines, leading to temporary local inflammation, which is perceived as a "danger signal" by the acquired immune system (65). However temporary, local inflammation is presumed to downregulate the tolerant state in the liver and in turn to promote the induction of liver-antigen-specific effector T cells.

The Switch from Tolerance to Danger Signal

If tolerance indeed prevails in the liver, then some mechanism must account for the long-lasting protection that the attenuated sporozoite model induces in rodents and humans. It is likely that the constitutive production of IL-10 by hepatocytes (reference 68, and K. Fedegin, personal communication) may be reversed by the release of accumulated schizonts, which can cause a proinflammatory local milieu. Such a reversal of tolerance has been achieved in mice expressing liver alloantigens in the presence of IL-2, and by immunization with bacteria (77). The "danger signal" may initiate the innate immunity required to overcome tolerance and lead to an induction of immune responses by T cells and macrophages residing in the liver. This may also be the critical event that determines the unique process of immunity induced with attenuated versus infectious sporozoites and which leads to such a strikingly different outcome: protection versus malaria infection.

Under physiological, noninfectious conditions, there are several types of mononuclear cells in the liver: the mainstream lymphocytes that are closely linked to the circulating mononuclear pool, which includes $CD4^+$ and $CD8^+$ T cells that arose from the intrathymic differentiation pathway (71); the alternative lymphocytes, consisting mainly of T cells expressing both T cell receptor of intermediate intensity and the $NK1.1^+$ surface marker (78,79); and monocytic cells, including Kupffer and dendritic cells. Since the liver is the initial target organ where intracellular development of the parasite occurs, this initial parasite–host intracellular interaction is marked by the presence of activated cells within the liver. Although the composition of these cells is fairly well established, we need to investigate whether the intrahepatic mononuclear cells represent (i) liver-resident cells, (ii) cells recruited from the periphery, or (iii) a combination of resident cells and cells recruited to the liver extravascular spaces by a pathogen with hepatic tropism.

Inflammation in the Liver

Most of the studies addressing the involvement of lymphocyte responses to Plasmodia antigens have examined peripheral blood mononuclear cells or spleen cells, and only recently has the search shifted toward analysis of liver lymphocytes. The early studies relied primarily on immunohistopathological techniques for the analysis of livers from animals immunized with sporozoites. Regions surrounding the developing parasites show infiltration by predominantly mononuclear cells and neutrophils (80). The composition of the cellular infiltrate and the kinetics of migration of the cells to the site of infection depend on the strain and pathogenicity of the parasite and also the method of immunization. Whereas cellular infiltrates and granuloma formation occur in the livers of attenuated sporozoite-immune mice challenged with infectious sporozoites, few, if any, infiltrates are detected in livers of sporozoite-naive mice challenged with infectious sporozoites (81). In animals immunized with attenuated sporozoites, infectious sporozoite challenge induces lymphocyte-rich infiltrates surrounding malaria-infected hepatocytes, whereas in immunologically naive mice the cellular response occurs at the time of the release of merozoites into the bloodstream and comprises predominantly inflammatory mononuclear cells with few T cells (82,83).

In frozen liver sections from attenuated sporozoite-immune rodents, probing with immunofluorescent labeling reveals the presence of $CD8^+$ and $CD4^+$ T cells and macrophages. The infiltrates show a significant (6-fold) increase in the number of $CD8^+$ T cells after sporozoite challenge, with no increase in the number of $CD4^+$ T cells (82). In a similar experiment, Khan et al. (80) demonstrated that protection induced with radiation-attenuated sporozoites correlated with the existence of cellular infiltrates in the liver. Attenuated sporozoite-immune and sporozoite-challenged mice have displayed moderate nonspecific histopathological changes in the liver parenchyma, but 35 % of the breakthrough schizonts have been infiltrated by inflammatory cells. Control mice as well as mice immunized with denatured sporozoites and challenged with live sporozoites have developed moderate nonspecific histopathological changes, since the surviving hepatic schizonts were not infiltrated by inflammatory cells. Cellular infiltration of breakthrough schizonts occurs much earlier in immune animals, indicating T cell–specific recognition of intact hepatocytes containing developing schizonts. Depletion of $CD4^+$ or $CD8^+$ T cells with specific monoclonal antibodies abrogates the inflammatory response after challenge immunization, suggesting that the infiltrates are secondary to an earlier induction of specific lymphocytes (80).

We have recently conducted a cytofluorometric analysis of lymphocytes residing in the liver. The results showed that immunization with attenuated *P. berghei* sporozoites induces lymphocytes to undergo blast transformation without causing an increase in the absolute number of liver lymphocytes in comparison to nonimmune naive control animals (R. Schwenk, M. Guebre-Xabier, and U. Krzych, manuscript in preparation). Similar observations have been made with a nonlethal strain of *P. yoelii* (84,85). The absolute numbers of $CD3^+$, $CD3^+CD4^-CD8^-$, and $CD3^+CD4^+$ T cells, as well as B cells, were comparable in immunized and naive mice, although the number of $CD3^+CD8^+$ T cells increased slightly after immunization with attenuated sporozoites. In contrast, mice that received infective sporozoites or parasitized red blood cells developed a self-healing hepatic and erythrocytic infection accompanied by an increase in the total number of mononuclear cells, including T lymphocytes (84). In a separate study, livers from sporozoite-naive mice challenged with a lethal strain of *P. berghei* also showed an increase in total cell number, but the percentage of $CD4^+$, $CD8^+$ T cells and B cells decreased significantly by day 4 after the challenge, and this decrease coincided with the detection of blood-stage parasites in these mice (R. Schwenk, M.Guebre-Xabier, and U. Krzych, manuscript in preparation). Taken together, these studies point to the $CD8^+$ T cells as the dominant intrahepatic T cell subset responding to Plasmodia antigens during protective immunity induced by attenuated sporozoites. This is in agreement with the widely accepted view that $CD8^+$ T cells are the central players mediating protection induced after immunization with attenuated sporozoites (86–88).

Memory $CD8^+$ T Cells in the Liver

In parallel with the above experiments, we have examined $CD4^+$ and $CD8^+$ T cells resident in the liver for the expression of CD45RB, a memory cell marker that is expressed either as $CD45RB^{hi}$ (bright) or as $CD45RB^{lo}$ (dim) depending on the degree of antigenic exposure and the state of cellular maturation (89). In immunologically naive mice, T cells express $CD45RB^{hi}$, and with increased antigenic exposure they switch to the $CD45RB^{lo}$ phenotype, indicating a mature stage of the primed T cells. We have observed that multiple immunizations with attenuated sporozoites are required to induce increased expression of $CD45RB^{lo}$ on $CD8^+$ T cells and that the memory marker is maintained on the $CD8^+$ T cells for at least 5 days after the challenge. In marked contrast, the switch from $CD45RB^{hi}$ to $CD45RB^{lo}$ on $CD4^+$ T cells occurred after the second immunization; expression, however, was transient, as by day 5 most of the $CD4^+$ T cells reverted to the RB^{hi} phenotype. This observation demonstrating separate kinetics of CD45RB expression on $CD4^+$ and $CD8^+$ T cells suggests that the (memory) $CD8^+$ T cells might depend on some inducing properties from the transiently activated $CD4^+$ T cells.

Regulatory Interaction between $CD4^+$ and $CD8^+$ T cells in the Liver

Based on observations demonstrating the importance of $CD8^+$ T cells during immunization with attenuated plasmodial sporozoites, we reasoned that this T cell subset might be distinguished by expression of other cell surface markers, most notably, IL-2R (CD25). A preliminary analysis of liver-resident T cells from C57Bl/6 mice after immunization with attenuated *P. berghei* sporozoites revealed upregulated expression of CD25 on $CD4^+$ T cells. In contrast, no changes in CD25 expression were noted on liver-resident $CD8^+$ T cells obtained from the same mice. Interestingly, challenge of sporozoite-immune mice with infectious sporozoites reversed the expression of CD25, which now appeared on $CD8^+$ T cells, while levels on $CD4^+$ T cells returned to baseline. This behavior is comparable to the expression of CD25 on naive mice receiving a challenge dose of infectious sporozoites. These results underscore the absolute requirement for liver-activated $CD8^+$ T cells during the effector phase of protective immunity to *P. berghei* sporozoites (86) and the need for $CD4^+$ T cells during the induction of protective immunity with attenuated sporozoites (90). Finally, these observations support the notion that intact and radiation-attenuated sporozoites might undergo unique antigen presentation that selectively favors activation of $CD8^+$ T cells and $CD4^+$ T cells.

The Role of $CD8^+$ T Cells—Cytolytic Responses

On the basis of observations from the attenuated-sporozoite model, it has now been widely accepted that cytolytic T lymphocytes (CTL) are the predominant anti-preerythrocytic-stage effector cells (87,91–93). $CD8^+$ CTL specific for class I MHC-associated peptides from CS protein and SSP2 have been found in both murine (13,14,87,92,93) and human (91,94) lymphocytes exposed to irradiated sporozoites, and CTL specific for LSA peptides have been shown in persons living in areas of malaria hyperendemicity (69). The involvement of $CD8^+$ T cells has been corroborated in studies showing that systemic depletion of these cells (87) interferes with protective immunity and conversely that adoptive transfer of $CD8^+$ T cell clones specific for CS protein (88,95) prevents parasitemia induced by infectious sporozoites. Furthermore, reduction of the parasite load has been noted in livers of protected animals in comparison to nonimmune controls (96). Upon adoptive transfer of CS protein-specific cloned $CD8^+$ T cells, it was observed that these cells homed to the liver and localized in direct apposition to an infected hepatocyte (95). Although the view favoring targeting of sporozoite-infected cells by cytolytic CD8+ T cells via a mechanism described for virally infected target cells has prevailed for more than a decade, it has recently begun to undergo certain modifications. An alternative hypothesis is advanced based on the concept of lymphokine-mediated parasite killing, involving mainly interferon-γ (INFγ), which leads to inducible nitric oxide synthetase (iNOS) (82) upregulation. Because the system is complex and may depend upon a network of integrated immune responses, more work is required before the mechanisms can be fully understood.

Cytokines in Liver-Stage Immunity

Although T cells and macrophages are the major effector cells providing parasite-specific immunity in the liver, it is likely that these cells mediate their effects in part through the elaboration of different cytokines. As a pro-inflammatory cytokine, IL-12 exerts potent effects that regulate T-cell-mediated immunity (97). It facilitates $CD8^+$ T cell responses (98) and induces expansion of $CD4^+$ Th1-type cells from naive T cells (99). The activated $CD4^+$ T cells produce IL-2 and IFNγ to accomplish cell-mediated responses, which ultimately regulate Th2-type reactivities by inhibiting production of IL-10. However, the regulatory interactions between IL-12 and IL-10 in the liver during immunization with Plasmodia sporozoites have not yet been addressed. Instead, studies have analyzed the effects of IL-12 administered in vivo on the course of protective immunity. Protection against *P. yoelii* sporozoites can be achieved by multiple treatments with recombinant IL-12 before challenge with infectious sporozoites (100). The timing of rIL-12 administration appears to be critical, as it is effective only if given before the challenge. This observation supports our hypothesis that in order to achieve protection, an inflammatory milieu in the liver must be established before sporozoite infection.

Although we are not privy to the mechanisms of IL-12 function, it is believed that regulation of IL-10 by IL-12 shifts the immunologically tolerant liver into an immunoreactive organ where induction of Plasmodia antigen-specific T cell responses can occur. The protective activity of IL-12 can be reversed by monoclonal antibody (mAb) to IFNγ, thus indicating that IL-12 acts through the production of IFNγ (100).

We have previously shown (101) that immunization with attenuated *P. berghei* sporozoites induces Th1-type cells to secrete IL-2 and IFNγ, and a recently published study (102) showed that systemic administration of rIL-12 resulted in acute liver graft rejection. According to these findings, IL-2 might be synergistic with IL-12, or IFNγ or both, in downregulating the effect of IL-10. The fate of the malaria parasite within the liver seems, therefore, to depend on the balance between IL-10/IL-12, INFγ, and IL-2 which temporarily biases the liver toward the establishment of a local inflammatory condition.

IFNγ was the first cytokine shown to inhibit, both *in vitro* and in vivo, the hepatic stages of rodent and human malaria. IFNγ appears to exhibit both a parasitostatic and a lytic effect on the developing liver-stage parasite (103). When injected in vivo, IFNγ can protect mice against sporozoite challenge (104), while administration of anti-IFNγ diminishes the level of protection observed after immunization with attenuated sporozoites (105). In addition, immunization with attenuated sporozoites does not generate protective immunity in IFNγ receptor knockout mice (106). The source of IFNγ could be $CD4^+$ T cells, because a $CD4^+$ T cell clone secreting IFNγ conferred protection against challenge with *P. berghei* sporozoites (76). The major source of IFNγ in *P. berghei* immune mice, however, is thought to be $CD8^+$ T cells in the liver. Secretion of IFNγ by these cells would preclude the need for direct lysis of hepatocytes by CTL and, moreover, could account for suppression of parasite growth in surrounding hepatocytes by the few $CD8^+$ T cells that encounter infected hepatocytes. IFNγ could contribute to protection, not only by its direct effect on the parasite, but also indirectly by upregulation of MHC class I and class II molecules and B7-1 and B7-2 costimulatory molecules on both Kupffer cells and hepatocytes. This, in turn, would further promote the activation of effector T cells.

Tumor Necrosis Factor-α (TNFα) is another inflammatory cytokine which, when injected in vivo, can suppress the development of exoerythrocytic forms of the malaria parasite (107). This cytokine does not appear to act directly on hepatocytes; rather, it induces nonparenchymal liver cells to secrete IL-6, which probably further stimulates the production of nitric oxide (NO), which in turn suppresses parasite development. TNFα could be derived from either activated T cells found in the liver or Kupffer cells. TNFα, like IFNγ, could also indirectly modulate parasite-specific immunity through the upregulation of MHC or costimulatory molecules or both.

IL-1 is a third cytokine known to have an inhibitory effect on preerythrocytic stages of *P. falciparum.* It functions, in part, via activation of acute-phase proteins in infected hepatocytes (107). In addition, IL-1, like TNFα, also mediates suppressive activity by stimulating the production of IL-6, and consequently, NO, in the liver. The source of IL-1 is probably activated Kupffer cells.

The β_2 Microglobulin Knockout Mouse Model

Much of the difficulty in determining definitively which effector mechanisms are directed at the infected hepatocytes is due to the fact that requirements for activation of protective T lymphocytes remain unknown. Mechanisms of T cell induction and recognition of exoerythrocytic or indeed any Plasmodia parasite antigens are also unknown. To address these issues, we adopted the β_2 microglobulin knockout mouse (β_2KO) to investigate whether MHC class I–restricted $CD8^+$ T cells are critical for protection induced by attenuated *P. berghei* sporozoites (86). We also investigated the requirements for activation of the $CD8^+$ T cells induced during immunization with attenuated sporozoites. β_2KO mice have previously been used to study autoimmunity, tumor immunity, and viral or protozoan infection, since $CD8^+$ T cells have been shown to be associated with either development of the disease or have been believed to mediate key immunological functions. In contrast to viral (108) and some protozoan infections (109), where other T cells have compensated for the absence of MHC class I–restricted $CD8^+$ T cells, we observed no compensatory cellular activity in preventing malaria infection. Unlike wild-type control mice, β_2KO mice became susceptible to malaria infection even though they received a full or hyperimmune dose of irradiated sporozoites (86).

To overcome the inability of the β_2KO mice to generate protective immunity to immunization with irradiated sporozoites, we adoptively transferred sporozoite-immune wild-type splenic cells containing sporozoite-specific $CD8^+$ effector T cells and a full complement of accessory cells. Adoptive transfer has been well described in the literature (88) and we reasoned that adoptively transferred donor cells, having been activated during immunization with attenuated sporozoites, presumably by liver-expressed antigens, would manifest their anti-parasite immune function upon sporozoite challenge. The adoptively transferred cells, however, failed to confer protection to β_2KO mice, despite a successful parallel transfer to a naive wild-type host. The simplest explanation for this failure rests on the inability of the infected host liver cells, either intrahepatic Kupffer APCs or alternative cell types, to engage donor T cells for activation of a productive anti-malaria response because they lack the MHC class I molecules. Assuming that irradiated sporozoites colonized the liver and developed into liver-stage parasites, the lack of class I expression on hepatocytes or on APCs in the liver either prevented the formation of the granuloma and hence recruitment and activation of the effector T cells, or interfered with the presentation of liver-stage antigens to the appropriate T cells. Even if the sporozoite-immune $CD8^+$ T cells traveled to the liver, they most likely appeared without upregulated CD25 molecules and hence remained refractory to the influences of $CD4^+$ T cells.

$NK1.1^+$ T Cells: Source of IL-4

Recent studies have shown that in addition to the intrathymic pathway of T cell differentiation, an extrathymic pathway exists in the liver (110). The extrathymic hepatic T cells, especially the $\alpha\beta$ TCR^+ T cells, are mainly double negative for CD4/CD8 ($CD4^-CD8^-$ phenotype), expressing both T cell receptors of intermediate intensity and the $NK1.1^+$ surface marker (78,79); therefore, they are commonly referred to as NK-T cells. They represent about 40% of mature T cells in the liver, but a very small percentage of these cells is found in other tissues, except bone marrow, which also contains a high percentage of NK-T cells. Their T cell receptor repertoire is highly restricted towards Vα14 coupled with Vβ8, Vβ7, or Vβ2 (78,79) and its expression requires MHC class I–like CD1 molecules (111,112). NK-T cells are potent cytotoxic effector cells in the liver (113), but one of their major features is the production of large amounts of cytokines, particularly interleukin-4 (IL-4) (114). Because they represent a high percentage of T cells in the liver, their activation might tip the outcome of specific T lymphocyte reactivities toward the development of T helper type 2 (Th2) responses. Although their function is still not fully understood, NK-T cells have been shown to have a compensatory role in MHC class II deficient mice (115). They have a major effect in regulation of immune responses to intracellular pathogens (115) and liver-associated tumors (116), and may also be involved in the induction of tolerance (79).

We have examined NK-T cell populations resident in liver of C57BL/6 naive mice and C57BL/6 mice immunized with attenuated *P. berghei* sporozoites after challenge with infectious sporozoites (M. Guebre-Xabier, R. Schwenk, and U. Krzych, manuscript in preparation). We found that $CD4^+$ NK-T cells declined during induction of protective immunity but returned to normal levels after challenge with infectious sporozoites. In naive control mice, challenge with infectious sporozoites resulted in malaria infection that was accompanied by a nearly complete disappearance of $CD4^+$ NK-T cells. When the mice developed hepatic and erythrocytic infection, however, natural killer cells were upregulated and were of the major cell type. Kaufman et al. (117), who showed that the IL-4-producing $CD4^+$ NK-TCR$\alpha\beta^{int}$ liver lymphocytes are downregulated early in listeriosis, speculated that the disappearance of these cells might promote the development of T helper type 1 (Th1) cells, which are known to be essential for protection against *Listeria* (118). In malaria, it has also been shown that initial infection with *P. chabaudi chabaudi* induces Th1-type cells and, after clearance of the acute phase, there is a switch to a Th2-type response (119). It is possible that downregulation of the prevailing NK-T cell activity in the liver is required to create a Th1 milieu during induction of protective immunity. Once immunity has been established, however, these cells might, by providing IL-4, participate in the generation and/or maintenance of a memory pool. We have shown that protective immunity induced in humans by attenuated *P. falciparum* sporozoites coincides with production of IL-4 by memory $CD45R0^+$ $CD4^+$ T cells (120).

The Role of Costimulatory Molecules in Sporozoite-Induced Immunity

For most conventional antigens, successful activation of antigen-naive T cells requires both an antigen-mediated signal conveyed via the clonally distributed T cell receptor (signal 1) and a costimulatory signal delivered via the CD28 molecule (signal 2). It is now widely accepted that signal 1 is delivered by metabolically derived antigenic peptides presented either by MHC class I to $CD8^+$ T cells or by class II to $CD4^+$ T cells, although exceptions have been observed for a few antigens, which can activate T cells without being internalized by APCs and metabolically degraded (121).

T cells receiving signal 1 in the absence of signal 2 tend to become unresponsive or anergic (122). Two costimulatory molecules that are ligands for CD28 have been identified on all professional APCs and have been designated B7-1 (CD80) and B7-2 (CD86) (123). At present it is not known whether attenuated sporozoites activate T cells in a manner analogous to conventional protein antigens and, therefore, whether costimulation is required for induction of sporozoite-specific immunity. Sporozoite antigens, although capable of activating previously immune T cells, do so without the need for cellular internalization and metabolic degradation by APCs

(124). Whether plasmodial sporozoites, however, are superantigens or another type of antigen capable of T cell activation by a still unknown mechanism remains unclear.

Of note, Kupffer cells express B7 on their surface (125) and there is evidence that infected hepatocytes are also $B7^{+}$ (126). Antibodies to B7 have been shown to inhibit the ability of Kupffer cells to act as APCs (125). Moreover, IL-10 has been shown to downregulate the expression of B7 on a variety of APCs, including Kupffer cells (125). It is conceivable, therefore, that constitutive IL-10 production by hepatocytes could be sufficient to cause a general downregulation of costimulatory molecules, and in doing so, to create conditions unfavorable for T cell activation. In contrast to IL-10, inflammatory cytokines such as IFNγ and TNFα have been shown to upregulate the expression of B7. It is likely, therefore, that the local inflammatory milieu in the granulomas surrounding attenuated sporozoite-infected hepatocytes could reverse the effects of IL-10 and promote expression of costimulatory molecules, leading to the effective activation of T cells. NK cells (Fig. 9.2B) and other components of the innate immune system, reacting to sporozoite-induced danger signals, could also be the initial source of these inflammatory cytokines, which lead to the subsequently acquired T cell immunity.

REQUIREMENTS FOR MAINTENANCE OF PROTECTIVE IMMUNITY

Liver Is the Depot for Attenuated Exoerythrocytic Forms

One of the cardinal rules for the induction of protection is the accumulation of threshold amounts of plasmodial antigens in the liver. This occurs during immunization with attenuated sporozoites because such forms lose their ability to infect red cells and, therefore, are either retained within the hepatocytes or are phagocytized by Kupffer cells or other APCs in the liver (Fig. 9.2B). The persistence of accumulated antigens in the liver is in turn critical for the maintenance of protective immunity (127). Treatment of mice with an antimalarial drug, primaquine, which interferes with the development of liver-stage parasites, results in lack of protective immunity (127).

At its simplest level, the failure of natural infection to confer complete long-lasting immunity may be due to an inadequate immunizing dose of antigen, because individuals rarely receive more than 300 infectious bites per year (128). Furthermore, individuals living in regions of low endemicity with high seasonal transmission periods develop poorer immunity than do persons living in areas of high endemicity, who receive multiple infectious bites per year. Even in the attenuated sporozoite model, protection was not achieved in volunteers exposed to fewer that 600 infectious bites during a 70–83 day period (128). Thus, it appears that an accumulation of a persisting antigen depot is required to induce and maintain a sustained memory response. Arrest of attenuated sporozoites at an early phase of their development in the liver probably favors accumulation of liver-stage antigens in this system. Zinkernagel et al. (129) have evidence to indicate that T cell memory is maintained only when there is a protracted restimulation of effector T cells, either by some form of persisting antigen or by cross-reacting environmental antigens. Hence, in malaria, when the depot of liver-stage antigens is eliminated, memory T cell activity would also subside.

Recognition of Liver and Blood-Stage Antigens by T Cells from Persons Immune to Attenuated Sporozoites

If, upon repeated immunizations, the developmentally arrested parasites accumulate in the liver and sustain expression of antigens normally associated with exoerythrocytic and erythrocytic-stage infection, then in principle they could activate T cells. Hence, we reasoned that effector/inducer T cells with a broad range of specificities might target this developmental stage of infection. We tested this hypothesis by examining human T lymphocytes from volunteers immunized with radiation-attenuated *P. falciparum* sporozoites for proliferative reactivities to parasitized red blood cells (pRBC) and recombinant proteins and synthetic peptides representing sporozoite-, liver-, and blood-stage antigens, all known to be present in the hepatic-stage parasite (44). Proliferative T cell responses revealed that patent parasitemia was not required for induction of T cells recognizing liver- and blood-stage antigens, because these T cells were detectable in persons immunized with attenuated sporozoites before the infectious sporozoite challenge (130). This is further emphasized by the inability to detect these T cells in persons who become parasitemic upon sporozoite challenge because they had not received the required number of immunizing bites for induction of protection, and hence most likely developed far fewer attenuated liver-stage parasites (Table 9.1).

In contrast to proliferative responses seen with Liver Stage Antigen (LSA), Merozoite Surface Protein (MSP)-1, MSP-2, and parasitized red blood cells (pRBC), we were unable to detect any proliferation on exposure to peptides of *P. falciparum* CS protein, regardless of the status of the lymphocytes with regard to sporozoite immunity (130). Similar observations were made in an analogous murine model by using irradiated *P. berghei* sporozoites (131). Although CS protein and LSA are both considered preerythrocytic antigens, LSA is synthesized only by the liver-stage infection and is secreted into the vacuole surrounding the parasite (6,60). CS protein is carried into the liver by sporozoites and is detectable on the liver parasite membrane, but is not thought to be synthesized by the liver-stage parasite (56). Antigens expressed de novo by the liver-stage may be present in greater quantities or processed and presented by hepatocytes differently from CS protein. In support of this hypothesis, we have observed that the lack of intracellular processing of *P. berghei* CS protein by splenic APCs could be responsible in part for the lack of *in vitro* reactivity to CS protein peptides in mice (124). This hypothesis is also in agreement with the currently held view that sporozoite infection of the liver occurs by a mechanism involving direct contact between hepatocytes and the CS protein on the sporozoites and, as such, it excludes the participation of Kupffer cells as APCs in interactions with sporozoites.

It could be argued that after sporozoite invasion of hepatocytes, the shed complexes of CS protein–heparan sulfate proteoglycans are most likely removed by Kupffer cells, processed intracellularly, and presented by MHC class I or class II molecules to $CD8^+$ or $CD4^+$ T cells resident in the liver. Even if this is the case, the low concentration of the CS protein found in these complexes and arising from very few infectious sporozoites might be inadequate for T cell activation. Moreover, intracellular proteolysis of such complexes might proceed quite differently from that of pro-

TABLE 9.1 Exposure to Radiation-Attenuated *P. falciparum* Sporozoites Generates Proliferative and Memory T Cell Responses to Selected Antigens Associated with Liver- and Blood-Stage Infections

Exposure to Plasmodia			Antigen-Specific Proliferative T Cells					
Attenuated SPZ (No. of Bites)	Infectious SPZ Challenge	Immune Status	CS	LSA	MSP-1	MSP-2	pRBC	$CD4^+CD45RO^+$ Memory T Cells
None	None		–	–	–	–	–	–
None	Yes	NP	–	–	nd	nd	+	–
600	None		–	–	–	–	–	nd
600	Yes	NP	–	–	–	–	+	nd
>1000	None		–	+	+	+	+	+
>1000	Yes	P	–	+	+	+	+	+

Peripheral blood mononuclear cells (PBMC) were obtained before and after the challenge with infectious *P. falciparum* sporozoites (SPZ) from volunteers previously exposed to the indicated number of bites from mosquitoes infected with attenuated *P. falciparum*. PBMC from persons naive to Plasmodia antigens served as controls. Parasitemia was determined by a thick blood smear and subjects were designated as protected (P) or not protected (NP). PBMC were evaluated for proliferative reactivity as previously described (130) to CS protein peptides, LSA peptides, proteins representing blood-stage infection, merozoite surface protein 1 (MSP-1) and merozoite surface protein 2 (MSP-2), and pRBC. Responses were determined by ^{3}[H]-thymidine incorporation; positive responses are indicated as (+) and responses that did not exceed control values are designated as negative (–). Responses which were not evaluated are designated as "nd." Isolated $CD4^+$ T cells were also evaluated for the expression of the CD45RO memory marker, as previously described (120). Increased expression of CD45RO is indicated as (+), unchanged expression as (–), and "nd" were not measured.

tein antigens. For example, such complexes might behave as superantigens, the exploration of which has only recently been reported (132).

Apparently contrasting results have been observed in studies of peripheral lymphocyte responses to CS protein among adult populations exposed to natural infection in endemic areas. The proliferative T cells had rather restricted specificity, in that the majority of the responses were directed either to peptides considered promiscuous (10) or to peptides representing cross-reactive responses, such as thrombospondin, among others. It has also been observed that malaria-naive lymphocytes can respond to these peptides upon stimulation *in vitro* (10). Additional studies are required to clarify whether CS protein responses seen among the naturally exposed populations are indeed Plasmodia antigen–specific or if they arise to cross-reactive self-antigens.

The role of hepatocytes themselves in antigen presentation has not been investigated, but given proper conditions, hepatocytes, in principle, can engage in the APC function. Although there is no evidence concerning Plasmodia antigen presentation by hepatocytes to T cells, conventional wisdom dictates that because so few hepatocytes become infected by the invading sporozoites, it is unlikely that they serve as competent APCs. Furthermore, the liver stage, although sufficiently long to engage hepatocytes in the APC function for some malaria species, such as *P. falciparum*, might be too short for *P. berghei* or *P. yoelli*, as the liver infection lasts only 2 days before the hepatocytes rupture and expel merozoites. Even given an optimal number of infected hepatocytes to function as APCs during sporozoite invasion, their entire intracellular function must be so drastically altered, presumably to benefit the parasite, that the role of antigen processing and presentation is most likely greatly diminished.

Memory T Cells Needed for Protection

The requirement for accumulation of antigen may simply signify a need for a threshold concentration to generate a T cell response, or it may suggest that the persistence of the T cell response (i.e., memory) depends on the presence of a certain concentration of the antigen. Is T cell memory required for the maintenance of protection to malaria infection? On the basis of evidence from our laboratory, $CD4^+$ T cells that express CD45RO, the marker thought to be involved in memory T cell responses, have been detected in the peripheral circulation of persons protected by immunization with attenuated *P. falciparum* sporozoites (Table 9.1). These cells are normally not induced during *in vitro* stimulation with antigens present on pRBC, but their level increases during protection and wanes as protective immunity decays (120). Currently, these cells represent the only *in vitro* marker associated with protective immunity induced by attenuated sporozoites.

We have also observed induction of memory T cells in the murine model of attenuated sporozoite–induced protection, except that $CD8^+$ T cells rather than $CD4^+$ T cells were detected in the liver after the challenge with infectious sporozoites. Although these memory T cells have been observed in two different systems under different conditions of detection, it could be postulated that the effector $CD8^+$ T cells decline after inflammation has subsided, but are maintained in a state of stasis within the liver if (i) sufficient levels of antigen persist in the liver and (ii) they are accompanied by memory $CD4^+$ T cells secreting IL-4 for their maintenance.

Apoptosis of $CD8^+$ T Cells in the Liver

If, during malaria infection, $CD8^+$ T cells are either induced in the liver or travel to the liver, the unusual immunology of the liver poses formidable challenges because, according to the responder trap hypothesis (71), the activated $CD8^+$ T cells that travel to the liver to kill infected hepatocytes will themselves be eliminated. One of the mechanisms of activation-induced cell death may involve Fas/FasL-mediated apoptosis (133,134), a mechanism that has been implicated in the allograft acceptance induced in the liver. Although Fas mRNA is not expressed in normal liver, it has been found within hepatocytes in inflammatory liver disease (134). It is also known that activated mainstream $CD8^+$ T cells express Fas and that alternative T cells, especially $CD4^+$ NK-T cells express FasL; hence, interactions of these cells may be responsible for the apoptosis of $CD8^+$ T cells induced in the liver (71).

If we accept the premise that Plasmodia-specific $CD8^+$ T cells are eliminated from the liver in order to maintain protection, they must be replaced. This presumably occurs by a constant ingress of naive $CD8^+$ T cells that can respond to residual parasite

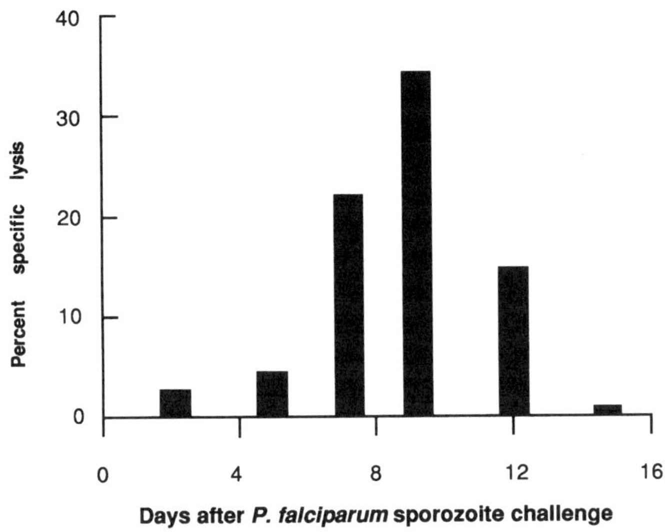

Figure 9.3. The appearance of cytolytic T cells parallels the development of liver-stage antigens after infection with *P. falciparum* sporozoites. Peripheral blood mononuclear cells (PBMC) were obtained at the indicated intervals (days) after the challenge with infectious *P. falciparum* sporozoites from volunteers immunized previously by repeated bites from mosquitoes infected with attenuated *P. falciparum*. PBMC were evaluated in a ^{51}Cr-release assay according to a published method (91) for the presence of cytolytic T cells specific for MHC class I–restricted epitopes on CS protein. The assays was performed using autologous B cells transformed by Epstein-Barr virus (EBV) and pulsed either with *P. falciparum* CS protein peptide known to contain cytolytic T cell epitope, amino acid 369–390 (10), or with irrelevant CS protein peptide. Nonpulsed autologous EBV-transformed B cells and heterologous EBV-transformed B cells pulsed with CS protein containing cytolytic T cell peptide were used as controls. Specific lysis, determined as described previously (86), is expressed as percent lysis.

antigens or those deposited by subsequent infections. Data from our laboratory suggest that CTLs do migrate in the irradiated-sporozoite model. We have detected CTL in the peripheral circulation of human volunteers but only between 5 and 12 days after booster immunizations (Fig. 9.3). Although the fate of these CTLs is unknown, they may have undergone activation-induced cell death in the liver. Alternatively, they may have converted to memory T cells, a subset dependent on the presence of continued antigenic stimulation for maintenance. This hypothesis is consistent with data from rodent models, where protection is dependent upon continued antigenic stimulation by persistent attenuated parasites in the liver (127).

Incomplete T Cell Activation

Currently, there is some evidence that the malaria sporozoite may not interact with antigen-presenting cells and/or T cells in a manner analogous to simple protein antigens. As described previously, in the absence of opsonization, sporozoites are not readily ingested by macrophages or Kupffer cells (25). In addition, splenic T cells from attenuated sporozoite-immunized mice do not respond to peptide antigens derived from the CS protein (131), whereas CS protein- (135) or CS protein peptide-immune T cells do so (U. Krzych, unpublished observations). These and similar results suggest that sporozoites may not undergo normal antigen processing and presentation (124). Hence, they may deliver only incomplete activation signals to T cells and consequently stimulate only transient T cell responses. The effects of sporozoite infection on other key parameters of T cell activation, such as the induction of costimulatory molecules, homing receptors, and chemokine production remain to be investigated. Taken together, these observations may also provide additional mechanisms to explain the lack of long-lived T cell memory to liver-stage antigens.

CONCLUDING REMARKS

The Plasmodia parasite is the causative agent of malaria, an infection that is prevalent in tropical areas, causing severe anemia, illness, and death in millions of people every year. The parasite is complex, and its biphasic life cycle requires an arthropod and a vertebrate host for its survival. The liver of the vertebrate host is the obligatory venue for the exponential amplification and molecular alterations of the parasite for invasion of red blood cells. It is believed that partly owing to constitutive production of IL-10 by hepatocytes, immunological tolerance persists in the liver and promotes parasite growth and development without causing pathology or a marked inflammatory response, a requisite for induction of antigen-specific cellular responses. Natural exposure to Plasmodia, therefore, results in an incomplete and short-lived immunity, which fails to prevent intermittent episodes of parasitemia. Antibody responses to blood-stage antigens rather than a cellular response to preerythrocytic stage antigens are thought to mediate immunity induced by natural exposure to infection.

In contrast, strong cellular responses consisting of $CD4^+$ and $CD8^+$ effector T cells arise to immunization with attenuated Plasmodia sporozoites and these confer protective immunity in humans and animal models. On the basis of ample evidence from both model systems, these responses are induced by antigens expressed on the aborted exoerythrocytic forms, which accumulate in the liver because they cannot invade red blood cells. The liver repository of Plasmodia antigens, designated as danger signal, causes a strong local inflammation, which temporarily abolishes the tolerant state; this local switch is the prerequisite for induction of immunological reactivities of antigen-specific T cells. The persistence of the aborted forms of Plasmodia antigens is required for maintenance of protective immunity, as it sustains the activity of effector T cells, either by memory T cell responses or activation of new immigrant T cells from the periphery.

It is hoped that investigations of these immunological events will become the primary focus of malaria research both in the laboratory and in the field. These responses are deemed to be of critical importance to the understanding of immunity induced by Plasmodia antigens and to development of strategies for the design of anti-malaria vaccines.

ACKNOWLEDGMENTS

With this chapter, U. Krzych would like to commemorate the late Dr. Helen R. Strausser, her professor at Rutgers University. The author would also like to thank all the members of her laboratory and particularly, Kate White, Pei Fang Sun, Robert Schwenk, Dupeh Palmer, Heidi Link Snyder, Terrie Jareed, and Mimi Guebre-Xabier, for all their exciting and valued contributions to the understanding of immune responses induced with Plasmodia antigens. She also would like to express her deep gratitude to her daughter, Malkah J. Bressler and her husband, Joseph P. Bressler, for all their love, support and most of all their patience during writing of this chapter.

All the authors would like to express their appreciations to the following persons: Ripley W. Ballou, the Chief of the Department of Immunology at WRAIR, for his constant support and unsurpassed encouragement for our efforts trying to learn the "ways of Plasmodia antigens"; Kate White, Pei Fang Sun, and Dupeh Palmer, our friends and colleagues, for many meaningful discussions about malaria and the liver; Konstanin Fedegin, Department of Pathology, for his insightful comments. Ann Lee Chen for skillful support; Patricia Stroy for the art work, and Pamela Talalay for editorial comments.

The views of the authors do not purport to reflect the position of the Department of the Army or the Department of Defense. The U.S. Government has the right to retain a nonexclusive, royalty-free license in and to any copyright covering this paper.

REFERENCES

1. Sturchler, D. 1989. How much malaria is there worldwide? *Parasitol. Today* 5:39.
2. World Health Organization. 1989. *Wkly. Epidemiol. Rec.* 32:241–247.
3. McGregor, I., and Wilson, R. In *Malaria: Principles and Practice of Malariology, Vol. 1.* Wernsdorfer, W., and McGregor, I., eds. New York: Livingston, pp 559–621.
4. Santoro, F., Cochrane, A.H., Nussenzweig, V., Nardin, E.H., Nussenzweig, R., Gwadz, W., and Ferreira, A. 1983. Structural similarities among the protective antigens of sporozoites from different species of malaria parasites. *J. Biol. Chem.* 258:3341–3345.
5. Nussenzweig V, and Nussenzweig R.S. 1989. Rational for the development of an engineered sporozoite malaria vaccine. *Adv. Immunol.* 45:283–334.
6. Guerin-Marchand, C., Druilhe, P., Galey, B., Londono, A., Patarapotikul, J., Beaudoin, R.L., Dubeaux, C., Tartar, A., Mercereau Puijalon, O., and Langsley, G. 1987. A liver-stage-specific antigen of *Plasmodium falciparum* characterized by gene cloning. *Nature* 329:164–167.
7. Holder, A.A. 1996. Preventing merozoite invasion of erythrocytes. In *Malaria Vaccine Development: A Multi-Immune Response Approach*, Hoffman, S.L., ed. Washington, DC: ASL Press pp 77–92.
8. Sim, B.K.L., Chitmus, C., Wasmiowska, K., Hadley, T., and Miller, L. 1994. Receptor and ligand domains for invasion of erythrocytes by *Plasmodium falciparum. Science* 264:1941–1944.
9. Day, K.P., and Marsh, K. 1991. Naturally acquired immunity to Plasmodium falciparum. *Immunol. Today* 12:A68–A71.

10. Nardin, E.H., and Nussenzweig, R.S. 1993. T cell responses to pre-erythrocytic stages of malaria. Role in protection and vaccine development against pre-erythrocytic stages. *Annu. Rev. Immunol.* 11:687.
11. Ponnudurai, T., Lensen, A.H.W., van Gemert, G.J.A., Bolmer, M.G., and Meuwissen, J.H.E.T. 1991. Feeding behavior and sporozoite ejection by infected *Anopheles stephensi. Trans. R. Soc. Trop. Med. Hyg.* 85:175–180.
12. Rosenberg, R., Wirtz, R.A., Schneider, I., and Burge, R. 1990. An estimation of the number of malaria sporozoites ejected by a feeding mosquito. *Trans. R. Soc. Trop. Med. Hyg.* 84:209–212.
13. Khusmith, S., Charoenvit, Y., Kumar, S., Sedegah, M., Beaudoin, R.L., and Hoffman, S.L. 1991. Protection against malaria by vaccination with sporozoite surface protein 2 plus CS protein. *Science* 252:715–718.
14. Khusmith, S., Sedegah, M., and Hoffman, S.L. 1994. Complete protection against *Plasmodium yoelii* by adoptive transfer of a $CD8^+$ cytotoxic T-cell clone recognizing sporozoite surface protein 2. *Infect. Immun.* 62:2979–2983.
15. Hadley, T.J. 1986. Invasion of erythrocytes by malaria parasites: A cellular and molecular overview. *Annu. Rev. Microbiol.* 40:451–477.
16. Meis, J.F.G.M., Verhave, J.P., Jap, P.H.K., and Meuwissen, J.H.E.T. 1983. An ultrastructural study on the role of Kupffer cells in the process of infection by *Plasmodium berghei* sporozoites in rats. *Parasitology* 86:231–242.
17. Richman, L., Klingenstein, R., Richman, J., Strober, W., and Berzofsky, J. 1979. The murine Kupffer cell, I. Characterization of the cell serving accessory function in antigen-specific T cell proliferation. *J. Immunol.* 123:2602–2609.
18. Shin, S.C.J., Vanderberg, J.P., and Terzakis, J.A. 1982. Direct infection of hepatocytes by sporozoites of *Plasmodium berghei. J. Protozool.* 29:448–454.
19. Sinnis, P. The malaria sporozoite's journey into the liver. *Infect. Agents Dis.* 5:182–189.
20. Leitner, W.W., and Krzych, U. 1997. *Plasmodium falciparum* malaria blood stage parasites preferentially inhibit macrophages with high phagocytic activity. *Parasite Immunol.* 19:103–110.
21. Sinden, R.E., and Smith, J.E. 1982. The role of the Kupffer cell in the infection of rodents by sporozoites of *Plasmodium:* Uptake of sporozoites by perfused liver and the establishment of infection in vivo. *Acta Trop.* 39:11–27.
22. Verhave, J.P., Meuwissen, J.H.E.T., and Golenser, J. 1980. The dual role of macrophages in the sporozoite-induced malaria infection. A hypothesis. *Int. J. Nuc. Med. Biol.* 7:149–156.
23. Vreden, S.G.S., Sauerwein, R.W., Verhave, J.P., Van Rooijen, N., Meuwissen, J.H.E.T., and Van Den Broek, M.F. 1993. Kupffer cell elimination enhances development of liver schizonts of *Plasmodium berghei* in rats. *Infect. Immun.* 61:1936–1939.
24. Vanderberg, J., Chew, S., and Stewart, M.J. 1990. *Plasmodium* sporozoite interactions with macrophages in vitro: A videomicroscopic analysis. *J. Protozool.* 37:528–536.
25. Seguin, M.C., Ballou, W.R., and Nacy, C.A. 1989. Interactions of *Plasmodium berghei* sporozoites and murine Kupffer cells in vitro. *J. Immunol.* 143:1716–1722.
26. Hollingdale, M.R., Leland, P., and Schwartz, A.L. 1983. *In vitro* cultivation of the exoerythrocytic stage of *Plasmodium berghei* in a hepatoma cell line. *Am. J. Trop. Med. Hyg.* 32:682–684.
27. Mazier, D., Beaudoin, R.L., Mellouk, S., et al. 1985. Complete development of hepatic stages of *Plasmodium falciparum* in vitro. *Science* 227:440–442.

28. Aley, S.B., Bates, M.D., Tam, J.P., and Hollingdale, M.R. 1986. Synthetic peptides from the circumsporozoite proteins of *Plasmodium falciparum* and *Plasmodium knowlesi* recognize the human hepatoma cell line HepG2-A16 in vitro. *J. Exp. Med.* 164:1915–1921.
29. Robson, K.J.H., Hall, J.R.S., Jennings, M.W., Harris, T., Marsh, K., Newbold, C., Tate, V., and Weatherall, D. 1988. A highly conserved amino-acid sequence in thrombospondin, properdin and in proteins from sporozoites and blood stages of a human malaria parasite. *Nature* 335:79–82.
30. Rogers, W.O., Rogers, M.D., Hedstrom, R.C., and Hoffman, S.L. 1992. Characterization of the gene encoding sporozoite surface protein 2, a protective *Plasmodium yoelii* sporozoite antigen. *Mol. Biochem. Parasitol.* 53:45–52.
31. Goundis, D., and Reid, K.B.M. 1988. Properdin, the terminal complement components, thrombospondin and the circumsporozoite protein of malaria parasites contain similar sequence motifs. *Nature* 355:82–85.
32. Klar, A., Baldassare, M., and Jessell, T.M. 1992. F-Spondin: A gene expressed at high levels in the floor plate encodes a secreted protein that promotes neural cell adhesion and neurite extension. *Cell* 69:95–110.
33. Leung-Hagestejin, C., Spence, A.M., Stern, B.D., Zhou, Y., Su, M., Hedgecock, E., and Culotti, J. 1992. UNC-5, a transmembrane protein with immunoglobulin and thrombospondin type 1 domains, guides cell and pioneer axon migrations in *C. Elegans*. *Cell* 71:289–299.
34. Clarke, L.E., Tomley, F.M., Wisher, M.H., Foulds, I.J., and Boursnell, M.E.G. 1990. Regions of an *Eimeria tenella* antigen contain sequences which are observed in circumsporozoite proteins from *Plasmodium* ssp. and which are related to the thrombospondin gene family. *Mol. Biochem. Parasitol.* 41:269–280.
35. Frevert, U., Sinnis, P., Cerami, C., Shreffler, W., Takacs, B., and Nussenzweig, V. 1993. Malaria circumsporozoite protein binds to heparan sulfate proteoglycans associated with the surface membrane of hepatocytes. *J. Exp. Med.* 177:1287–1298.
36. Cerami, C., Frevert, U., Sinnis, P., Takas, B., Clavijo, P., Santos, M., and Nussenzweig, V. 1992. The basolateral domain of the hepatocyte plasma membrane bears receptors for the circumsporozoite protein of *Plasmodium falciparum* sporozoites. *Cell* 70:1021–1033.
37. Robson, K.J.H., Frevert, U., Reckmann, I., et al. 1995. Thrombospondin-related adhesive protein (TRAP) *of Plasmodium falciparum:* Expression during sporozoite ontogeny and binding to human hepatocytes. *EMBO J* 14:3883–3894.
38. Cerami, C., Frevert, U., Sinnis, P., Takacs, B., and Nussenzweig, V. 1994. Rapid clearance of malaria circumsporozoite protein (CS) by hepatocytes. *J. Exp. Med.* 55:604–608.
39. Pancake, S.J., Holt, G.H., Mellouk, S., and Hoffman, S.L. 1992. Malaria sporozoites and circumsporozoite proteins bind specifically to sulfated glycoconjugates. *J. Cell. Biol.* 6:1351–1357.
40. Frevert, U. 1994. Malaria sporozoite–hepatocyte interactions. *Exp. Parasitol.* 79:206–210.
41. Stewart, M.J., Nawrot, R., Schulman, S., and Vanderberg, J.P. 1986. *Plasmodium berghei* sporozoite invasion is blocked in vitro by sporozoite-immobilizing antibodies. *Infect. Immun.* 51:859–864.
42. Stewart, M.J., and Vanderberg, J.P. 1988. Malaria sporozoites leave behind trails of circumsporozoite protein during gliding motility. *J. Protozool.* 35:389–393.
43. Stewart, M.J., and Vanderberg, J.P. 1992. Electron microscopic analysis of circumsporozoite trail formation by gliding malaria sporozoites. *J. Protozool.* 39:663–671.

44. Szarfman, A., Lyon, J.A., Walliker, D., et al. 1988. Mature liver stages of cloned *Plasmodium falciparum* share epitopes with proteins from sporozoites and asexual blood stages. *Parasite Immuol.* 10:339–351.

45. Rogers, W.O., Malik, A., Mellouk, S., Nakamura, K., Rogers, M., Szarfman, A., Gordon, D., Mussler, A., Aikawa, M., and Hoffman, S. 1992. Characterization of *Plasmodium falciparum* sporozoite surface protein 2. *Proc. Natl. Acad. Sci. U.S.A.* 89:9176–9180.

46. Hollingdale, M.R., Sinden, R.E., and van Pelt, J.F. 1993. Sporozoite invasion. *Nature* 362:26.

47. Aikawa, M., Schwartz, A., Uni, S., Nussenzweig, R., and Hollingdale, M. 1984. Ultrastructure of in vitro cultured exoerythrocytic stage of *Plasmodium berghei* in a hepatoma cell line. *Am. J. Trop. Med. Hyg.* 33:792–799.

48. Hollingdale, M.R. 1988. Malaria and the liver. In *The Liver: Biology and Pathobiology*, Arias, I.M., ed. New York: Raven, pp 1195–1211.

49. Meis, J.F., Rijntjes, P.J., Verhave, J.P., Ponnudurai, T., Hollingdale, M.R., Smith, J.E., Sinden, R.E., Jap, P.H., Meuwissen, J.H., and Yap, S.H. 1986. Fine structure of the malaria parasite *Plasmodium falciparum* in human hepatocytes in vitro. *Cell Tissue Res.* 244:345–350.

50. Krotoski, W.A., Garnham, P.C., Bray, R.S., Krotoski, D.M., Killick Kendrick, R., Draper, C.C., Targett, G.A., and Guy, M.W. 1982. Observations on early and late post-sporozoite tissue stages in primate malaria, I. Discovery of a new latent form of *Plasmodium cynomolgy* (the hypnozoite), and failure to detect hepatic forms within the first 24 hours after infection. *Am. J. Trop. Med. Hyg.* 31:24–35.

51. Garnham, P.C.C. 1980. Malaria in its various vertebrate hosts. In *Malaria, Vol. 1: Epidemiology, Chemotherapy, Morphology, and Metabolism*, Kreier, J., ed. New York: Academic pp 96–144.

52. Meis, J.F., Ponnudurai, T., Mons, B., Van Belkum, van Eerd, PM, Druilhe, P., and Schellekens, H. 1990. *Plasmodium falciparum:* Studies on mature exoerythrocytic forms in the liver of the chimpanzee, Pan troglodytes. *Exp. Parasitol.* 70:1–11.

53. Atkinson, C.T., Hollingdale, M.R., and Aikawa, M. 1992. Localization of a 230-kd parasitophorous vacuole membrane antigen of *Plasmodium berghei* exoerythrocytic schizonts (LSA-2) by immunoelectron and confocal laser scanning microscopy. *Am. J. Trop. Med. Hyg.* 46:533–537.

54. Renia, L., Mattei, D., Gonna, J., Pied, S., Dubois, P., Miltgen, F., Nussler, A., Matile, H., Menegaux, F., Gentilini, M., and Mazier, D. 1990. A malaria heat-shock-like determinant expressed on the infected hepatocyte surface is the target of antibody-dependent cell-mediated cytotoxic mechanisms by nonparenchymal liver cells. *Eur. J. Immunol.* 20:1445–1449.

55. Terzakis, J.A., Vanderberg, J.P., Foley, D., and Shustak, S. 1979. Exoerythrocytic merozoites of *Plasmodium berghei* in rat hepatic Kupffer cells. *J. Protozool.* 26:385–389.

56. Atkinson, C.T., Aikawa, M., Aley, B., and Hollingdale, M.R. 1989. Expression *of Plasmodium berghei* circumsporozoite antigen on the surface of exoerythrocytic schizonts and merozoites. *Am. J. Trop. Med. Hyg.* 41:9–17.

57. Aikawa, M., Atkinson, C.T., Beaudoin, L.M., Sedegah, M., Charoenvit, Y., and Beaudoin, R. 1990. Localization of CS and non-CS antigens in the sporogonic stages of *Plasmodium yoelii. Bull. World Health Org.* 68(suppl.):165–171.

58. Rogers, W.O., Malik, A., Mellouk, S., Nakamura, K., Rogers, M.D., Szarfman, A., Gordon, D.M., Nussler, A.K., Aikawa, M., and Hoffman, S.L. 1992. Characterization of *Plasmodium falciparum* sporozoite surface protein 2. *Proc. Natl. Acad. Sci. U.S.A.* 89:9176–9180.

59. Fidock, D.A., Gras Masse, H., Lepers, J.P., et al. 1994. *Plasmodium falciparum* liver stage antigen-1 is well conserved and contains potent B and T cell determinants. *J. Immunol.* 153:190–204.

60. Zhu, J., and Hollingdale, M.R. 1991. Structure of *Plasmodium falciparum* liver stage antigen-1. *Mol. Biochem. Parasitol.* 48:223–226.

61. Charoenvit, Y., Mellouk, S., Sedegah, M., Toyoshima, T., Leef, M.F., De la Vega, P., Beaudoin, R.L., Aikawa, M., Fallarme, V., and Hoffman, S.L. 1995. *Plasmodium yoelii:* 17-kDa hepatic and erythrocytic stage protein is the target of an inhibitory monoclonal antibody. *Exp. Parasitol.* 80:419–429.

62. Fidock, D.A., Sallenave Sales, S., Sherwood, J.A., Gachihi, G.S., Ferreira da Cruz, M.F., Thomas, A.W., and Druihe, P. 1994. Conservation of the *Plasmodium falciparum* sporozoite surface protein gene, STARP, in field isolates and distinct species of Plasmodium. *Mol. Biochem. Parasitol.* 67:255–267.

63. Hoffman, S.L., Franke, E.D., Hollingdale, M.R., and Druilhe, P. 1996. Attacking the infected hepatocyte. In *Malaria Vaccine Development: A Multi-Immune Response Approach*, Hoffman, S.L., ed. Washington, DC: American Society for Microbiology, pp 35–75.

64. Suhrbier, A., Winger, L., O'Dowd, C., Hodivala, K., and Sinden, R.E. 1990. An antigen specific to the liver stage of rodent malaria recognized by a monoclonal antibody. *Parasite Immunol.* 12:473–481.

65. Matzinger, P. 1994. Tolerance, danger and the extended family. *Annu. Rev. Immunol.* 12:991–1045.

66. Rajan, T.V. 1997. Why does *Plasmodium* have a pre-erythrocytic cycle? *Parasitol. Today* 13:284–286.

67. Ferber, I., Schonrich, G., Schenkel, J., Mellor, A.L., Hammerling, G., and Arnold, B. 1994. Levels of peripheral T cell tolerance induced by different doses of tolerogen.*Science* 263:674–676.

68. Alfrey, E.J., Mast, D., Wang, X., Lee, L.K., Holm, B., Kreiger, N.R., Sibley, R.K., Huie, P., and Dafoe, D.C. 1995. Interferon-gamma and interleukin-10 messenger RNA are upregulated after orthotopic liver transplantation in tolerant rats: Evidence for cytokine-medicated immune dysregulation. *Surgery* 118:399–405.

69. Hill, A., Elvin, J., Willis, A.C., et al. 1992. Molecular analysis of the association of HLA-B53 and resistance to severe malaria. *Nature* 360:434–439.

70. Hill, A., Allsopp, C.E.M., Kwiatkowski, D., et al. 1991. Common West African HLA antigens are associated with protection from severe malaria. *Nature* 352:595–600.

71. Crispe, I.N., and Mehal, W.Z. Strange brew: T cells in the liver. *Immunol. Today* 17:522–525.

72. Lalvani, A., Hurt, N., Aidoo, M., Kibatala, P., Tanner, M., and Hill, A.V.S. 1996. Cytotoxic T lymphocytes to *Plasmodium falciparum* epitopes in an area of intense and perennial transmission in Tanzania. *Eur. J. Immunol.* 26:773–779.

73. Clyde, D.F., Most, H., McCarthy, V.C., and Vanderberg, J.P. 1973. Immunization of man against sporozoite-induced *falciparum* malaria. *Am. J. Med. Sci.* 266:169–177.

74. Rieckmann, K.H., Beaudoin, R.L., Cassells, J.S., and Sell, D.W. 1979. Use of attenuated sporozoites in the immunization of human volunteers against falciparum malaria. *Bull World Health Org.* 57(suppl. 1):261–265.

75. Nussenzweig, R.S., Vanderberg, J., Most, H., and Orton, C. 1967. Protective immunity produced by the injection of X-irradiated sporozoites of *Plasmodium berghei. Nature* 216:160–162.

76. Tsuji, M., Romero, P., Nussenzweig, R., and Zavala, F. 1990. $CD4^+$ cytolytic T cell clones confers protection against murine malaria. *J. Exp. Med.* 172:1353–1357.

77. Hammerling, G. 1997. Tolerance and autoimmunity. Presented at the Keystone Symposia on Molecular and Cellular Biology. Keystone, Co. April 13, 1997. Abstract. Keystone symposia, Silverthorne. p 5.

78. Mac Donald, H.R. 1995. $NK1.1^+$ T cell receptor $\alpha\beta^+$ cells: New clues to their origin, specificity and function. *J. Exp. Med.* 182:633–638.

79. Vicari, P., and Zlotnik, A.P. 1996. Mouse $NK1.1^+$ T cells: A new family of T cells. *Immunol. Today* 17:71–76.

80. Khan, Z.M., and Vanderberg, J.P. 1992. Specific inflammatory cell infiltration of hepatic schizonts in BALB/c mice immunized with attenuated *plasmodium yoelii* sporozoites. *Int. Immunol.* 4:711.

81. Hoffman, L.H., Isenbarger, D., Long, G.W., Sedegah, M., Szarfman, A., Waters, L., Hollingdale, M.R., Van Der Meide, P.H., Finboom, D.S., and Ballou, W.R. 1989. Sporozoite vaccine induces genetically restricted T cell elimination of malaria from hepatocytes. *Science* 244:1078–1081.

82. Scheller, L.F., Green, S.J., and Azad, A.F. 1997. Inhibition of nitric oxide interrupts the accumulation of $CD8^+$ T cells surrounding malaria infected hepatocytes. *Infect. Immun.* 65:3882–3888.

83. Khan, Z.M., and Vanderberg, J.P. 1991. Eosinophil-rich, granulomatous inflammatory response to *plasmodium berghei* hepatic schizonts in non-immunized rats is age-related. *Am. J. Trop. Med. Hyg.* 45:190–201.

84. Faure, P., Marussig, M., Goossens, P., Miltgen, F., and Mazier, D. 1994. Characterization of liver lymphomyeloid cells in mice infected with *Plasmodium yoelii* sporozoites. *Immunology* 82:645–650.

85. Faure, P., Hulier, E., Miltgen, F., Renia, L., and Mazier, D. 1995. Protective immunity against malaria: Cellular changes in the liver vary according to the method of immunization. *Parasite Immunol.* 17:469–477.

86. White, K.L., Link-Snyder, H., and Krzych, U. 1996. MHC class I-dependant presentation of exoerythrocytic antigens to $CD8^+$ T lymphocytes is required for protective immunity against *Plasmodium berghei*. *J. Immunol.* 156:3374–3381.

87. Weiss, W.R., Sedegah, M., Beaudoin, L., Miller, L., and Good, M. 1988. $CD8^+$ T cells (cytotoxic/suppressors) are required for protection in mice immunized with malaria sporozoites. *Proc. Natl. Acad. Sci. U.S.A.* 185:573–576.

88. Romero, P., Maryanski, J.L., Corradin, G., Nussenzweig, R.S., Nussenzweig, V., and Zavala, F. 1989. Cloned cytotoxic T cells recognize an epitope in the circumsporozoite protein and protect against malaria. *Nature* 341:323–326.

89. Lee, W.T., Yin, X.M., and Vivetta, E.S. 1990. Functional and ontogenic analysis of murine $CD45R^{hi}$ and $CD45R^{lo}$ $CD4^+$ T cells. *J. Immunol.* 144:3288–3295.

90. Weiss ,W.R., Sedegah, M., Berzofsky, J.A., and Hoffman, S.L. 1993. The role of $CD4^+$ T cells in immunity to malaria sporozoites. *J. Immunol.* 151:2690–2698.

91. Malik, A., Egan, J.E., Houghten, R.A., Sadoff, J.C., and Hoffman, S.L. 1991. Human cytotoxic T lymphocytes against the *Plasmodium falciparum* circumsporozoite protein. *Proc. Natl. Acad. Sci. U.S.A.* 88:3300–3304.

92. Kumar, S., Miller, L.H., Quakyi, A., Keister, D.B., Houghten, R.A., Maloy, W.L., Moss, B., Berzofsky, J.A., and Good, M.F. 1988. Cytotoxic T cells specific for the circumsporozoite protein of *Plasmodium falciparum*. *Nature* 334:258–260.

93. Krzych, U., White, K., Link, H.T., Sadoff, J., Lanar, D., Ballou, W.R., Jareed, T., and Agarwal, A. 1990. Role of circumsporozoite protein-specific T-cells in protective immunity against *Plasmodium berghei. Bull World Health Org.* 68(Suppl.):88–93.

94. Wizel, B., Houghten, R., Church, P., Tine, J.A., Lanar, D.E., Gordon, D.M., Ballou, W.R., Sette, A., and Hoffman, S.L. 1995. HLA-A2-restricted cytotoxic T lymphocyte responses to multiple *Plasmodium falciparum* sporozoite surface protein-2 epitopes in sporozoite-immunized volunteers. *J. Immunol.* 155:766–775.

95. Rodrigues, M., Nussenzweig, R.S., Romero, P., and Zavala, F. 1992. The in vivo cytotoxic activity of $CD8^+$ T cell clones correlates with their levels of expression of adhesion molecules. *J. Exp. Med.* 175:895–905.

96. Weiss, W.A., Mellouk, S., Houghten, R.A., Sedegah, M., Kumar, S., Good, M.F., Berzofski, J.A., Miller, L.H., and Hoffman, S.L. 1990. Cytotoxic T cells recognize a peptide from the circumsporoaoite protein on malaria infected hepatocytes. *J. Exp. Med.* 171:763–773.

97. Trinchieri, G., and Scott, P. 1995. Immunoregulation by interleukin-12. *Res. Immunol.* 146:423–651.

98. Gately, M.K., Wolitzky, A.G., Quinn, P.M., and Chizzonite, R. 1992. Regulation of human cytolytic lymphocyte responses by interleukin-12. *Cell. Immunol.* 143:127–142.

99. Hsieh, C., Macatonia, S.E., Tripp, C.S., Wolf, S.F., O'Garra, A., and Murphy K.M. 1993. Listeria induced Th1 development in $\alpha\beta$ TCR transgenic $CD4^+$ T cells occurs through macrophage production of IL-12. *Science* 260:547–549.

100. Sedegah, M., Finkelman, F., and Hoffman, S.L. 1994. Interleukin-12 induction of interferon-γ-dependent protection against malaria. *Proc. Natl. Acad. Sci. U.S.A.* 91:10700–10702.

101. White, K.L., Jarboe, D.L., and Krzych, U. 1994. Immunization with irradiated *Plasmodium berghei* sporozoites induces IL-2 and IFN-γ but not IL-4. *Parasite Immunol.* 16:479–491.

102. Qian, S., Lu, L., Fu, F., Li, Y., Li, W., Starzl, T.E., Fung, J.J., and Thomson A.W. 1997. Apoptosis within spontaneously accepted mouse liver allografts. *J. Immunol.* 158:4654–4661.

103. Mellouk, S., Maheshwari, R., Rhodes-Feuillette, A., et al. 1987. Inhibitory activity of interferons and interleukin-1 on the development of *Plasmodium falciparum* in human hepatocyte cultures. *J. Immunol.* 139:4192–4195.

104. Ferreira, A., Schofield, L., Enea, V., Schellekens, H., Vandermeide, P., Collins, W., Nussenzweig, R., and Nussenzweig, V. 1986. Inhibition of development of exoerythrocytic forms of malaria parasites by γ-interferon. *Science* 232:881–884.

105. Schofield, L., Villaquiran, J., Ferreira, A., Schellekens, H., Nussenzweig, R., and Nussenzweig, V. 1987. γ-interferon, $CD8^+$ T cells and antibodies are required for immunity to malaria sporozoites. *Nature* 330:664–666.

106. Tsuji, M., Miyahira, Y., Nussenzweig, R., Aguet, M., Reichel, M., and Zavala, F. 1995. Development of antimalaria immunity in mice lacking IFN-γ receptor. *J. Immunol.* 154:5338–5344.

107. Suhrbier, A. 1991. Immunity to liver stages of malaria. *Parasitology Today* 7:160–163.

108. Muller, D., Koller, B.H., Whitton, J.L., LaPan, K.E., Brigman, K.K., and Frelinger, J.A. 1992. LCMV-specific, class II-restricted cytotoxic T cells in β_2-microglobulin-deficient mice. *Science* 255:1576–1578.

109. Denkers, E.Y., Gazzinelly, R.T., Martin, D., and Sher, A. 1993. Emergence of $NK1.1^+$ cells as effectors of IFN-γ-dependent immunity to *Toxoplasma gondii* in class I-deficient mice. *J. Exp. Med.* 178:1465–1472.

110. Ohteki, T., Seki, S., Abo, T., and Kumogai, K. 1990. Liver is a possible site for the proliferation of abnormal $CD3^+4^-8^-$ double-negative lymphocytes in autoimmune MRL-lpr/lpr mice. *J. Exp. Med.* 172:7–12.

111. Bendelac, A. 1995. Positive selection of mouse NK1.1$^+$ T cells by CD1-expressing cortical thymocytes. *J. Exp. Med.* 182:2091.

112. Ohteki, T., and MacDonald, H.R. 1994. Major histocompatibility complex class I related molecules control the development of $CD4^+8^-$ and $CD4^-8^-$ subsets of NK1.1$^+$ T cell receptor-α/β^+ cells in the liver of mice. *J. Exp. Med.* 180:699–704.

113. Hashimoto, W., Takeda, K., Anzai, R., Ogasawara, K., Sakihara, H., Sugiura, K., Seki, S., and Kumagai, K. 1995. Cytotoxic NK1.1 Ag$^+$ $\alpha\beta$ T cells with intermediate TCR induced in the liver of mice by IL-12. *J. Immunol.* 154:4333–4340.

114. Yoshimoto, T., and Paul, W.E. 1994. $CD4^{pos}$, NK1.1^{pos} T cells promptly produce interleukin-4 in response to in vivo challenge with anti-CD3. *J. Exp. Med.* 179:1285–1295.

115. Denkers, E.Y., Scharton-Kersten, T., Barbieri, S., Caspar, P., and Sher, A. 1996. A role for CD4+ NK1.1+ T lymphocytes as major histocompatibility complex class II independent helper cells in the generation of CD8$^+$ effector function against intracellular infection. *J. Exp. Med.* 184:131–139.

116. Takeda, K., Seki, S., Ogasawara, K., Anzai, R., Hashimoto, W., Sugiura, K., Takahashi, M., Satoh, M., and Kumagai, K. 1996. Liver NK1.1$^+$ CD4$^+$ $\alpha\beta$ T cells activated by IL-12 as a major effector in inhibition of experimental tumor metastasis. *J. Immunol.* 156:3366–3373.

117. Emoto, M., Emoto, Y., and Kaufman, S.H.E. 1995. Interleukin-4 producing CD4$^+$ NK1.1$^+$ TCR$\alpha\beta^{intermediate}$ liver lymphocytes are down regulated by listeria monocytogenes. *Eur. J. Immunol.* 25:3321–3325.

118. Kaufman, S.H.E. 1993. Immunity to intracellular bacteria. *Annu. Rev. Immunol.* 11:129.

119. Langhorne, J., Gillard, S., Simon, B., Slade, S., and Eichmann, K. 1989. Frequencies of CD4$^+$ T cells reactive with *Plasmodium chabaudi chabaudi*, I. Distinct response kinetics of cells with Th1 and Th2 characteristics during infection. *Int. Immunol.* 1:416–424.

120. Bergmann, E.S., Ballou, R.W., and Krzych, U. 1997. Detection of CD4$^+$ C D45RO$^+$ T Lymphocytes producing IL-4 in response to antigens on *Plasmodium falciparum erythrocytes*: An *in vitro* correlate of a protective immunity induced with attenuated *Plasmodium falciparum* sporozoites *Cell. Immunol.* 180:143–152.

121. Vergelli, M., Pinet, V., Vogt, A.B., Kalbus, M., Malnati, M., Riccio, P., Long, E.O., and Martin R. 1997. HLA-DR-restricted presentation of purified myelin basic protein is independent of intracellular processing. *Eur. J. Immunol.* 27:941–951.

122. Schwartz, R. 1996. Models of T cell anergy: Is there a common molecular mechanism? *J. Exp. Med.* 184:1–8.

123. Boussiotis, V., Freeman, G., Gribben, J., and Nadler, L. 1996. The role of B7-1/B7-2: CD28/CTLA-4 pathways in the prevention of anergy, induction of protective immunity and down-regulation of immune responses. *Immunol. Rev.* 153:5–26.

124. Link, H.T., White, K., and Krzych, U. 1993. *Plasmodium berghei*-specific T cells respond to nonprocessed sporozoites presented by B cells. *Eur. J. Immunol.* 23:2263–2269.

125. Lohse, A.W., Knolle, P.A., Bilo, K., Uhrig, A., Waldmann, C., Ibe, M., Schmitt, E., Gerken, G., Mayer, Z., and Buschenfelde, K.H. 1996. Antigen presenting function and B7 expression on murine Kupffer cells. *Gastroenterology* 110:1175–1181.

126. Mochizuki, K., Hayashi, N., Katayama, K., et al. 1997. B7 expression and hepatitis activity in liver tissues of patient with chronic hepatitis C. *Hepatology* 25:713–718.

127. Scheller, L.F., and Azad, A.F. 1995. Maintenance of protective immunity against malaria by persistent hepatic parasites derived from irradiated sporozoites. *Proc. Natl. Acad. Sci. U.S.A.* 92:4066.

128. Egan, J., Hoffman, S., Haynes, D., Sadoff, J.C., Schneider, I., Grau, G.E., Hollingdale, M.R., Ballou, W.R., and Gordon, D.M. 1993. Humoral immune responses in volunteers immunized with irradiated *Plasmodium falciparum* sporozoites. *Am. J. Trop. Med. Hyg.* 49:166–173.

129. Zinkernagel, R., Bachman, M., Kundig, T., Kundig, T.M., Oehen, S., Pirchet, M., and Hengartner, H. 1996. On immunological memory. *Annu. Rev. Immunol.* 14:333–367.

130. Krzych, U., Lyon, J.A., Jareed, T., Schneider, I., Hollingdale, M., Gordon, D., and Ballou, W.R. 1995. T lymphocytes from volunteers immunized with irradiated *Plasmodium falciparum* sporozoites recognize liver and blood stage malaria antigens. *J. Immunol.* 155:4072–4077.

131. Link, H., Ballou, W.R., and Krzych, U. 1990. Immune response to *Plasmodium berghei* sporozoite antigens, I. Evaluation of murine T cell repertoire following immunization with irradiated sporozoites. *Am. J. Trop. Med. Hyg.* 43:452–458.

132. Pied, S., Voegtle, D., Marussig, M., Renia, L., Miltgen, F., Mazier, D., and Cazenave, P. 1996. Evidence for superantigenic activity during murine malaria infection. *Int. Immunol.* 9:17–25.

133. Lynch, D.H., Ramsdell, F., and Alderson, M.R. 1995. Fas and FasL in the homeostatic regulation of immune responses. *Immunol. Today* 16:569–574.

134. Galle, P.R., Hofman, W.J., Walczak, H., Schaller, H., Otto, C., Stremmel, W., Krammer, P.H., and Runkel, L. 1995. Involvement of the CD95 (APO-1/Fas) receptor and ligand in liver damage. *J. Exp. Med.* 182:1223–1230.

135. Krzych, U., Jareed, T., Link, H.T., Loomis, L.D., and Ballou, W.R. 1992. Distinct T cell specificities are induced with the authentic versus recombinant *Plasmodium berghei* circumsporozoite protein. *J. Immunol.* 148:2530–2538.

CHAPTER 10

T CELLS AND AUTOIMMUNE LIVER DISEASE

JUDY VAN DE WATER and M. ERIC GERSHWIN
University of California, Davis School of Medicine, Davis, CA

INTRODUCTION

While their pathogenic mechanisms remain a mystery, there are several liver diseases that are considered to be autoimmune in nature. Among these are primary biliary cirrhosis (PBC), primary sclerosing cholangitis (PSC), and autoimmune hepatitis (AIH). Autoimmune diseases are believed to be caused by a failure of the immune system to distinguish between self, for which there exists a state of natural immune tolerance, and non-self. Failure of immune tolerance often results in adverse consequences, including tissue and organ destruction due to abnormalities of both humoral and cell-mediated immune responses. The role of T cells and inflammation and the influence of immunogenetics, in these diseases has been studied extensively during the past few years. In this chapter we will review these factors relative to three well-known autoimmune diseases of the liver, PBC, PSC, and AIH.

T CELLS AND INFLAMMATION

The immunopathogenesis of autoimmune liver disease is poorly understood. While autoantibodies to ubiquitous intracellular antigens are present in most of these diseases, the reason for the specificity of damage to the liver remains unknown. The presence of lymphocytic infiltrates is one of the histological hallmarks of these chronic autoimmune liver diseases.

Immunohistochemical studies have shown that equal numbers of $CD8^+$ and $CD4^+$ T cells can be found in such infiltrates (1–6). The role of these infiltrating T cells in

T Lymphocytes in the Liver: Immunobiology, Pathology, and Host Defense, Edited by I. Nicholas Crispe
ISBN 0-471-19218-X

autoimmune liver disease has been studied extensively, yet there has been no definitive correlation made between T cell infiltrates and liver pathology in diseases such as primary biliary cirrhosis (PBC), primary sclerosing cholangitis (PSC), and autoimmune hepatitis (AIH).

Autoimmune Hepatitis (AIH)

Although the pathogenic mechanisms underlying the development and progression of AIH are still unclear, several characteristics of the disease suggest that it is an immunologically mediated disease process. The presence of a number of autoantibodies against intracellular structures, such as nuclear and microsomal antigens, cytoskeleton, and cytosol, in the sera of such patients are used as diagnostic markers for AIH. It has also been demonstrated that one such microsomal antigen, cytochrome P450IID6, is expressed on the surface of hepatocytes (7).

Immunohistological studies in AIH patients show a predominance of $CD4^+$ T cells in addition to B cells and plasma cells within dense lymphocytic infiltrates (8,9) (Table 10.1). In contrast to chronic viral hepatitis, there are few activated macrophages or cytotoxic $CD4^+$ and $CD8^+$ T cells (8). When T cells are isolated from the liver of patients with AIH, there is a predominance of T helper type 1 (Th1)-cytokine-releasing $CD4^+$ T cells. However, there is also an increase in the frequency of Th2 $CD4^+$ T cells producing interleukin-4 (IL-4) (10).

It has been recently demonstrated that liver-infiltrating T cell clones from patients with type II AIH recognize a recombinant LKM-1 antigen that contains the immunodominant region of cytochrome P450IID6 antigen. Moreover, activated LKM-specific T cells were shown to release IFNγ but little or no IL-4. Interestingly, $CD4^+$ T cells isolated from peripheral blood of three AIH patients secreted large amounts of IFNγ upon stimulation with autologous irradiated LKM-P1-specific T cell lines. This suggests the existence of specific regulatory cells. Also, the sequence homologies of greater than 70% between the aa 254–285 LKM-1 region and hepatitis C virus antigens suggest the possibility of molecular mimicry (11). While a correlation between

TABLE 10.1 Phenotypic Characteristics of Liver-derived T Cells from Patients with PBC, PSC, and AIH

Characteristic	PBC	PSC	AIH
Known T cell Antigens	PDC-E2, PDC-E1	Unknown	LKM-1
T cell phenotype	Predominantly $CD4^+$	Predominantly $CD4^+$	Predominantly $CD4^+$
Lymphokine profile	IL-2, IL-4, and IFNγ	n.d.*	IFNγ, IL-4
T cell receptor			
phenotype	α/β	α/β, γδ	α/β
Vβ usage	Heterogeneous	n.d.	Restricted, Vβ3 association
$CD45RO^+$ (memory)	10–30%	n.d.	n.d.

*n.d.: not determined.

T cell reactivity to LKM and disease activity has been suggested (11), there has been no direct correlation between either antibody reactivity or T cell responsiveness to the LKM antigen and the pathogenesis of this disease.

Cytokines released by activated T cells are crucial for the development of a chronic inflammatory response such as that seen in autoimmune liver disease. The cytokine response of non-antigen-specific T cells isolated from the livers of patients with AIH has been shown to be predominately IL-4 (Table 10.1). This is in contrast to viral hepatitis, where IFNγ is the predominant cytokine (6,10).

On a more molecular level, the pattern of T cell receptor (TCR) usage by liver-infiltrating T cells has recently been extensively investigated in several liver diseases. The TCR, a heterodimer which is composed of α and β, or γ and δ chains, is present on the surface of most T cells and is responsible for the recognition of antigenic peptide fragments in association with the major histocompatibility complex (MHC) molecules. The TCR β chain contains four distinct regions; the variable (V), diversity (D), junctional (J), and constant (C) regions. There is an accumulation of diversity within the V, D, and J regions, and additional diversity is generated by random insertion or deletion of nucleotides in the V-D-J junction region. This region is known as the complimentarity-determining region 3 (CDR3), and is thought to be the site of contact with antigenic peptides (12). Analysis of T cell receptor β chain V region usages and CDR3 sequences of the TCR has been considered an important factor in understanding the immune mechanisms of the T cell response in autoimmune liver disease. In fact, this approach has been used intensively to investigate several autoimmune diseases, including multiple sclerosis (13).

Analysis of the T cell receptor β chain has recently been performed on liver-infiltrating T cells from patients with AIH (14). In one such study, all four of the patients analyzed showed a remarkable bias for the usage of Vβ3 (Table 10.1). Moreover, V$\beta 3^+$ Jβ 1.2^+ T cell clones with a particular Asp-Arg-Pro motif in the CDR3 were shown to be closely associated with human leukocyte antigen DR4 (HLA-DR4) (14). While this study was done on a relatively small number of patients, it does offer an interesting clue as to the relationship between a particular DR allele and the antigen-binding site of the TCR.

Primary Sclerosing Cholangitis (PSC)

Primary sclerosing cholangitis (PSC) is a chronic cholestatic liver disease, the cause of which has not yet been ascertained. It leads to progressive obliterating fibrosis of the bile ducts, with the eventual development of biliary cirrhosis followed by liver failure (15,16). Although the evidence that PSC is an autoimmune disease is less compelling than for primary biliary cirrhosis (PBC), immunological damage to the biliary tree remains the most likely cause of PSC (17,18). As in PBC, PSC is characterized by lymphocytic infiltration and bile duct destruction, hypergammaglobulinemia, and an association with other autoimmune disorders, including inflammatory bowel disease (IBD), thyroiditis, and arthritis (19). In fact, 70% to 80% of PSC cases are associated with IBD (20). However, in contrast to PBC and AIH, the presence of classic autoantibodies such as antimitochondrial, antinuclear, or antimicrosomal antibodies is less frequent in patients with PSC (21). More recent studies have found a high incidence of circulating anti-colon antibodies, anti-neutrophil nuclear antibodies, and anti-neutrophil cytoplasmic antibodies (ANCAs) (22–24). While the presence of such antibodies indicates an interesting link with IBD, there is the possibility that they are merely an epiphenomenon and have no relation to the etiopathogenesis of PSC. This statement, of course, could be applied to any of the three diseases discussed in this chapter. However, the presence of autoantibodies is often one of the few clues that we have to suggest an immunological disregulation in a patient with a disease of unknown etiology.

There are also several abnormalities found in the cellular immune system in patients with PSC. For instance, several studies have reported a significant increase in the CD4/CD8 ratio due to a decrease in the CD8 population of T cells (25,26) (Table 10.1). There was also a correlation made between cirrhosis and an increase in this ratio; those patients with no cirrhosis had more $CD8^+$ T cells in peripheral blood (25). The important of this decrease in $CD8^+$ T cells remains to be clarified. However, it does suggest a possible decrease in a regulatory T cell population. Alternatively, it is possible that this decrease is correlated with a sequestration of these cells in the portal tract, and an increase in $CD8^+$ T cells has been demonstrated in the portal lesions of PSC patients in conjunction with infiltration of the bile duct epithelium (27). This suggests that the bile duct epithelium is in fact a target of the immune response in PSC. No studies showing specificity of these portal T cells towards a particular antigen or against bile duct epithelial cells have been performed to date. Thus, there is as yet no solid evidence of the role of these infiltrating T cells in PSC.

More recently, an immunohistochemical study of liver infiltrating lymphocytes reported an elevation in the percentage and absolute numbers of $\gamma\delta$ T cells in the portal areas of patients with PSC (10.55%), and a less dramatic increase in persons with AIH (7.16%) and PBC (5.57%), when compared with controls (2.23%) (28) (Table 10.1). The authors suggest that these $\gamma\delta$ T cells play a role in the immune damage of these autoimmune liver diseases. However, it is also a possibility, given the recent evidence of the proposed regulatory role of these cells, that their presence indicates an attempt at downregulation of the local inflammatory response (29,30). It has been speculated that $\gamma\delta$ T cells produce downregulatory factors that mediate T cell suppression. In addition, these cells are present at high frequency in the intestinal tract and are thus thought to be the cells involved in the development of oral tolerance.

Primary Biliary Cirrhosis (PBC)

Primary biliary cirrhosis is the quintessential example of an organ-specific autoimmune disease, a group of disorders in which the antigen is broadly distributed to virtually all nucleated cells, but the immune destruction is specifically targeted to a relatively few tissues. The autoantigens recognized in PBC are predominantly components of normal mitochondria, although less commonly components of the nucleus and cytoplasm are also recognized. How a mitochondrial antigen, physically sheltered from the immune system by two membrane barriers, can elicit an immune response or, once tolerance is broken, how this "self-reactive" immunity causes tissue damage in only some cells, is still unknown. Undeniably, however, the immune damage in PBC is almost exclusively directed against the intrahepatic biliary epithelium (31,32).

Autoimmune mechanisms have been implicated in the pathogenesis of this disease, which is characterized by the presence of high titers of autoantibodies to mitochondrial antigens (AMA) (33) with the immunodominant response directed at the E2 component of pyruvate dehydrogenase (PDC-E2) (34,35). The presence of T cell infiltrates in the portal tract has led to much speculation concerning the role of these cells in the pathogenesis of PBC. Due to the strong autoimmune association and intense portal infiltrates, a great deal of study has been concentrated on T cells in PBC. Early studies focused on the phenotypic characterization of these liver-infiltrating T cells. The $CD3^+$, $CD4^+$ or $CD8^+$ T lymphocyte expressing the TCR Vβ chain is the predominant cell type surrounding the portal triads in late-stage PBC. There is a long-standing controversy regarding whether $CD4^+$ or $CD8^+$ T cells are the dominant cell type in portal tract lesions. Some studies (36) indicate that the $CD8^+$ T lymphocyte is the predominant cell type. In one study, the authors found that the CD4/CD8 ratio was decreased, the relative activation of T cell subsets and NK cells was increased, the suppressor-inducer T subset was depressed, and the primed memory T subset was increased. The cytotoxic T cell subset ($CD11b^-$) dominated within the $CD8^+$ population (37). In contrast, Krams et al. (4) reported that the predominant cell type in the mononuclear infiltrate is the $CD3^+$, $CD4^+$ T lymphocyte bearing the T cell receptor αβ (Table 10.1). In addition, Leon et al. described a marked shift towards the CD45RO high RA^- "memory" phenotype in the liver-infiltrating $CD4^+$ T cells in PBC patients. Cells within the $CD4^+$ memory subpopulation were further subgrouped according to expression of CD45RB, whose level of expression has been associated with functional differences in the memory subset. A statistically significant difference in the distribution of these memory subsets, with an increased memory-2/memory-1 ratio was observed in the liver-infiltrating $CD4^+$ T cells of PBC patients, especially when compared with those from alcoholic cirrhosis patients (38). In another investigation, it was found that liver tissue and peripheral blood T cells of patients with PBC were dominated by $CD4^+$ $TCR\alpha\beta^+$ T helper/inducer cells. This was in contrast to patients with chronic viral hepatitis, where an enrichment of $CD8^+$ $TCR\alpha\beta^+$ cytotoxic/suppressor T cells was observed (6). The above conflicting results emphasize the need to develop functional assays to analyze the inflammatory infiltrates in PBC.

It has been hypothesized that the destruction of the biliary tract in PBC is mediated by autoreactive liver-infiltrating T cells exerting cytotoxic activity or lymphokine release. Although it has been suggested that the infiltrating T cells are oligoclonal, there have been several reports on the characterization of PDC-E2-specific cloned T cells lines (1,39–41). In an early study by Meuer et al. (42), phenotypic and functional analysis of human liver T lymphocytes in patients with PBC demonstrated a heterogeneous cell population. However, when compared to peripheral blood lymphocytes of the same patients, a marked enrichment for $CD8^+$ cytotoxic T cells was found to exist in the liver of these patients. From this data, the authors suggested that liver cell injury in PBC may be mediated by an immunological mechanism that was most likely executed by cells of the T lineage.

A study by Van de Water et al. (41) using cloned T cell lines from liver biopsies from patients with PBC demonstrated for the first time that clones reacting with PDC-E2 and/or branched-chain ketoacid dehydrogenase (BCKD-E2) were present in the livers of patients with PBC but not in the livers of controls with chronic active hepatitis. In addition, these clones were found to be $CD4^+$, $CD8^-$, $TCR\alpha\beta^+$ and produced IL-2 specifically in response to PDC-E2 or BCKD-E2 (43) (Table 10.1). In a related study, liver-infiltrating T cells were also shown to be specific for the bovine pyruvate dehydrogenase complex (PDC), the purified E2 subunit (PDC-E2), and a crude preparation of human liver mitoplasts (HLM; i.e., mitochondria depleted of their outer membranes, ref. 39). Peripheral blood lymphocytes (PBL) from 11 of 15 patients (73.3%) with PBC showed an HLA class II–restricted proliferative response to the PDC complex. These results were in contrast to those from patients with chronic viral hepatitis, autoimmune hepatitis, or extrahepatic cholestatic icterus, and to healthy controls. In addition, 13 of 15 patients with PBC (86.6%) and 3 of 9 patients with autoimmune hepatitis (33.3%) had PBL that reacted with the crude HLM preparation, whereas no reactivity was found with control PBL. Analysis of 115 liver-infiltrating T cell clones derived from two diagnostic liver biopsies of patients with PBC revealed a predominance of activated $CD4^+CD8^-$ T helper cells. Nine of the 115 T cell clones responded to the PDC complex but not to the purified subunit of PDC (PDC-E2) when the antigen was presented by autologous B cell lines. Reactivities of 6 of 42 tested T cell clones to the HLM preparation were HLA-DR dependent. Of these 6 T cell clones, 3 were also responsive to PDC. The authors concluded that among liver-infiltrating T cells in PBC, there are autoreactive T cells that recognize some epitopes on the inner mitochondrial membranes that seem to be located in part on the PDC complex (39).

The immunodominant epitope of PBC, PDC-E2, contains two lipoic acid binding regions, the inner (E2L1) and outer (E2L2) lipoic domains, which share a 63% sequence homology (44). In a study by Surh et al., sera from patients with PBC were tested for antibody activity against these two lipoyl domains, and 80% to 90% of patients show activity to both domains (44). However, antibody titers to the inner domain (E2L2) are frequently 100-fold greater. Previous data suggested that the B cell epitopes for these two domains had partial cross-reactivity based on selective absorption data (45). When the peripheral T cell response to these antigens was examined (46), 54% of patients showed a response to the outer lipoic acid binding region (E2L2), while only 36% responded to the inner lipoyl domain. Thus, the peripheral T cell response appears to be directed against two entirely separate regions of the PDC-E2 molecule. Surprisingly, only 4 of the 10 patients who responded to the E2L1 and E2L2 domains also reacted to the full-length PDC-E2 molecule. This may indicate the presence of an epitope within the full-length PDC-E2 molecule that overlaps the E2L1 and E2L2 proteins and is not present on either of the smaller lipoyl domains.

Antigen-specific T cell clones derived from the livers of patients with PBC have also been examined. These clones demonstrated specificity for PDC-E2, PDC-E1, and the E2L1 and E2L2 domains of PDC-E2 (46). The majority of the clones responded to the inner lipoic acid domain, E2L2. The difference in T cell specificity between patients was quite remarkable. For example, 25% of the cloned T cell lines from one patient showed specificity for PDC-E1, while none of the T cell clones from another patient showed similar specificity. These differences could be attributed to chance during cloning or could be due to a difference in the stage of the liver at the time of transplant. A final possibility could be MHC differences and their ability to recognize and present the various antigens. This data raises the issue of whether there is preferential homing of the E2L2-reactive T cells to the liver and whether the epitope recognized by these E2L2-specific T cells may cross-react with a non-PDC antigen, as has been suggested by previous histological studies (47). As these studies suggest, there is in fact more than one T cell epitope on the PDC-E2 antigen and some of these epitopes may be shared while others are unique to the two lipoyl regions.

Due to the high incidence of recurrent urinary tract infection in patients with PBC, it has been hypothesized that PBC may have a bacterial etiology (31,48). PDC-E2 peptides are evolutionarily highly conserved among various species, especially at the lipoic binding sites (49). Furthermore, the sera from patients with PBC has been shown to react with both human PDC-E2 and *E. coli* PDC-E2 (50). However, a contradictory study involving the measurement of the functional reactivity of serum autoantibodies by means of an enzyme inhibition assay against pyruvate dehydrogenase complex from different sources including mammalian, *Saccharomyces cerevisiae*, and *E. coli*, reported that the PBC sera were highly inhibitory for mammalian PDC (10 of 10 inhibitory; mean level of inhibition, 99%), moderately inhibitory for yeast pyruvate dehydrogenase complex (10 of 10 inhibitory; mean level, 70%), and only weakly inhibitory for *E. coli* pyruvate dehydrogenase complex (4 of 10 inhibitory; mean level, 26%). Thus, using a functional assay that depends on epitope recognition of PBC sera, cross-reactivity between mammalian and bacterial pyruvate dehydrogenase complex enzymes was low and the concept of "molecular mimicry," at least at the B lymphocyte level, was not supported (51).

Still, a mechanism of "molecular mimicry" has been proposed as a possible cause of PBC at the T cell level (52) (Fig. 10.1). According to this hypothesis, the T cells would first recognize the lipoyl domain of *E. coli* PDC-E2 containing EGDKA sequences. These T cells would then cross-react to self-peptides containing AVDKA sequences from the HLA DR α chain of ETDKA sequences from human PDC-E2 by aberrantly expressed class II HLA molecules on biliary epithelial cells (53). Finally, this reactivity would initiate the autoimmune cascade leading to the destruction of the bile ducts in which AMA and/or autoreactive T cells specific for mitochondrial Ags may play a pathogenic role. At this final stage, the autoimmune process would take place in the absence of the exogenous antigens, such as *E. coli* PDC-E2, which initiated the original immune response. In some animal models of autoimmune diseases, such as experimental allergic encephalomyelitis and autoimmune oophoritis, the "molecular mimicry" mechanism has been demonstrated to operate *in vivo* (54–59).

In a study by Shimoda et al. (60), the demonstration of T cell clones specific for human PDC-E2 163–176 (GDLLAEIETDKATI) which cross-react with the lipoic acid binding site of *E. coli* PDC-E2 (EQSLITVEGDKASM) suggests that "molecular mimicry" between human and *E. coli* PDC-E2 can be operative at the T cell clonal level in PBC. However, none of these PDC-E2-specific T cell clones cross-reacted with the HLA DR α chain peptide 82–95 (QGALANIAVDKANL), or the human

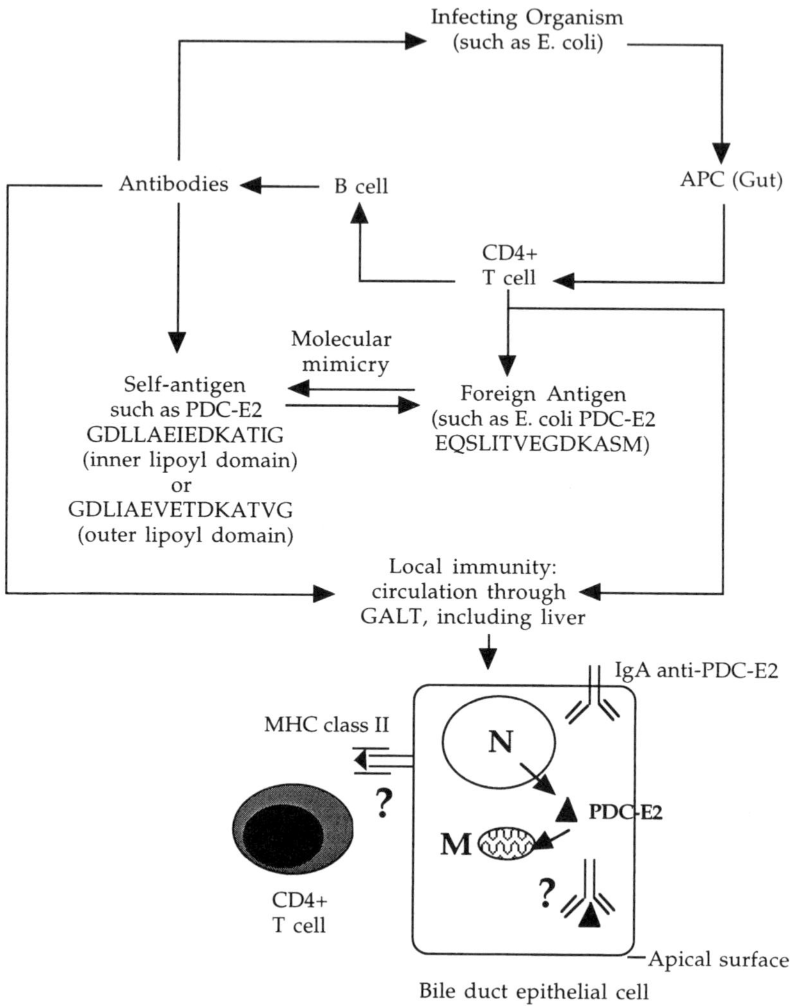

Figure 10.1. What role, if any, does molecular mimicry play in autoimmune liver disease? Diagram of hypothetical relationship between a foreign antigen (*E. coli* PDC-E2) and a self–intracellular protein (PDC-E2). PBC was used for this example; however, this hypothesis could apply to any of the autoimmune diseases discussed herein. N = nucleus and M = mitochondria.

glycogen phosphorylase b peptide 354–367 (LVDLERMDWDKAWD), both of which have some amino acid homology with PDC-E2 but lack the requisite EXDK sequence. Moreover, it is important to note that clone T-pep-11-2 cross-reacted to *E. coli* PDC-E2 (EQSLITVEGDKASM) but not to *P. putida* PDC-E2 (DELLATIET-DKIDI), which not only has EXDK sequences but also has a higher degree of amino acid homology with human PDC-E2 163–176 than with *E. coli* PDC-E2 (EQS-LITVEGDKASM). Interestingly, the T cell epitope of the PDC-E2 peptide 163–176 almost completely overlaps the B cell epitope that was previously identified as part of the inner lipoyl domain of PDC-E2 (PDC-E2 165–184, with lipoic acid located at aa174 [K]) (34,50). In addition, all of the T cell clones specific for the PDC-E2 peptide 163–176 cross-reacted with the PDC-E2 peptide 36–49, which corresponds to the outer lipoyl domain of PDC-E2. This PDC-E2 outer lipoyl domain was also shown to be a B cell epitope of PDC-E2, which cross-reacts with the immunodominant B cell epitope of the inner lipoyl domain of PDC-E2, although to a much lesser degree (34,50,61). Recently, "universal" T cell epitopes of certain viruses have been found to be located near the B cell epitopes, indicating that the regions containing both T and B cell epitopes can be highly immunogenic (62). Although there have been no reports showing the exact relationship between T and B cell epitopes of self-antigens, these results may indicate the possibility that peptides of self-antigens containing both T and B cell epitopes could be highly immunogenic autoepitopes.

Several TCR Vβ usage studies have been performed on liver-derived T cells from patients with PBC (Table 10.1). Moebius et al. (63) generated non-antigen-specific T cell clones from liver biopsies of three patients with chronic active hepatitis B and two patients with primary biliary cirrhosis. These T cell clones (n = 84) were analyzed by means of T cell receptor (TCR) β gene rearrangements to determine whether the infiltrate consisted of a polyclonal or oligoclonal T cell population. The majority (62 of 64) of T cell clones from three different patients with chronic active hepatitis B showed no identical rearrangements of the TCR Vβ chain genes. In contrast, both patients with PBC had T cell clones of limited diversity. Thus identical TCR Vβ gene rearrangements were found in 5/10 and 2/10 T cell clones from one patient and 3/9 and 2/9 T cell clones from the second patient, respectively. The authors have suggested that a clonal dominance is characteristic for local T cell responses in autoimmune liver disease such as primary biliary cirrhosis, whereas in virus-induced chronic active hepatitis T cell activation occurs polyclonally.

Tsai et al. (64) analyzed the TCR Vβ usage in different regions of the livers removed during transplantation from two PBC patients. Using reverse transcription and polymerase chain reaction (RT-PCR), a limited heterogeneity of rearranged TCR Vβ transcripts was demonstrated in different locations of the same liver. Sequence analysis of the Vβ-Dβ-Jβ (CDR3: the third complementarity determining region) showed the presence of conserved residues, no random non-germline encoded (N) region additions, and a common motif within the CDR3. The authors suggested from these results that T cells homing to PBC liver may be antigen driven (64).

A recent study by Van de Water et al. supports the notion of antigen-specific T cells homing to the liver, but reports that the T cell receptor Vβ repertoire utilized by PDC-reactive clones infiltrating the liver was remarkable in its heterogeneity (46). This heterogeneity was especially apparent within subsets that responded to particular domains. For example, in two patients with PBC, PDC-E2L2-reactive (inner lipoyl domain) T cell clones utilized multiple different Vβs and only a few examples of repetitive Vβ usage were noted. This contrasts greatly with studies of peripheral blood cloned T cell lines in multiple sclerosis (65), but is consistent with other studies (66). A few Vβs were also noted to be possibly overutilized, but the relatively small number of clones used to estimate total repertoire limits any definite conclusions. The reason for the markedly heterogeneous repertoire is unclear. The E2L2 domain is 113 amino acids long, and it is possible that multiple different peptide epitopes are present within this region. Since the patients studied were advanced in their disease process, additional epitopes may have elicited responses related to the tissue damage, by a process analogous to the determinant spreading defined in experimental allergic encephalomyelitis (EAE) (56,57). It is also possible that the multiple class II molecules present in these human patients may contribute to the diverse T cell repertoire.

IMMUNOGENETICS AND AUTOIMMUNE LIVER DISEASE

One cannot thoroughly discuss the role of T cells in autoimmune liver disease without acknowledging the importance of HLA molecules in this process. While many autoimmune diseases have a genetic predisposition, this relationship is not as clear with regard to autoimmune liver diseases, such as AIH, PSC, and PBC. Moreover, immunohistochemical evidence of aberrant MHC class II molecules on bile duct epithelium has been noted in several of these diseases. What role, if any, this class II expression plays in the disease process is still unknown. Whether it is merely a secondary phenomenon, due to local inflammation, or this expression of MHC class II molecules plays a more active role in the pathogenesis of disease is still under investigation. There have been few studies in autoimmune liver disease which have addressed the binding of specific autoepitopes to the MHC class II molecules expressed on target tissue such as bile duct epithelium. However, significant progress has been made in the association of certain HLA alleles with a particular autoimmune liver disease. For example, it has been shown that most autoimmune diseases have been associated with overrepresentation of the HLA A1-B8-DR3 haplotype (68). Indeed, it would appear that AIH, PSC, and PBC have all had some association with DR3 (Table 10.2).

The recognition of peptide fragments in the context of MHC class II molecules by T cells is a central event in the development of immune responses (69). Proteolytic fragments of peptides processed by APCs that match the physiochemical character of the peptide-binding grooves formed by α and β chains of MHC class II molecules are expressed on the surface of APC and are recognized by T cells (69). The structural motifs of peptides capable of binding to HLA-DR have been determined on the basis of the peptide sequences eluted from purified DR complexes (70) or phage peptide libraries (71). These reports indicated that only certain residues are involved in allele-specific peptide binding, while the other residues are promiscuous (70). An analysis of the crystal structure of HLA DRB1 0101 protein complexed with an influenza virus peptide demonstrated the exact structural explanation for the MHC class II–peptide-TCR interaction at the molecular level (72). Because polymorphic

TABLE 10.2 Immunogenetic Characteristics of Patients with PBC, PSC, and AIH

Disease	MHC Association
PBC	DR3, Drw8, DR4 (?), DR2
PSC	B8, DR3, DR3$^-$/DR2$^{+/}$DR4$^-$, DRw52 (associated with DR3 or DR6)
AIH	A1, B8, DR3, DR4 and DR4$^-$/DR2$^+$ (Japanese population)

residues of DR alleles are scattered within the peptide-binding grooves, different DR molecules are capable of binding peptides with different structural motifs, and this phenomenon contributes to the HLA-linked polymorphism of the immune response. For example, DRB1 0405 confers increased susceptibility to rheumatoid arthritis (RA) but not to insulin autoimmune syndrome (IAS), whereas DRB1 0406 conversely confers susceptibility to IAS but not to RA (73).

To date, motifs for binding peptides have been reported in various DR molecules including DR1 (DRB1 0101), DR2 (DRB1 1501), DR3 (DRB1 0301), DR4 (DRB1 0401, DRB1 0405, DRB1 0406), DR11 (DRB1 1101), DR7 (DRB1 0701), and DR8 (DRB1 0801) (74). These results indicate that two or three hydrophobic amino acids are necessary for the binding of the peptide to HLA hydrophobic pockets. However, no peptide-binding motif of HLA DRB4 0101 has yet been reported.

Autoimmune hepatitis has been associated with certain HLA alleles including A1, B8, DR3, and DR4 (10,75) (Table 10.2). In Japanese patients, a strong correlation between AIH and HLA-DR4 has been noted, while AIH patients who were DR4 negative were HLA-DR2 positive (76).

Historically, there has been a strong association between HLA-B8 and HLA-DR3 in patients with PSC (77,78) (Table 10.2). This was more recently confirmed in a study of Europeans (79,80). In DR3-negative patients with PSC, a second positive association with DR2 and a negative association for DR4 is reported (81). In addition, the HLA class antigen DRw52a was found in 100% of 29 patients with PSC who had been evaluated for transplantation, whereas only 35% of the normal population had this haplotype (81,82). DRw52a is encoded by the gene locus DRB3 and is only present in those patients who are $DR3^+$ or $DR6^+$.

In Caucasians, PBC has been reported to be associated with HLA-DR3 (83), HLA DRw8 (82), and possibly HLA DR4 (84) (Table 10.2). An association with HLA DR2 (85) and DP B1 0501 (86) has been reported in Japanese patients with PBC. In other studies, no such disease associations with HLA antigens were found (87). Thus, no consensus seems to exist concerning the associations between PBC and HLA. In the recent study by Shimoda et al. (88), T cell clones from four different patients with PBC recognized human PDC-E2 peptide 163–176 in the context of the same HLA allele, HLA DRB4 0101, indicating that the PDC-E2 peptide 163–176 may play a central role in the patients with PBC who have the HLA DRB4 0101 allele. However, the frequency of the HLA DRB4 0101 allele among patients with PBC is approximately 77%, which is similar to that among the control Japanese population (89), indicating that the possession of HLA DRB4 0101 may not be a genetic predisposition for PBC. In contrast to the high degree of polymorphism of HLA DRB1, polymorphism of HLA DRB4 0101 has not yet been reported. Therefore, it is possible that the HLA DRB4 0101–binding PDC-E2 peptide identified in the Shimoda study (88) could provide important information for the development of peptide-specific immunotherapy in the majority of patients with PBC who have an HLA DRB4 0101 allele. Although the precise analysis of the peptide-binding motif of HLA DRB4 0101 is now underway, using HLA DRB4 0101–transfected L cells and various modified peptides based on PDC-E2 peptide 163–176 (GDLLAEIETDKATI), a preliminary study indicates that LXXIXXD is an HLA DRB4 0101 binding motif. If this is the case, E and

K at positions 170 and 173 may be crucial TCR binding sites, and the amino acid at position 169 (I for human and *P. putida* PDC-E2, and V for *E. coli* PDC-E2) may be important for the structure of the TCR binding site.

The identification of the immunodominant autoepitopes and HLA molecules involved in the immune response to mitochondrial antigens may also provide insight into the pathogenesis of PBC. Shimoda et al. also found PDC-specific T cells circulating in the peripheral blood of Japanese patients with PBC, and that T cell lines specific for the entire PDC complex also proliferated in response to PDC-E2 (88). In addition, PDC-E2-specific T cell clones were generated using various peptides from PDC-E2 as clone-selecting antigens. The characterization of six PDC-E2-specific T cell clones successfully generated in this study showed that minimal T cells autotypes of T cells clones specific for PDC-E2 were all located in the same region of PDC-E2 peptide 163–176 (GDLLAEIETDKATI), which corresponds to the inner lipoyl domain of human PDC-E2. Furthermore, all T cell clones specific for human PDC-E2 163–176 were restricted by the same MHC molecule, HLA DRB4 0101; the amino acids E, D, and K (at positions 170, 172, and 173, respectively) are essential amino acid residues for this T cell epitope; and all T cell clones specific for human PDC-E2 163–176 also reacted to the PDC-E2 peptide 36–49 (GDLIAEVETDKATD), which corresponds to the outer lipoyl domain of human PDC-E2. One T cell clone (T-pep-11-2) cross-reacted to the exogenous antigen, *E. coli* PDC-E2 peptide 31–44/134–147/235–248(EQSLITVEGDKASM), which contains the sequence EXDK. However, none of the T cell clones cross-reacted to the *P. putida* BCOADC peptide 104–117 (DELLATIETDKIDI), which also has EXDK sequences, and none of the T cell clones cross-reacted to self-peptides derived from human glycogen phosphorylase b or HLA-DR α chain, both of which contain some amino acid homology with human PDC-E2 163–176 but do not contain EXDK sequences.

As more evidence for the genetic association of particular autoimmune diseases becomes known, our knowledge of the etiology and pathogenesis of immune-mediated diseases will also expand.

CONCLUSIONS

One factor that each of the above autoimmune liver diseases has in common is the presence of lymphocytic infiltrates. The physiological mechanism by which those cells accumulate in the liver is similar, regardless of the disease. Chemokines are required for the trafficking of inflammatory cells to a particular site and cytokines are required for the activation and proliferation of these cells once they reach their destination. Yet what drives the autoimmune response of T cells directed against an intracellular antigen in an organ-specific disease is still a subject of intense investigation. Recent advances in molecular immunology, together with other emerging technologies (such as affinity mass spectrometry), have been of cardinal importance in elucidating the identity of the autoantigens and the epitopes on the molecules targeted by T and B cell responses in autoimmune liver disease. Nonetheless, the primary event that leads to such diseases remains unknown. To a large extent, the present difficulties in better understanding the effector mechanisms involved in the pathogenesis of diseases such as PBC, PSC, and AIH, stem from our inability to examine the disease in its earliest stages and throughout its evolution. When patients first come to the attention of the clinician, the disease is believed to have been present for years to decades. Thus, when we come to dissect the immune response, we are observing the end-stages of a process, and many of the immune responses we can detect may result from 'bystander' or secondary responses to cellular components released from dying cells.

An age-old question in autoimmunity is: How does one lose tolerance to self-proteins? For any autoimmune disease, one must consider the inherent structural constraints for binding of a peptide to MHC class II molecules to help answer this question. Such parameters at the site of TCR recognition are dependent upon the efficient generation of the antigenic determinant during natural processing of the whole protein antigen (90). Strikingly, only a minor fraction of such potential determinants on an antigen are presented in an immunodominant manner, while the remaining peptides are silent (cryptic). Why one determinant is selected while the majority are neglected is still unresolved. Features of the antigen remote from the actual determinant are thought either to steer processing toward disclosure or revelation of a determinant, or to interfere with the binding of peptides to MHC. Different MHC molecules can compete for determinants at an early stage of processing when the antigen is close to its original length. There are shifts in the hierarchy of display of dominant and cryptic determinants, and these shifts relate to local inflammatory states, to changes in the state or composition of the APC population, and to aspects of exogenous versus endogenous processing. It has been suggested that the cryptic peptides of autoantigens may become expressed at sites of inflammation (90). This can lead to the engagement of T cells potentially directed against cryptic self-determinants that escaped tolerance induction in the thymus, a process leading to induction and/or perpetuation of autoimmune reactivity. This self-directed T cell repertoire can also be activated silently to induce memory and participate unexpectedly in responses to foreign antigens, and may be responsible for molecular mimicry (91). It has been suggested by studies using $CD4^+$ T cell responses to two different strains of mycobacteria that T cell cross-reactive epitopes can exist in proteins even with little linear sequence homology (92). These seemingly nonhomolgous cross-reactive epitopes could represent conformational or structural epitopes. The potential of cross-reactive epitopes for unsuspected cross-sensitization may play a role in the maintenance of T cell memory, in the pathogenesis of autoimmune diseases, and possibly in a wider range of host immune responses to infectious pathogens (92). Therefore, to explain these phenomena of cross-reactivity at the T cell clonal level, it would be necessary to dissect the molecular mechanism of MHC class II–peptide-TCR interaction and to identify both linear and structural epitopes.

What are the possibilities of oral tolerance for treatment in these diseases? The definition of specific target antigens would expedite this process. However, using the technique of "bystander tolerance," where the oral antigen merely targets the tolerogenic T cells to the site of immune destruction, creates more realistic therapeutic possibilities in diseases such as PSC and AIH, where the T cell epitopes have not been defined. Even for PBC, where we have information regarding the epitopes of liver infiltrating T cells, a more generic approach to therapy may be more effective, as the exact role of these T cells has yet to be defined. Perhaps the use of bile duct– or liver-specific toleragen would be useful for such therapy.

The continued study of the role of T cells in autoimmune liver disease will help answer some of the above dilemmas. In addition, identification of the genetic factors involved in these diseases, whether it is at the MHC class I or class II level, or both, is a difficult but necessary component of such studies. Looking at what role, if any, environmental factors play in disease pathogenesis is another important consideration. Comparison of the similarities and differences among the various autoimmune liver diseases could provide important clues as to their etiology.

REFERENCES

1. Meuer, S.C., Moebius, U., Manns, M.M., Dienes, H.P., Ramadori, G., Hess, G., Hercend, T., and Meyer zum Buschenfelde, K.H. 1988. Clonal analysis of human T lymphocytes infiltrating the liver in chronic active hepatitis B and primary biliary cirrhosis. *Eur. J. Immunol.* 18:1447–1452.
2. Montano, L., Aranguibel, F., Boffill, M., Goodall, A.H., Janossy, G., and Thomas, H.C. 1983. An analysis of the composition of the inflammatory infiltrate in autoimmune and hepatitis B virus-induced chronic liver disease. *Hepatology* 3:292–296.
3. Pape, G.R., Rieber, E.P., Eisenburg, J., Hoffmann, R., Balch, C.M., Paumgartner, G., and Riethmuller, G. 1983. Involvement of the cytotoxic/suppressor T-cell subset in liver tissue injury of patients with acute and chronic liver diseases. *Gastroenterology* 85:657–662.
4. Krams, S.M., Van de Water, J., Coppel, R.L., Esquivel, C., Roberts, J., Ansari, A., and Gershwin, M.E. 1990. Analysis of hepatic T lymphocyte and immunoglobulin deposits in patients with primary biliary cirrhosis. *Hepatology* 12:306–313.
5. Husby, G., Blomhoff, J.P., Elgjo, K., and Williams, R., Jr. 1982. Immunohistochemical characterization of hepatic tissue lymphocyte subpopulations in liver disease. *Scand. J. Gastroenterol.* 17:855–860.
6. Lohr, H.F., Schlaak, J.F., Gerken, G., Fleischer, B., Dienes, H.P., and Meyer zum Buschenfelde, K.H. 1994. Phenotypical analysis and cytokine release of liver-infiltrating and peripheral blood T lymphocytes from patients with chronic hepatitis of different etiology. *Liver* 14:161–166.
7. Loeper, J., Descatoire, V., Maurice, M., Beaune, P., Belghiti, J., Houssin, D., Ballet, F., Feldmann, G., Guengerich, F.P., and Pessayre, D. 1993. Cytochromes P-450 in human hepatocyte plasma membrane: Recognition by several autoantibodies. *Gastroenterology* 104:203–216.
8. Eggink, H.F., Houthoff, H.J., Huitema, S., Gips, C.H., and Poppema, S. 1982. Cellular and humoral immune reactions in chronic active liver disease, I. Lymphocyte subsets in liver biopsies of patients with untreated idiopathic autoimmune hepatitis, chronic active hepatitis B and primary biliary cirrhosis. *Clin. Exp. Immunol.* 50:17–24.
9. Bach, N., Thung, S.N., and Schaffner, F. 1992. The histological features of chronic hepatitis C and autoimmune chronic hepatitis: A comparative analysis. *Hepatology* 15:572–577.
10. Schlaak, J.F., Lohr, H., Gallati, H., Meyer zum Buschenfelde, K.H., and Fleischer, B. 1993. Analysis of the in vitro cytokine production by liver-infiltrating T cells of patients with autoimmune hepatitis. *Clin. Exp. Immunol.* 94:168–173.

11. Lohr, H.F., Schlaak, J.F., Lohse, A.W., Bocher, W.O., Arenz, M., Gerken, G., and Meyer Zum Buschenfelde, K.H. 1996. Autoreactive CD4+ LKM-specific and anticlonotypic T-cell responses in LKM-1 antibody-positive autoimmune hepatitis. *Hepatology* 24:1416–1421.
12. Davis, M.M., and Bjorkman, P.J. 1988. T-cell antigen receptor genes and T-cell recognition. *Nature* 334:395–402.
13. Wucherpfennig, K.W., Ota, K., Endo, N., Seidman, J.G., Rosenzweig, A., Weiner, H.L., and Hafler, D.A. 1990. Shared human T cell receptor Vβ usage to immunodominant regions of myelin basic protein. *Science* 248:1016–1019.
14. Hoshino, Y., Enomoto, N., Izumi, N., Kurosaki, M., Marumo, F., and Sato, C. 1995. Limited usage of T-cell β chains and sequences of the complementarity determining region 3 of lymphocytes infiltrating in the liver of autoimmune hepatitis. *Hepatology* 22:142–147.
15. Chapman, R.W., Arborgh, B.A., Rhodes, J.M., Summerfield, J.A., Dick, R., Scheuer, P.J., and Sherlock, S. 1980. Primary sclerosing cholangitis: A review of its clinical features, cholangiography, and hepatic histology. *Gut* 21:870–877.
16. Wiesner, R.H. 1994. Current concepts in primary sclerosing cholangitis. [Review]. *Mayo Clin. Proc.* 69:969–982.
17. Chapman, R.W., and Jewell, D.P. 1985. Primary sclerosing cholangitis—an immunologically mediated disease? *West. J. Med.* 143:193–195.
18. Crippin, J.S., and Lindor, K.D. 1992. Primary sclerosing cholangitis: Etiology and immunology. *Eur. J. Gastroenterol. Hepatol.* 4:261–265.
19. Wiesner, R.H., LaRusso, N.F., Ludwig, J., and Dickson, E.R. 1985. Comparison of the clinicopathologic features of primary sclerosing cholangitis and primary biliary cirrhosis. *Gastroenterology* 88:108–114.
20. Wiesner, R.H., and LaRusso, N.F. 1980. Clinicopathologic features of the syndrome of primary sclerosing cholangitis. *Gastroenterology* 79:200–206.
21. Chapman, R.W., Cottone, M., Selby, W.S., Shepherd, H.A., Sherlock, S., and Jewell, D.P. 1986. Serum autoantibodies, ulcerative colitis and primary sclerosing cholangitis. *Gut* 27:86–91.
22. Snook, J.A., Chapman, R.W., Fleming, K., and Jewell, D.P. 1989. Anti-neutrophil nuclear antibody in ulcerative colitis, Crohn's disease and primary sclerosing cholangitis. *Clin. Exp. Immunol.* 76:30–33.
23. Das, K.M., Vecchi, M., and Sakamaki, S. 1990. A shared and unique epitope(s) on human colon, skin, and biliary epithelium detected by a monoclonal antibody. *Gastroenterology* 98:464–469.
24. Lo, S.K., Fleming, K.A., and Chapman, R.W. 1992. Prevalence of anti-neutrophil antibody in primary sclerosing cholangitis and ulcerative colitis using an alkaline phosphatase technique. *Gut* 33:1370–1375.
25. Lindor, K.D., Wiesner, R.H., Katzmann, J.A., LaRusso, N.F., and Beaver, S.J. 1987. Lymphocyte subsets in primary sclerosing cholangitis. *Dig. Dis. Sci.* 32:720–725.
26. Chapman, R.W., Kelly, P.M., Heryet, A., Jewell, D.P., and Fleming, K.A. 1988. Expression of HLA-DR antigens on bile duct epithelium in primary sclerosing cholangitis. *Gut* 29:422–427.
27. Snook, J.A., Chapman, R.W., Sachdev, G.K., Heryet, A., Kelly, P.M., Fleming, K.A., and Jewell, D.P. 1989. Peripheral blood and portal tract lymphocyte populations in primary sclerosing cholangitis. *J. Hepatol.* 9:36–41.

28. Martins, E.B., Graham, A.K., Chapman, R.W., and Fleming, K.A. 1996. Elevation of gamma delta T lymphocytes in peripheral blood and livers of patients with primary sclerosing cholangitis and other autoimmune liver diseases. *Hepatology* 23:988–993.

29. Yong, K., Pearce, K., Lake, J.P., Ziegler, H.K., and Kapp, J.A. 1997. γδ T lymphocytes regulate the induction and maintenance of oral tolerance. *J. Immunol.* 158:3610–3518.

30. Wildner, G., Hunig, T., and Thurau, S.R. 1996. Orally induced, peptide-specific g/d TCR+ cells suppress experimental autoimmune uveitis. *Eur. J. Immunol.* 26:2140–2148.

31. Kaplan, M.M. 1987. Primary biliary cirrhosis. [Review]. *N. Engl. J. Med.* 316:521–528.

32. Ahrens, E., Jr., Payne, M.A., Kunkel, H.G., Eisenmenger, W.J., and Blondheim, S.H. 1994. Primary biliary cirrhosis. 1950 [classical article]. *Medicine* 73:264–278.

33. Walker, J., G., Doniach, D., Roitt, I.M., and Sherlock, S. 1965. Serological tests in the diagnosis of primary biliary cirrhosis. *Lancet* 1:827–830.

34. Van de Water, J., Gershwin, M.E., Leung, P., Ansari, A., and Coppel, R.L. 1988. The autoepitope of the 74-kD mitochondrial autoantigen of primary biliary cirrhosis corresponds to the functional site of dihydrolipoamide acetyltransferase. *J. Exp. Med.* 167:1791–1799.

35. Fussey, S.P., Guest, J.R., James, O.F., Bassendine, M.F., and Yeaman, S.J. 1988. Identification and analysis of the major M2 autoantigens in primary biliary cirrhosis. *Proc. Natl. Acad. of Sci. U.S.A.* 85:8654–8658.

36. Hoffmann, R.M., Pape, G.R., Spengler, U., Rieber, E.P., Eisenburg, J., Dohrmann, J., Paumgartner, G., and Riethmuller, G. 1989. Clonal analysis of liver-derived T cells of patients with primary biliary cirrhosis. *Clin. Exp. Immunol.* 76:210–215.

37. Bjorkland, A., Festin, R., Mendel-Hartvig, I., Nyberg, A., Loof, L., and Totterman, T.H. 1991. Blood and liver-infiltrating lymphocytes in primary biliary cirrhosis: Increase in activated T and natural killer cells and recruitment of primed memory T cells. *Hepatology* 13:1106–1111.

38. Leon, M.P., Spickett, G., Jones, D.E., and Bassendine, M.F. 1995. CD4+ T cell subsets defined by isoforms of CD45 in primary biliary cirrhosis. *Clin. Exp. Immunol.* 99:233–239.

39. Lohr, H., Fleischer, B., Gerken, G., Yeaman, S.J., Meyer zum Buschenfelde, K.H., and Manns, M. 1993. Autoreactive liver-infiltrating T cells in primary biliary cirrhosis recognize inner mitochondrial epitopes and the pyruvate dehydrogenase complex. *J. Hepatol.* 18:322–327.

40. Si, L., Whiteside, T.L., Schade, R.R., Starzl, T.E., and Van Thiel, D.H. 1984. T-lymphocyte subsets in liver tissues of patients with primary biliary cirrhosis (PBC), patients with primary sclerosing cholangitis (PSC), and normal controls. *J. Clin. Immunol.* 4:262–272.

41. Van de Water, J., Ansari, A.A., Surh, C.D., Coppel, R., Roche, T., Bonkovsky, H., Kaplan, M., and Gershwin, M.E. 1991. Evidence for the targeting by 2-oxo-dehydrogenase enzymes in the T cell response of primary biliary cirrhosis. *J. Immunol.* 146:89–94.

42. Meuer, S.C., Moebius, U., Manns, M.M., Dienes, H.P., Ramadori, G., Hess, G., Hercend, T., and Meyer zum Buschenfelde, K.H. 1988. Clonal analysis of human T lymphocytes infiltrating the liver in chronic active hepatitis B and primary biliary cirrhosis. *Eur. J. Immunol.* 18:1447–1452.

43. Van de Water, J., Ansari, A.A., Surh, C.D., Coppel, R., Roche, T., Bonkovsky, H., Kaplan, M., and Gershwin, M.E. 1991. Evidence for the targeting of 2-oxo-dehydrogenase enzymes in the T cell response of primary biliary cirrhosis. *J. Immunol.* 146:89–94.

44. Surh, C.D., Ahmed-Ansari, A., and Gershwin, M.E. 1990. Comparative epitope mapping of murine monoclonal and human autoantibodies to human PDH-E2, the major mitochondrial autoantigen of primary biliary cirrhosis. *J. Immunol.* 144:2647–2652.

45. Surh, C.D., Coppel, R., and Gershwin, M.E. 1990. Structural requirement for autoreactivity on human pyruvate dehydrogenase-E2, the major autoantigen of primary biliary cirrhosis. Implication for a conformational autoepitope. *J. Immunol.* 144:3367–3374.

46. Van de Water, J., Ansari, A., Prindiville, T., Coppel, R., Ricalton, N., Kotzin, B.L., Liu, S., Roche, T.E., Krams, S.M., Munoz, S., and Gershwin, M.E. 1995. Heterogeneity of autoreactive T cell clones specific for the E2 component of the pyruvate dehydrogenase complex in primary biliary cirrhosis. *J. Exp. Med.* 181:723–733.

47. Van de Water, J., Turchany, J., Leung, P.S., Lake, J., Munoz, S., Surh, C.D., Coppel, R., Ansari, A. Nakanuma, Y., and Gershwin, M.E. 1993. Molecular mimicry in primary biliary cirrhosis. Evidence for biliary epithelial expression of a molecule cross-reactive with pyruvate dehydrogenase complex-E2. *J. Clin. Invest.* 91:2653–2664.

48. Butler, P., Hamilton-Miller, J., Baum, H., and Burroughs, A.K. 1995. Detection of M2 antibodies in patients with recurrent urinary tract infection using an ELISA and purified PBC specific antigens. Evidence for a molecular mimicry mechanism in the pathogenesis of primary biliary cirrhosis? *Biochem. Mol. Biol. Int.* 35:473–485.

49. Yeaman, S.J., Fussey, S.P., Danner, D.J., James, O.F., Mutimer, D.J., and Bassendine, M.F. 1988. Primary biliary cirrhosis: Identification of two major M2 mitochondrial autoantigens. *Lancet* 1:1068–1070.

50. Fussey, S.P., Ali, S.T., Guest, J.R., James, O.F., Bassendine, M.F., and Yeaman, S.J. 1990. Reactivity of primary biliary cirrhosis sera with Escherichia coli dihydrolipoamide acetyltransferase (E2p): Characterization of the main immunogenic region. *Proc. Natl. Acad. Sci. U.S.A.* 87:3987–3991.

51. Teoh, K.L., Mackay, I.R., Rowley, M.J., and Fussey, S.P. 1994. Enzyme inhibitory autoantibodies to pyruvate dehydrogenase complex in primary biliary cirrhosis differ for mammalian, yeast and bacterial enzymes: Implications for molecular mimicry. *Hepatology* 19:1029–1033.

52. Burroughs, A.K., Butler, P., Sternberg, M.J., and Baum, H. 1992. Molecular mimicry in liver disease. *Nature* 358:377–378.

53. Joplin, R., Lindsay, J.G., Hubscher, S.G., Johnson, G.D., Shaw, J.C., Strain, A.J., and Neuberger, J.M. 1991. Distribution of dihydrolipoamide acetyltransferase (E2) in the liver and portal lymph nodes of patients with primary biliary cirrhosis: An immunohistochemical study. *Hepatology* 14:442–447.

54. Fujinami, R.S., and Oldstone, M.B.A. 1986. Amino acid homology and cross-reacting immune responses between the encephalitogenic site of myelin basic protein and virus: Virus-induced autoimmunity. In *Vaccine 86: Modern Approaches to Immunizations*. New York: Cold Spring Harbor Laboratory, pp 247–251.

55. Oldstone, M.B. 1987. Molecular mimicry and autoimmune disease [published erratum appears in *Cell* 51(5):878, Dec. 4, 1987]. *Cell* 50:819–820.

56. Lehmann, P.V., Forsthuber, T., Miller, A., and Sercarz, E.E. 1992. Spreading of T-cell autoimmunity to cryptic determinants of an autoantigen. *Nature* 358:155–157.

57. Gautam, A.M., Lock, C.B., Smilek, D.E., Pearson, C.I., Steinman, L., and McDevitt, H.O. 1994. Minimum structural requirements for peptide presentation by major histocompatibility complex class II molecules: Implications in induction of autoimmunity. *Proc. Natl. Acad. Sci. U.S.A.* 91:767–771.

58. Nickowitz, R.E., and Worman, H.J. 1993. Autoantibodies from patients with primary biliary cirrhosis recognize a restricted region within the cytoplasmic tail of nuclear pore membrane glycoprotein Gp210. *J. Exp. Med.* 178:2237–2242.

59. Luo, A.M., Garza, K.M., Hunt, D., and Tung, K.S. 1993. Antigen mimicry in autoimmune disease sharing of amino acid residues critical for pathogenic T cell activation. *J. Clin. Invest.* 92:2117–2123.

60. Shimoda, S., Nakamura, M., Ishibashi, H., Hayashida, K., and Niho, Y. 1995. HLA DRB4 0101-restricted immunodominant T cell autoepitope of pyruvate dehydrogenase complex in primary biliary cirrhosis: Evidence of molecular mimicry in human autoimmune diseases. *J. Exp. Med.* 181:1835–1845.

61. Matsui, M., Nakamura, M., Ishibashi, H., Koike, K., Kudo, J., and Niho, Y. 1993. Human monoclonal antibodies from a patient with primary biliary cirrhosis that recognize two distinct autoepitopes in the E2 component of the pyruvate dehydrogenase complex. *Hepatology* 18:1069–1077.

62. Graham, S., Wang, E.C.Y., Jenkins, O., and Borysiewicz, L.K. 1993. Analysis of the human T-cell response to picornaviruses: Identification of T-cell epitopes close to B cells epitopes in poliovirus. *J. Virol.* 67:1627–1637.

63. Moebius, U., Manns, M., Hess, G., Kober, G., Meyer zum Buschenfelde, K.H., and Meuer, S.C. 1990. T cell receptor gene rearrangements of T lymphocytes infiltrating the liver in chronic active hepatitis B and primary biliary cirrhosis (PBC): Oligoclonality of PBC-derived T cell clones. *Eur. J. Immunol.* 20:889–896.

64. Tsai, S.L., Lai, M.Y., and Chen, D.S. 1996. Analysis of rearranged T cell receptor (TCR) V beta transcripts in livers of primary biliary cirrhosis: Preferential V beta usage suggests antigen-driven selection. *Clin. Exp. Immunol.* 103:99–104.

65. Kotzin, B.L., Karuturi, S., Chou, Y.K., Lafferty, J., Forrester, J., Better, M., Nedwin, G.E., Offner, H., and Vandenbark, A.A. 1991. Preferential T-cell receptor b-chain variable gene use in myelin basic protein-reactive T cell clones from patients with multiple sclerosis. *Proc. Natl. Acad. Sci. U.S.A.* 88:9161–9165.

66. Meinl, E., Weber, F., Drexler, K., Movelle, C., Ott, M., Saruhan-Direskeneli, G., Goebels, N., Erte, B., Jechart, G., Giegerich, G., Shonbeck, S., Bannwarth, W., Wekerle, H., and Hohlfeld, R. 1993. Myelin basic protein-specific T lymphocyte repertoire in multiple sclerosis. *J. Clin. Invest.* 92:2633–2643.

67. Lehmann, P.V., Sercarz, E.E., Forsthuber, T., Dayan, C.M., and Gammon, G. 1993. Determinant spreading and the dynamics of the autoimmune T-cell repertoire [see comments]. *Immunol. Today* 14:203–208.

68. Donaldson, P., Doherty, D., Underhill, J., and Williams, R. 1994. The molecular genetics of autoimmune liver disease. *Hepatology* 20:225–239.

69. Jorgensen, J.L., Reay, P.A., Ehrich, E.W., and Davis, M.M. 1992. Molecular components of T-cell recognition. *Annu. Rev. Immunol.* 10:835–873.

70. Kropshofer, H., Max, H., Muller, C.A., Hesse, F., Stevanovic, S., Jung, G., and Kalbacher, H. 1992. Self-peptide released from class II HLA-DR1 exhibits a hydrophobic two-residue contact motif. *J. Exp. Med.* 175:1799–1803.

71. Hammer, J., Valsasnini, P., Tolba, K., Bolin, D., Higelin, J., Takacs, B., and Sinigaglia, F. 1993. Promiscuous and allele-specific anchors in HLA-DR-binding peptides. *Cell* 74:197–203.

72. Stern, L.J., Brown, J.H., Jardetzky, T.S., Gorga, J.C., Urban, R.G., Strominger, J.L., and Wiley, D.C. 1994. Crystal structure of the human class II MHC protein HLA-DR1 complexed with an influenza virus peptide. *Nature* 368:215–221.

73. Matsushita, S., Takahashi, K., Motoki, M., Komoriya, K., Ikagawa, S., and Nishimura, Y. 1994. Allele specificity of structural requirement for peptides bound to HLA-DRB1*0405

and -DRB1*0406 complexes: Implication for the HLA-associated susceptibility to methimazole-induced insulin autoimmune syndrome. *J. Exp. Med.* 180:873–883.

74. Wucherpfennig, K.W., Sette, A., Southwood, S., Oseroff, C., Matsui, M., Strominger, J.L., and Hafler, D.A. 1994. Structural requirements for binding of an immunodominant myelin basic protein peptide to DR2 isotypes and for its recognition by human T cell clones. *J. Exp. Med.* 179:279–290.
75. Manns, M.P., and Kruger, M. 1994. Immunogenetics of chronic liver diseases. [Review]. *Gastroenterology* 106:1676–1697.
76. Seki, T., Ota, M., Furuta, S., Fukushima, H., Kondo, T., Hino, K., and Mizuki, N. 1992. HLA class II molecules and autoimmune hepatitis susceptibility in Japanese patients. *Gastroenterology* 103:1041–1047.
77. Chapman, R.W., Varghese, Z., Gaul, R., Pates, G., Kokinon, N., and Sherlock, S. 1983. Association of primary sclerosing cholangitis with HLA-B8. *Gut* 24:38–41.
78. Schrumpf, E., Fausa, O., Forre, O., Dobloug, J.H., Ritland, S., and Thorsby, E. 1982. HLA antigens and immunoregulatory T cells in ulcerative colitis associated with hepatobiliary disease. *Scand. J. Gastroenterol.* 17:187–191.
79. Magrin, S., Nouri Aria, K.T., Donaldson, P.T., Wilkinson, M.L., Portmann, B.C., Williams, R., and Eddleston, A.L. 1989. The relationship between HLA-DR3 and T-cell regulation of immunoglobulin production in primary sclerosing cholangitis. *Clin. Immunol. Immunopathol.* 50:205–212.
80. Donaldson, P.T., Farrant, J.M., Wilkinson, M.L., Hayliar, K., Portmann, B.C., and Williams, R. 1991. Dual association of HLA DR2 and DR3 with primary sclerosing cholangitis. *Hepatology* 13:129–133.
81. Farrant, J.M., Doherty, D.G., Donaldson, P.T., Vaughan, R.W., Hallar, K.M., Welsh, K.I., Eddelston, A.L.W.F., and Williams, R. 1992. Amino acid substitutions at position 38 of the DRb polypeptide confer susceptibility and protection from primary sclerosing cholangitis. *Hepatology* 16:390–395.
82. Prochazka, E.J., Terasaki, P.I, Park, M.S., Goldstein, L.I., and Busuttil, R.W. 1990. Association of primary sclerosing cholangitis with HLA-DRw52a. *N. Engl. J. Med.* 322:1842–1844.
83. Ercilla, G., Pares, A., Arriaga, F., Bruguera, M., Gastillo, R., Rodes, J., and Vives, J. 1979. Primary biliary cirrhosis associated with HLA-DRw3. *Tissue Antigens* 14:449–452.
84. Johnston, D.E., Kaplan, M.M., Miller, K.B., Connors, C.M., and Milford, E.L. 1987. Histocompatibility antigens in primary biliary cirrhosis. *Am. J. Gastroenterol.* 82:1127–1129.
85. Miyamori, H., Kato, Y., Kobayashi, K., and Hattori, N. 1983. HLA antigens in Japanese patients with primary biliary cirrhosis and autoimmune hepatitis. *Digestion* 26:213–217.
86. Seki, T., Kiyosawa, K., Ota, M., Furuta, S., Fukushima, H., Tanaka, E., Yoshizawa, K., Kumagai, T., Mizuki, N., Ando, A., et al. 1993. Association of primary biliary cirrhosis with human leukocyte antigen DPB1*0501 in Japanese patients. *Hepatology* 18:73–78.
87. Bassendine, M.F., Dewar, P.J., and James, O.F. 1985. HLA-DR antigens in primary biliary cirrhosis: Lack of association. *Gut* 26:625–628.
88. Shimoda, S., Nakamura, M., Ishibashi, H., Hayashida, K., and Niho, Y. 1995. HLA DRB4 0101-restricted immunodominant T cell autoepitope of pyruvate dehydrogenase complex in primary biliary cirrhosis: Evidence of molecular mimicry in human autoimmune diseases. *J. Exp. Med.* 181:1835–1845.
89. Imanishi, T., Akaza, T., Kimura, A., Tokunaga, K., and Gojobori, T. 1991. Allele and haplotype frequencies for HLA and complement loci in various ethic groups. In *HLA 1991*,

Tsuiji, K., Aizawa, M., and Sasazuki, T., eds. Oxford: Oxford University Press, pp 1065–1220.

90. Sercarz, E.E., Lehmann, P.V., Ametani, A., Benichou, G., Miller, A., and Moudgil, K. 1993. Dominance and crypticity of T cell antigenic determinants. *Annu. Rev. Immunol.* 11:729–766.

91. Moudgil, K.D., and Sercarz, E.E. 1994. The T cell repertoire against cryptic self determinants and its involvement in autoimmunity and cancer. *Clin. Immunol. Immunopathol.* 73:283–289.

92. Harris, D.P., Vordermeier, H.M., Singh, M., Moreno, C., Jurcevic, S., and Ivanyi, J. 1995. Cross-recognition by T cells of an epitope shared by two unrelated mycobacterial antigens. *Eur. J. Immunol.* 25:3173–3179.

CHAPTER 11

HEPATIC T CELLS IN PRIMARY SCLEROSING CHOLANGITIS AND AUTOIMMUNE HEPATITIS

WAJAHAT Z. MEHAL
Yale University School of Medicine, New Haven, CT

INTRODUCTION

Hepatic T cell numbers, phenotype, and function are of interest as they may provide insight into the immune process responsible for initiating and maintaining autoimmune liver diseases. The first attempts to characterize the hepatic T cell populations in autoimmune hepatitis (AIH) and primary sclerosing cholangitis (PSC) date back to 1975 (1), and since then over 30 studies have directly addressed this issue. Any attempt to synthesize these studies into a coherent model of the T cell populations in AIH and PSC has to contend with many confounding factors: A paucity of human liver tissues requires assimilation of data from a number of studies conducted many years apart. For studies prior to the general availability of hepatitis C serology in 1992, it is unclear how much of a role this viral infection had in the liver tissues studied, particularly because infection with hepatitis C is more likely in patients with liver disease due to their multiple transfusions and procedures. Furthermore, the subdivision of AIH into types I to III in 1987, means that the early studies have an uncertain composition with regard to this categorization (2). The stage of the liver disease is also a confounding factor, with many of the liver samples obtained from patients with relatively advanced disease. This presents difficulties in discriminating the changes due to the primary disease process, from those due to bouts of bacterial cholangitis common in PSC, as well as those due to drug reactions.

Technical considerations also add to the complexity of establishing hepatic T cell numbers and phenotypes. Quantification of T cell populations in histological sections

T Lymphocytes in the Liver: Immunobiology, Pathology, and Host Defense, Edited by I. Nicholas Crispe
ISBN 0-471-19218-X

can only provide relative information, allowing comparison of cellular populations. For data on total cell numbers it is necessary to extract the intrahepatic lymphocytes (IHLs), and variations in the digestion and purification procedures have significant effects on the final yield of T cell subpopulations. Pronase, collagenase I, and collagenase IV (3–5) have been used for digestion, and these enzymes probably result in similar degrees of digestion due to their cross-specificity. A much more important variable is whether the liver is perfused with these enzymes, or incubated after mechanical disruption only. We have found that perfusion with collagenase liberates approximately four times as many IHL as mechanical disruption followed by digestion, but this procedure is clearly not possible when liver biopsies are being studied. An equally important variable is the purification step. Lymphocytes have been purified on density gradients of Ficoll and sucrose (4,5), but the two have not been directly compared. A comparison of Ficoll with metrizamide in the purification of mouse intrahepatic lymphocytes (IHLs) demonstrated that a Ficoll density gradient resulted in the loss of an activated $CD8^+$ T cell population (6). A final point to consider is the known sampling variation of liver biopsies, with two biopsies taken at the same time from the same entry site having a diagnostic correlation of only 35% (7).

THE NORMAL NONPARENCHYMAL CELL POPULATION

The nonparenchymal cells (NPCs) consist of endothelial cells, Kupffer's cells, Ito cells, and a complex mixture of IHL containing T cell receptor αβ cells ($TCR\alpha\beta^+$) $CD4^+$ cells, $TCR\alpha\beta^+CD8^+$ cells, $TCR\gamma\delta^+$ cells, classical natural killer (NK) cells, and NK cells with the TCRαβ receptor (NK-T). The relative contribution of these populations to the NPC population has been studied in a pronase-digested rat liver suspension of NPCs. Kupffer's cells were identified by fluorescence-activated cell sorter (FACS) analysis utilizing their ability to endocytose latex beads and FITC-conjugated albumin to distinguish them from endothelial cells, which can endocytose only the FITC-conjugated albumin (8). This led to an estimated contribution to the NPCs of 25% from Kupffer's cells and 50% from endothelial cells, which correlates well with an earlier morphometric study of NPC volumes (9). Since Ito cells do not survive pronase digestion, the remaining 25% were assumed to be IHL.

Data on NPCs or IHLs from normal and near-normal human livers is extremely limited. Hata et al. (4) provide data on four normal liver wedge resections, which were processed by mechanical disruption, collagenase IV digestion, and purified on two Ficoll-Hypaque gradients with overnight adherence on cell culture flasks. The mean yield of the nonadherent population was 73×10^4 cells per gram of liver tissue, of which 42% were $TCR\alpha\beta^+$ as analyzed by FACS, and 62% were $CD56^+$ (an NK cell marker). The percentage obtained for the NK contribution was slightly higher than the percentage of cells with NK cell morphology (large granular lymphocytes, range 38–52%). CD56 is, however, known to be expressed on T cells as well as NK cells. Isolation of IHLs from livers with fatty infiltration, by mechanical disruption and collagenase IV digestion without a further purification step, gave a yield of only 0.54×10^4 cells per gram of tissue (3). The TCRαβ percentage of this population is not available, but this low yield can probably be attributed to the fatty infiltration of the liver, and 73 × 10^4 cells per gram of liver is the better of these estimates for the normal human liver. However, this is almost certainly an underestimate, because we have found that isolation of murine IHLs by mechanical disruption followed by collagenase IV digestion gives a yield of 5.7 × 10^6 TCR$\alpha\beta^+$ cells per gram, as compared to digestion by collagenase perfusion which isolates 14.4 × 10^6 TCR$\alpha\beta^+$ cells per gram. If a similar improvement in yield occurs for human liver the actual number of T cells in the human liver is nearer 1.8 × 10^6 per gram.

FACS analysis is a valuable tool in identifying the relative proportions of cellular populations based on their cell surface phenotype. We have performed three-color FACS analysis of murine IHLs purified on a metrizamide gradient. This purification removes most endothelial and Kupffer cells, and revealed approximately 20% of the IHLs to be TCR$\alpha\beta$, 20% NK, and 50% to be NK-T. A similar figure of 60% for NK-T cells has been obtained for human IHLs from patients who underwent partial hepatectomy for malignant and benign tumors (10). Human hepatic NK and NK-T cells have the characteristic MHC unrestricted NK activity against various cell lines (11), but the presence of class I MHC inhibitory receptors has not been investigated.

CD4 and CD8 expression on TCR$\alpha\beta^+$ cells identifies T cell populations with different functions. TCR$\alpha\beta^+$CD8$^+$ cells have a primarily cytotoxic function on activation, whereas TCR$\alpha\beta^+$CD4$^+$ cells can have a Th1 (inflammatory) or a Th2 (helper) function. Estimations of the CD4/CD8 ratio of human hepatic TCR$\alpha\beta^+$ cells are much higher 1.7 (36) when immunohistological techniques are used, compared to FACS analysis of 0.2 (4), 0.4 (10), and 0.5 (3). FACS scanning has been validated against quantitative immunohistochemistry as an accurate method for estimation of lymphocyte subsets (12), and this difference is probably due to the inclusion of CD4 on Kupffer cells during histological analysis. During FACS analysis Kupffer cells can be gated out because of their greater size and granularity. TCR$\gamma\delta^+$ cells at 2.2% ± 0.7% are a small proportion of normal hepatic T cells, and are predominantly CD4$^+$ and CD8$^+$ (13). The subdivisions of the human NPC populations are presented in Figure 11.1.

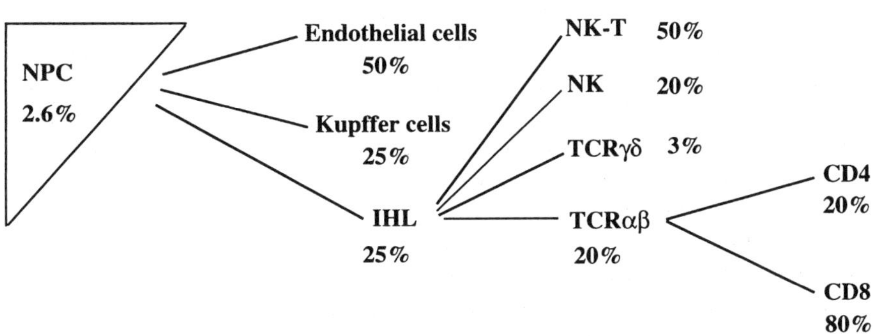

Figure 11.1. Distribution of human intrahepatic cell subpopulations, based on cell isolation and immunohistochemical studies. Nonparenchymal cells (NPC), intrahepatic lymphocytes (IHL), natural killer cells with the T cell receptor (NK-T), conventional natural killer cells (NK).

PRIMARY SCLEROSING CHOLANGITIS AND AUTOIMMUNE HEPATITIS

Primary sclerosing cholangitis (PSC) is characterized by a chronic inflammatory and fibrotic process in intra- and extrahepatic segments of the biliary tree, and usually occurs in association with ulcerative colitis (UC). This results in progressive narrowing or obliteration of the bile ducts, with clinical and biochemical evidence of cholestasis. In some cases the condition progresses to secondary biliary cirrhosis, hepatic failure, and cholangiocarcinoma. The diagnosis is based on the demonstration of segmental narrowing and dilatation of the biliary system or the histological changes in the absence of other causes of biliary pathology. PSC was originally considered to be a very rare condition, but a systematic review of the liver function test of UC patients followed by endoscopic evaluation of the biliary system suggests that it affects between 3.9% and 4.5% of patients with UC, and there is a stronger association with pancolitis compared with distal colitis (14). The clinical features of PSC are male predominance, variable clinical course, high frequency of UC, rarity of association with Crohn's disease, elevated serum immunoglobulin M (IgM), absence of anti-mitochondrial antibody and presence of anti-neutrophil cytoplasmic antibodies (ANCA) (15,16). There is also an association with the HLA haplotype A1, B8, DR3, Dw52a (17,18). Of these alleles, the association with Dw52a is the strongest, but it is not 100% as was originally reported (19,20). An independent association with the allele HLA DR2 was demonstrable when the strong association with HLA DR3 was controlled for (21). In addition HLA DR4, although not associated with PSC, was shown to identify patients with a more rapid progression to end-stage disease (22). The demonstration of an HLA association was a major step in the study of PSC. For the first time it demonstrated a genetic component to the pathogenesis of the disease, and immediately identified a subpopulation of individuals with UC who were at high risk of developing PSC. In addition it provided evidence for the importance of the immune response in disease pathogenesis. Many diseases that are accepted as having an autoimmune basis possess such HLA associations and commonly this association is with the haplotype HLA A1, B8, DR3, Cw7, Dw52a (23).

Anti-mitochondrial antibodies are not present in PSC, but anti-nuclear and anti–smooth muscle antibodies have been reported in 5% to 10% of patients (15,16). Recently, anti-neutrophil cytoplasmic antibodies (ANCA) have been demonstrated in the serum of the majority of patients with PSC and appear to be relatively specific for this condition (24,25). The ANCA response is mostly IgG, and is directed against a protease-sensitive target distinct from myeloperoxidase or a serine proteinase, which are the targets of the p-ANCA and c-ANCA antibody responses that occur in patients with Wegener's granulomatosis.

The histological hallmarks of PSC are concentric rings of periductal fibrosis (onion skin fibrosis), bile duct proliferation, periductal inflammation, and ductopenia (Fig. 11.2B) (26). The inflammation can affect any portion of the biliary tree and results in infiltration of the submucosal and serosal areas with mononuclear and inflammatory cells, while the mucosal surface is relatively normal until a late stage in the fibrotic process (27,28). In the context of an autoimmune process, this suggests that the mucosal surface is not the location of the target antigen(s).

Autoimmune hepatitis is characterized by limiting plate necrosis (piecemeal necrosis), lobular necrosis, and multinucleated hepatocytes in association with a

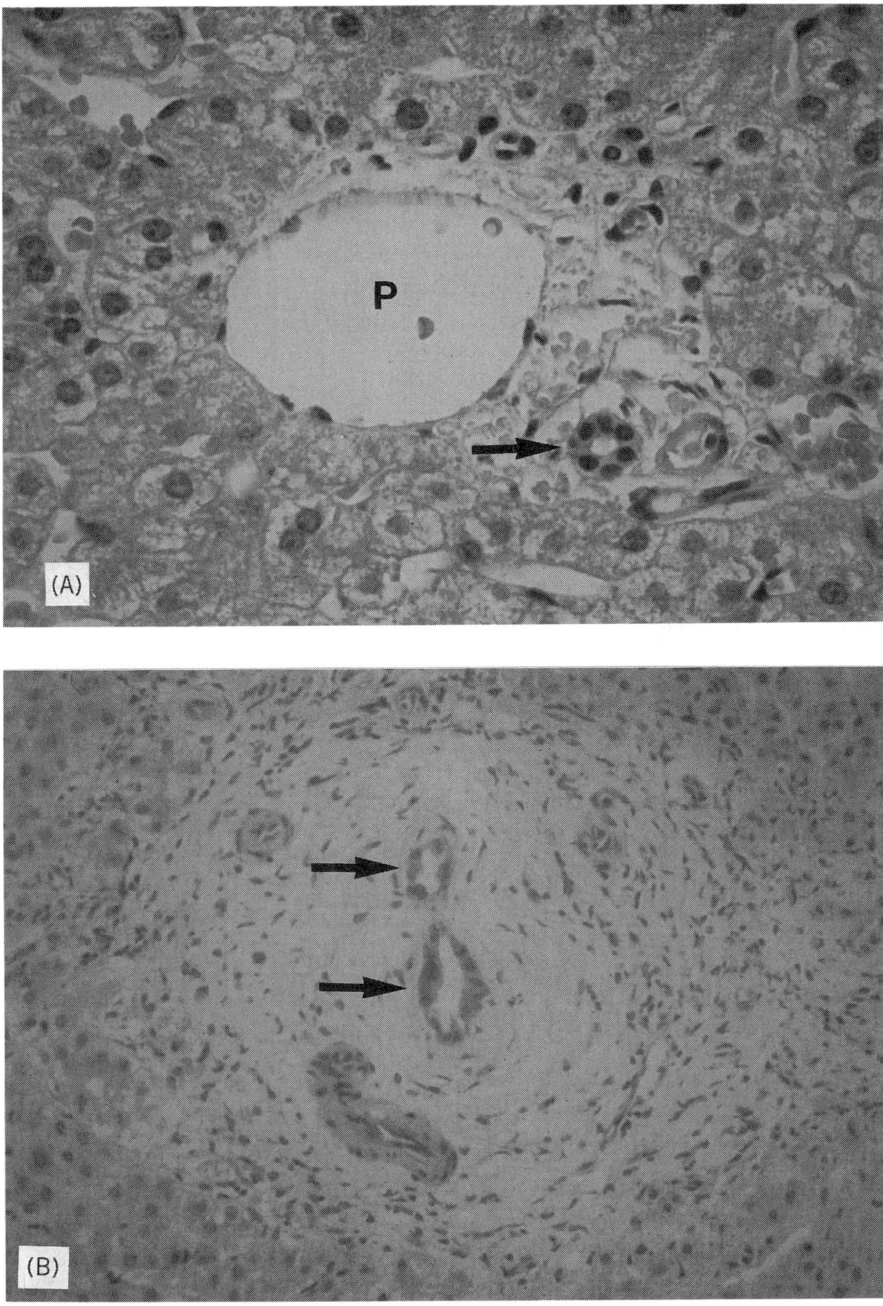

Figure 11.2. (**A**). (Haematoxylin and eosin, × 400) Normal portal area demonstrating a large-diameter vessel, which is a branch of the portal vein (P), and a smaller diameter bile duct lined by cuboidal epithelium (filled black arrow). Note the lack of fibrosis and lymphocytes. (**B**). (H & E × 200) Portal tract from a patient with PSC. Note the loss of normal architecture due to concentric rings of fibrosis around two bile ducts (filled black arrows), as well as an extensive lymphocytic infiltrate.

range of autoantibodies (29,30). These criteria are, however, present in a range of liver conditions varying from viral hepatitis to drug-induced liver injury, and a diagnosis of AIH is one of exclusion of other possible causes of liver injury. Three subgroups of hepatitis can be identified; type 1 is the oldest recognized form and accounts for 70% to 80% of AIH (31). The clinical features of type 1 AIH are the presence of anti-nuclear or anti–smooth muscle antibodies, an association with the HLA haplotype A1,B8,DR3 with a secondary association with DR4, a female predominance, hypergammaglobulinemia, and the presence of other immunological diseases, such as autoimmune thyroiditis and rheumatoid arthritis. Type II AIH shares most of the features of type I AIH, but is further characterized by the presence of antibodies to liver kidney microsomes type 1 (anti-LKM1) (32). Patients with type II AIH are usually much younger, with age ranges of 2–14 years, and are more likely to progress to cirrhosis. The target of the humoral response has been identified as the hepatocyte membrane surface protein cytochrome monooxygenase P450 IID6 (33), and although these antibodies will neutralize the enzyme *in vitro*, there is no evidence for a pathogenic role *in vivo*. Type III AIH again share most of the features of type I AIH, and is characterized by the presence of antibodies against soluble liver antigen, which are directed against cytokeratins 8 and 18 (34,35). Virtually all patients with type III AIH are female, but in terms of HLA profile, clinical course, and response to steroids, type III and type I are not distinguishable.

HEPATIC TCRαβ CELLS IN PSC AND AIH

Immunohistochemistry reveals that TCRαβ$^+$ cells are the major population of the mononuclear cell infiltrates present in PSC and AIH. However, very little data is present on exact percentages of TCRαβ$^+$ cells. Immunochemistry showed that 56% of IHL from PSC livers, and 55% from AIH livers, were T cells (36). FACS analysis of isolated IHL gives similar figures (4). These values are very close to those for IHL from normal human livers. The increase in total TCRαβ$^+$ cells in PSC and AIH as assessed by a quantitative immunohistochemistry varies widely, ranging from 1.6 to 7.5 times the estimated 1.8×10^6 cells per gram in a normal human liver. None of these studies address the question of what proportion of these cells are NK-T cells by double staining for CD56 and a T cell marker, but analysis of independent staining for CD56 and CD3 shows that in end-stage PSC there are approximately 30% fewer CD56$^+$ cells than in normal livers (37). The increase in TCRαβ$^+$ cells and the decrease in CD56$^+$ cells suggest that the major population infiltrating the liver in PSC and AIH are conventional TCRαβ$^+$ T cells and not NK-T cells.

There has been much interest in the relative proportions of CD4$^+$ and CD8$^+$ T cells in PSC and AIH, and immunohistochemical studies in PSC report CD4/CD8 T cells ratios of 0.52 (39), 1.2 (4), 1.5 (40), and for AIH 0.6 (38) and 2.0 (40). Unfortunately none of these studies double stained for T cells as well as CD4, so that they are likely to be overestimating the number of CD4$^+$ T cells due to the presence of CD4 on Kupffer cells. Of these studies, three had normal liver controls, and two found a significantly lower CD4/CD8 ratio in persons with PSC compared to normals (36,39). In the third study no significant difference was found between AIH and control groups (3). The single FACS study reports a CD4/CD8 ratio of 0.6 for PSC, which was not significantly different from controls, but the PSC sample size was only 3 (4). It is difficult to reach firm conclusions, but there is probably a lower CD4/CD8 ratio in PSC and AIH compared to normals, with an absolute increase in both $CD4^+$ and $CD8^+$ T cells. There is a consensus that the T cells immediately surrounding proliferating bile ducts, and occasionally infiltrating the biliary epithelium, as well as those associated with areas of piecemeal necrosis are $CD8^+$ (36,39,40).

The increased numbers of $CD8^+$ T cells fits well with a model of activated, clonally expanded effector $CD8^+$ T cell populations mediating antigen specific cytotoxicity. Other possibilities are that many of the $CD8^+$ cells present are naive and have not received a primary stimulatory response. The $CD8^+$ T cells could also be memory T cells remaining after an immune response, or the poorly characterized suppressor cells, which may mediate suppression by direct cytotoxicity towards activated T cells or by cytokines such as transforming growth factor β (TGFβ). The functions of activated $CD4^+$ T cells are more varied, with the Th1 or inflammatory response leading to recruitment and activation of Kupffer cells, these being the effector cells against intracellular pathogens. In addition Th1 T cells have a limited ability to kill cells directly by the production of tumor necrosis factor α (TNFα) and interferon-γ (IFNγ). The Th2 or helper T cells are necessary for the activation of specific B cells and the development of a humoral immune response. Although a range of autoantibodies are produced in PSC and AIH, there is no evidence that any of them are pathogenic, and it is difficult to form a model in which the primary changes occur with the Th2 pathway but lead to the production of a self-damaging cellular immune response.

Attempts at identifying whether the hepatic T cells are naive or activated have focused on the isoforms of CD45, which is one of the most abundant glycoproteins on the surface of T cells. The cytoplasmic domain of CD45 has two tyrosine phosphatase sites, and the extracellular domain contains a variable number of O-linked carbohydrate attachment sites (42). The variation of the extracellular domain is due to alternative splicing of exons 4, 5, and 6, which can produce a total of 8 mRNAs, of which 6 have been identified in human T cells (43,44). The largest isoform containing exons 4, 5, and 6 is CD45RA, which is almost twice the size of the isoform lacking all three of these exons, CD45RO (45). The closely regulated expression of CD45 isoforms in T cell development and activation makes them candidate markers for functional T cell populations. Most information on CD45 isotypes was obtained from $CD4^+$ cells. The $CD4^+CD45RO^+$ subset of mature T cells responds maximally to previously seen antigens and provides help for B cell IgG synthesis. In contrast the $CD4^+CD45RA^+$ subset responds poorly to previously seen antigens, and lacks helper function (46–49). Following activation, $CD4^+CD45RA^+$ T cells downregulate CD45RA and express a higher density of CD45RO (50). This apparent switch of CD45 isoforms and the preferential responsiveness of $CD4^+CD45RO^+$ cells to previously seen antigens has led to the concept that $CD45RA^+$ cells are "naive," and that following activation they convert to an "activated" or "memory" phenotype (51). This paradigm has a number of limitations. First, after activation, CD45RA expression is downregulated but not completely lost, and some 30% to 50% of T cells continue to express CD45RA (52). In addition the CD45RA-expressing cells that have undergone phenotypic changes to a CD45RO-expressing phenotype are able to provide only minimal help to B cells, suggesting that the CD45RA population remains functionally distinct even after activation (53). Other cell adhesion molecules cosegregate with the CD45 isoforms, particularly CD29 (the β1 chain of very late activation antigen (VLA)-5, which is present at high levels in $CD4^+CD45RO^+$ T cells. The limited data on $CD8^+$ cells is analogous to that on $CD4^+$ T cells, with unstimulated $CD8^+$ cells expressing CD45RA, and the loss of at least exon 4 in activated/memory cells resulting in a smaller isoform (54).

$CD4^+$ and $CD8^+$ T cells are relatively rare on immunohistochemical examination of normal human liver, and they are fairly evenly divided between CD45RA- and CD45RO-expressing cells. There are no studies in which large numbers of livers from PSC and AIH have been examined, but the smaller studies reach the same conclusion. In PSC, AIH, and other liver diseases such as primary biliary cirrhosis and chronic hepatitis B infection, virtually all the parenchymal and periportal $CD4^+$ and $CD8^+$ T cells expressed the $CD45RO^+$ isoform, while immunostaining for CD45RA was not present (55,56). In addition the $CD45RO^+$ cells expressed high levels of CD29, also a marker of an activated phenotype (56). An increase in total $CD8^+$ cell number along with an activated phenotype suggests that a $CD8^+$-mediated cytotoxic response is at least partly responsible for the immune-mediated damage.

Although there is a decrease in the CD4/CD8 ratio, there is an absolute increase in hepatic $CD4^+$ T cells in PSC and AIH. Attempts to understand their function have focused on their division into Th1 and Th2 subtypes. The Th1/Th2 division is, however, much less distinct in humans than in mice, and there are no cell surface markers to identify these subtypes. Cloning of IHLs followed by analysis of the cytokine profiles of the clones has been attempted. Cloning by spontaneously outgrowing IHLs in recombinant interleukin-2 (rIL-2) from patients with AIH, followed by stimulation with phytohemagglutinin (PHA), revealed that 80% of the $CD4^+$ clones produced IFNγ and IL-4 representing a Th0 phenotype, 14% Th1, and 6% Th2 (57). The available controls were IHLs from patients with hepatitis, mostly of the viral origin, and among these 72% of clones were Th0, 28% TH1, and none were TH2. The ratio of IFNγ to IL-4 varied from 0.16 to 3.9, but was conspicuously higher (at 35) from anti-LKM^+ IHL. In non-AIH clones the ratio was 3.4. A second study in which T cells were cloned by serial dilution after PHA stimulation also found a mixed cytokine profile, with on average approximately eight times more IFNγ being produced than IL-4 (58). The Th1 cells certainly have cytotoxic potential as well as helper function, but whether the Th0 can also be cytotoxic is unclear. The major limitation of such cloning strategies is that the cloned cells may not be representative of the parent IHL populations, and this is suggested by the fact that the CD4/CD8 ratio of the cloned cells was 2.8 and 2.9 (57,58), which is substantially higher than estimates of hepatic CD4/CD8 ratios by immunohistochemistry or FACS analysis.

Direct evidence for the cytotoxicity of $CD4^+$ and $CD8^+$ IHLs is present from IHL clones from four patients with type II or LKM^+ AIH. Ninety percent of $CD8^+$ and 30% of $CD4^+$ clones lysed autologous as well as allogenic B cell lines transformed by Epstein-Barr virus or K562 cells. For 5 of the 26 $CD8^+$ clones, this cytotoxic response was inhibited by anti–class I, but not anti–class II antibodies, a result which suggests a specific autoimmune response (59). Control data from normal IHLs was not available, and the antigenic specificity of these clones was not known. From the same individuals, 5 of 139 $CD4^+$ IHL clones proliferated specifically to recombinant liver kidney microsomes (LKM) antigen in a class II–restricted manner. A similar response was found from peripheral blood leukocytes (PBLs) of 3 of the 4 patients but none of 46 normal controls. Subsequently an 18 amino-acid peptide of the LKM was identified as a sufficient epitope for the generation of these proliferative responses, and PBL from 50% of patients with type I AIH were also shown to proliferate to this peptide. This was surprising, since patients with type I AIH did not have anti-LKM antibodies, and suggests that the LKM antigen may be the target of a broader T cell immune response in AIH than was originally inferred from the presence of auto-antibodies (60). Similar data showing PBL and hepatic T cell proliferation are present for the asialoglycoprotein receptor. Peripheral blood lymphocytes from approximately half of the studied patients with AIH proliferated in response to, and spontaneously produced antibodies to the asialoglycoprotein receptor, and the antibody production was lost in T cell–depleted PBL cultures (61). The ability to produce anti-asialoglycoprotein antibodies was restored by coculturing with hepatic $CD4^+$ $TCR\alpha\beta^+$ clones, which proliferated in response to asialoglycoprotein, but not by the addition of supernatants from the same $CD4^+$ clones. This complements the Th2 cytokine profiles of some of the $CD4^+$ T cell clones by demonstrating a helper function. In addition, since the anti-LKM response was present in $CD4^+$ cells from type I and type II AIH, and the anti-asialoglycoprotein response was present in PBC as well as type I AIH, the epitopes for the Th2 $CD4^+$ T cell response in these conditions may represent a mosaic of commonly occurring hepatic proteins. It remains to be answered whether the cytotoxic T cell response ($CD4^+$ or $CD8^+$) has an equally heterogeneous specificity, or whether each of the subtypes of AIH and PSC will be eventually defined at the T cell level by cytotoxic responses to distinct immunodominant epitopes.

Information on the heterogeneity of the T cell response is potentially available by studying the degree of clonality at the level of the TCR. This was attempted by extraction of total RNA from the livers of four patients with AIH, followed by reverse transcription of the TCRβ chain C region, and the detection of a total of 21 Vβ gene usages by separate amplifications (62). A variety of Vβ regions were amplified in the four patients, with Vβ3 being the only one that was present in all patients, and 6 being the maximum number present in any one patient. This compared with amplification of 19 out of 21 Vβ regions from the liver of a patient with hepatitis C infection and all 21 from the PBL of normal individuals. A similar approach was employed by Tanaka et al. (63) with successful amplification of all 20 Vβ regions from six patients with AIH, and three patients with viral hepatitis. The lack of amplification of the earlier study may be due to different amplification efficiencies of the Vβ primers, which were able to amplify from PBL cDNA, but not from the poorer IHL cDNA samples. Tanaka et al. went on to study the PCR products by polyacrylamide gel electrophoresis to show that each amplification product contained a mixture of VDJ rearrangements based on differences in size of a few base pairs (63). The total number of VDJ recombinations detected using primers for all 20 Vβ regions varied between 75 and 141 for the IHL of patients with AIH. This was not significantly less than the numbers present in the amplified DNA from PBLs of the same patients or viral hepatitis controls. To identify subpopulations of VDJ recombinations within the IHLs, which were common to IHLs from different regions of the liver, the PCR products from IHLs in two different parts of the same liver were compared. Between 21 and 58 VDJ region recombinations were common between the two populations of IHLs as detected by this amplification protocol, and again this was not significantly less than the VDJ regions present in the viral hepatitis livers. It was not technically feasible to sort IHLs by CD4 and CD8 to see if the TCR clones common to both regions of the livers were $CD4^+$ or $CD8^+$, but for each patient between 5 and 9 amplification products identical in size to those obtained from IHL cDNA were produced from PBL cDNA. By sorting PBLs for $CD4^+$ and $CD8^+$ before Vβ amplification it was shown that PBL clones with VDJ recombinations common to two regions of the liver were predominantly $CD8^+$. This was not true of the control patients with hepatitis C infection, whose $CD4^+$ and $CD8^+$ PBLs contained VDJ recombinations identical to those common to two regions of the liver. This was interpreted as an oligoclonal response of $CD8^+$T cells to a limited set of antigens distributed diffusely in the liver. Unfortunately, in over 70% of normal individuals oligoclonality of $CD8^+$ PBLs is present, and until it can be shown that a similar situation does not exist for IHLs, the above findings may be a normal feature of the human immune system (64,65).

IHL proliferation and cytotoxicity data are not available from PSC livers, but a 40-kD molecule has been identified that is specifically recognized by IgG purified from ulcerative colitis colonic tissue, but not by IgG extracted from Crohn's disease colonic tissue and IgG present in normal serum (66,67). A monoclonal antibody (7E12H12) to the 40-kD molecule was used to screen tissues, and showed staining of the basolateral membranes of colon, gallbladder, biliary ducts, and epidermis (68). The fairly selective biliary and colonic distribution is highly relevant to the tissue damage present in patients with PSC, most of whom also have UC. Subsequently 60% of patients with PSC were shown to contain antibodies to an epitope on sections of bile ducts and gallbladder that could be displaced by 7E12H12 (69). Similar reactivity was not present in the sera of patients with PBC and secondary biliary strictures. Information on non-PSC UC sera was not available. By using an enzyme-linked immunosorbent assay (ELISA) against 7E12H12-reactive protein, 93% of patients with PSC were shown to have antibodies against this antigen, suggesting that a polyclonal response against this antigen was present in virtually all PSC patients. The identity of this antigen, and the presence of any T cell responses to it are not yet known.

MODELS OF AUTOIMMUNE HEPATITIS

Due to the very limited experimental manipulations possible on human tissues, there is an obvious need for animal models of autoimmune liver disease. Hepatic inflammatory responses have been induced by hepatotoxins, lypopolysaccharides from gram-negative bacteria in galactosamine-sensitized mice, and anti-CD3 antibodies to nonspecifically activate T cells (70,71). The best-characterized model of AIH uses concanavalin A (Con-A), a plant lectin known to induce polyclonal activation and proliferation of T cells. Thirty minutes after intravenous injection there is liver endothelium–specific binding of Con-A, with minimal or no binding in the lungs or renal tissues. By 4 hours after injection, large numbers of leukocytes are adherent to the sinusoidal endothelium, and by 8 hours a dose-dependent transaminitis occurs (72,73). Necrosis of hepatocytes is visible by light microscopy, but the parenchymal lymphocyte infiltrate is minimal. In addition to infiltration by lymphocytes, infiltration by neutrophils, and erythrocyte agglutination are prominent features. Simultaneous with these changes there is an elevation in the serum concentration of a number of cytokines known to be produced by T cell activation including IL-2, IL-1a, granulocyte-macrophage colony stimulating factor (GM-CSF), and tumor necrosis factor (TNF).

The model of Con-A-induced liver injury, like the others, provides very little information about the processes that initiate the immune response in AIH. It does, however, provide an opportunity to dissect out the effector components of immune-mediated liver injury induced by hepatic sinusoid adhesion and polyclonal activation of T cells. The requirement of functioning lymphocytes was demonstrated very early by the demonstration that in SCID mice, lacking T cells, and in athymic mice with immature lymphocytes, the degree of hepatitis after Con-A injection was minimal (72). This was confirmed by depletion of T cells by Thy 1.2 antibodies, and the T cell dependence was localized to $CD4^+$ T cells by selective depletion of $CD4^+$ and $CD8^+$ T cells. Since the elevation in the above cytokines occurs before the hepatocyte injury, they were the first candidates in determining the molecular process responsible for the hepatitis. Anti-TNF antiserum neutralized Con-A induced elevation in TNF and protected against hepatitis without affecting serum levels of other cytokines (73,74). Coculture of lymph node T cells and hepatic NPCs, which were over 80% macrophages, demonstrated that both were required for maximal production of TNF in response to Con-A (73). These results lead to a model of polyclonal T cell activation, and sinusoidal localization by the agglutination properties of Con-A, followed by $CD4^+$ T cell–dependent TNF production and hepatocyte damage. The dependence of TNF production on $CD4^+$ T cells does not necessarily mean that they are the source of the TNF. Most likely, Kupffer cells are producing the TNF, but require a strong Th1 $CD4^+$ T cell response for maximal production. Other candidates for TNF production are hepatic NK-T cells. An unexpected finding was the ability of recombinant IL-6 to protect against Con-A-induced hepatitis (74). The protective effects of IL-6 were associated with a reduction in the elevation in TNF. The mechanism of the modulation of TNF by IL-6 is not established, but the recent demonstration of IL-6 leading to a Th2 response by the production of IL-4 (75) suggests that in the presence of IL-6 the Con-A-induced $CD4^+$ T cell activation is shifted towards a Th2 helper, rather than a Th1 inflammatory T cell response.

In a coculture system of hepatocytes and $CD4^+$and $CD8^+$ splenocytes, the addition of Con-A resulted in hepatocyte lysis as measured by the lactate dehydrogenase activity of the supernatant (76). Hepatocytes from CD95 (Fas) deficient mice were susceptible to this splenocyte-mediated cytotoxicity, but splenocytes from perforin-deficient mice were unable to lyse normal hepatocytes. Depletion of $CD4^+$ and $CD8^+$ T cells identified $CD8^+$ T cells as the effectors of this CD95-independent, perforin-dependent cytotoxicity. This coculture system did not contain any Kupffer cells or NK-T cells and is probably reproducing the *in vivo* effects of Con-A distinct from the $CD4^+$ T cell, Kupffer cell and TNF dependent pathway discussed above. Injection of Con-A in CD95-deficient, and perforin-deficient mice produce hepatitis in the CD95-deficient mice, but there was significantly reduced liver damage in the perforin-knockout mice. The occurrence of hepatitis in CD95-deficient mice is not surprising if TNF-induced apoptosis is a major feature of Con-A-induced hepatitis. The lack of hepatitis in the perforin-knockout animals is at odds with the requirement of $CD4^+$ but not $CD8^+$ T cells in the production of Con-A hepatitis in normal mice, since $CD4^+$ T cells are not recognized as mediators of perforin-induced cytotoxicity. TNF production was not assayed in the perforin-knockout mice, and it is possible that in addition to losing the $CD8^+$ T cell perforin mediation cytotoxicity, the livers of perforin-knockout mice have reduced numbers of the cell populations responsible for TNF production in normal mice (e.g., NK-T).

SUMMARY

PSC and AIH are both characterized by an infiltrate of lymphocytes, most of which are conventional T cells with TCRαβ. There is a preferential increase in $CD8^+$ T cells, but total numbers of $CD4^+$ T cells are also increased. Based on analysis of CD45 isoforms, virtually all the T cells have an activated or memory phenotype. Further subdivision of $CD4^+$ cells by cloning, using limiting dilution, has shown a majority to have a Th0 cytokine profile, with Th1 and Th2 represented in 14% and 6% of the clones, respectively. $CD8^+$ and $CD4^+$ clones from AIH livers have shown cytotoxicity against various cell lines, along with proliferation in response to LKM and asialoglycoprotein receptor. Oligoclonality of the T cell response is present in AIH, particularly for $CD8^+$ cells, but interpretation is limited by the lack of data from normal human livers. Two alternative models could explain these findings. In one, cytotoxic $CD4^+$ or $CD8^+$ T cell clones of very limited specificity are primed by an unknown antigen, and subsequently cross-react with a single hepatic epitope (molecular mimicry). The trigger for the second model of AIH need not be a specific antigen that primes cross-reactive T cell clones, but a range of stimuli varying from hepatitis A to drug reactions. These stimuli, in a host with the appropriate HLA background, lead to localized breakdown of tolerance and result in a polymorphic, chronic, self-priming cellular response against a variety of hepatic proteins. The available data, particularly from T cell proliferation in response to LKM and asialoglycoprotein receptor, favors the second hypothesis.

ACKNOWLEDGMENTS

I am grateful to Dr. James Crawford for providing Figures 2A and B.

This work was supported by the Howard Hughes Medical Institute, The National Institute of Health, and the Liver Center at Yale University.

REFERENCES

1. Husby, G., Strickland, R.G., Caldwell, J.L., and Williams, R.C.J. 1975. Localization of T and B cells and alpha fetoprotein in hepatic biopsies from patients with liver disease. *J. Clin. Invest.* 56:1198–1209.
2. Maddrey, W.C. 1987. Subdivisions of idiopathic autoimmune chronic active hepatitis. *Hepatology* 7:1372–1375.
3. Li, X.M., Jeffers, L.J., Reddy, K.R., de Medina, M., Silva, M., Villanueva, S., Klimas, N.G., Esquenazi, V., and Schiff, E.R. 1991. Immunophenotyping of lymphocytes in liver tissue of patients with chronic liver diseases by flow cytometry. *Hepatology* 14:121–127.
4. Hata, K., Zhang, X.R., Iwatsuki, S., Van Thiel, D.H., Herberman, R.B., and Whiteside, T.L. 1990. Isolation, phenotyping, and functional analysis of lymphocytes from human liver. *Clin. Immunol. Immunopathol.* 56:401–419.
5. Bjorkland, A., Festin, R., Mendel-Hartvig, I., Nyberg, A., Loof, L., and Totterman, T.H. 1991. Blood and liver-infiltrating lymphocytes in primary biliary cirrhosis: Increase in activated T and natural killer cells and recruitment of primed memory T cells. *Hepatology* 13:1106–1111.
6. Huang, L., Sye, K., and Crispe, I.N. 1994. Proliferation and apoptosis of B220+CD4-CD8-TCR$\alpha/\beta^{intermediate}$ T cells in the liver of normal mice: Implication for *lpr* pathogenesis. *Int. Immunol.* 6:533.
7. Maharaj, B., Maharaj, R.J., Leary, W.P., Cooppan, R.M., Naran, A.D., Pirie, D., and Pudifin, D.J. 1986. Sampling variability and its influence on the diagnostic yield of percutaneous needle biopsy of the liver. *Lancet* 1:523–525.
8. Doolittle, M., Bohman, R., Durstenfeld, A., and Cascarano, J. 1987. Identification and characterization of liver nonparenchymal cells by flow cytometry. *Hepatology* 7:696–703.
9. Blouin, A., Bolender, R.P., and Weibel, E.R. 1977. Distribution of organelles and membranes between hepatocytes and nonhepatocytes in the rat liver parenchyma. A stereological study. *J. Cell. Biol.* 72:441–455.
10. Winnock, M., Lafon, M.E., Boulard, A., Ferrer, A.M., Saric, J., Dubuisson, L., Bioulac-Sage, P., and Balabaud, C. 1991. Characterization of liver-associated natural killer cells in patients with liver tumors. *Hepatology* 13:676–682.
11. Winnock, M., Garcia Barcina, M., Lukomska, B., Huet, S., Saric, J., Balabaud, C., and Bioulac-Sage, P. 1995. Human liver-associated lymphocytes: An overview. *J. Gastroenterol. Hepatol.* 10(Suppl. 1):S43–S46.
12. Garcia, C.F., Weiss, L.M., Lowder, J., Komoroske, C., Link, M.P., Levy, R., and Warnke, R.A. 1987. Quantitation and estimation of lymphocyte subsets in tissue sections. Comparison with flow cytometry. *Am. J. Clin. Pathol.* 87:470–477.
13. Martins, E.B., Graham, A.K., Chapman, R.W., and Fleming, K.A. 1996. Elevation of gamma delta T lymphocytes in peripheral blood and livers of patients with primary sclerosing cholangitis and other autoimmune liver diseases. *Hepatology* 23:988–993.
14. Olsson, R., Danielsson, A., Jarnerot, G., Lindstrom, E., Loof, L., Rolny, P., Ryden, B.O., Tysk, C., and Wallerstedt, S. 1991. Prevalence of primary sclerosing cholangitis in patients with ulcerative colitis. *Gastroenterology* 100:1319–1323.
15. Chapman, R.W., Arborgh, B.A., Rhodes, J.M., Summerfield, J.A., Dick, R., Scheuer, P.J., and Sherlock, S. 1980. Primary sclerosing cholangitis: A review of its clinical features, cholangiography, and hepatic histology. *Gut* 21:870–877.

16. Wiesner, R.H., and LaRusso, N.F. 1980. Clinicopathologic features of the syndrome of primary sclerosing cholangitis. *Gastroenterology* 79:200–206.
17. Chapman, R. W., Varghese, Z., Gaul, R., Patel, G., Kokinon, N., and Sherlock, S. 1983. Association of primary sclerosing cholangitis with HLA-B8. *Gut* 24:38–41.
18. Manns, M.P., and Kruger, M. 1994. Immunogenetics of chronic liver diseases. *Gastroenterology* 106:1676–1697.
19. Prochazka, E.J., Terasaki, P.I., Park, M.S., Goldstein, L.I., and Busuttil, R.W. 1990. Association of primary sclerosing cholangitis with HLA-DRw52a. *N. Engl. J. Med.* 322:1842–1844.
20. Mehal, W.Z., Wordsworth, B.P., Taylor, C.J., Bell, J.I., Fleming, K.A., and Chapman, R.W. 1991. Inability to attribute susceptibility to primary sclerosing cholangitis to specific amino acid positions of the HLA-DRw52a allele. *N. Engl. J. Med.* 325:1251–1252.
21. Donaldson, P.T., Farrant, J.M., Wilkinson, M.L., Hayllar, K., Portmann, B.C., and Williams, R. 1991. Dual association of HLA DR2 and DR3 with primary sclerosing cholangitis. *Hepatology* 13:129–133.
22. Mehal, W.Z., Lo, Y.M., Wordsworth, B.P., Neuberger, J.M., Hubscher, S.C., Fleming, K.A., and Chapman, R.W. 1994. HLA DR4 is a marker for rapid disease progression in primary sclerosing cholangitis. *Gastroenterology* 106:160–167.
23. Svejgaard, A., and Ryder, L.P. 1979. HLA markers and disease. *Prog. Clin. Biol. Res.* 32:523–543.
24. Lo, S.K., Fleming, K.A., and Chapman, R.W. 1992. Prevalence of anti-neutrophil antibody in primary sclerosing cholangitis and ulcerative colitis using an alkaline phosphatase technique. *Gut* 33:1370–1375.
25. Bansi, D.S., Fleming, K.A., and Chapman, R.W. 1996. Importance of antineutrophil cytoplasmic antibodies in primary sclerosing cholangitis and ulcerative colitis: Prevalence, titre, and IgG subclass. *Gut* 38:384–389.
26. Ludwig, J., Barham, S.S., LaRusso, N.F., Elveback, L.R., Wiesner, R.H., and McCall, J.T. 1981. Morphologic features of chronic hepatitis associated with primary sclerosing cholangitis and chronic ulcerative colitis. *Hepatology* 1:632–640.
27. Kimmelstiel, P., Large, H.L., and Verner, H.D. 1952. Liver damage in ulcerative colitis. *Am. J. Path.* 28:259–290.
28. Vinnik, I.E., and Kern, F. 1963. Liver disease in ulcerative colitis. *Arch. Intern. Med.* 112:87–95.
29. Czaja, A.J. 1984. Natural history, clinical features, and treatment of autoimmune hepatitis. *Semin. Liver Dis.* 4:1–12.
30. Czaja, A.J. 1996. Autoimmune liver disease. In *Hepatology A Textbook of Liver Disease*, Zakim D., and Boyer, J.D., eds. Philadelphia: W.B. Saunders.
31. Czaja, A.J. 1993. Chronic active hepatitis: The challenge for a new nomenclature. *Ann. Intern. Med.* 119:510–517.
32. Homberg, J.C., Abuaf, N., Bernard, O., Islam, S., Alvarez, F., Khalil, S.H., Poupon, R., Darnis, F., Levy, V.G., and Grippon, P. 1987. Chronic active hepatitis associated with antiliver/kidney microsome antibody type 1: A second type of "autoimmune" hepatitis. *Hepatology* 7:1333–1339.
33. Manns, M.P., Johnson, E.F., Griffin, K.J., Tan, E.M., and Sullivan, K.F. 1989. Major antigen of liver kidney microsomal autoantibodies in idiopathic autoimmune hepatitis is cytochrome P450db1. *J. Clin. Invest.* 83:1066–1072.

34. Manns, M., Gerken, G., Kyriatsoulis, A., Staritz, M., and Meyer zum Buschenfelde, K.H. 1987. Characterisation of a new subgroup of autoimmune chronic active hepatitis by autoantibodies against a soluble liver antigen. *Lancet* 1:292–294.
35. Manns, M.P. 1991. Cytoplasmic autoantigens in autoimmune hepatitis: Molecular analysis and clinical relevance. *Semin. Liver Dis.* 11:205–214.
36. Whiteside, T.L., Lasky, S., Si, L., and Van Thiel, D.H. 1985. Immunologic analysis of mononuclear cells in liver tissues and blood of patients with primary sclerosing cholangitis. *Hepatology* 5:468–474.
37. Hata, K., Van Thiel, D.H., Herberman, R.B., and Whiteside, T.L. 1991. Natural killer activity of human liver-derived lymphocytes in various liver diseases. *Hepatology* 14:495–503.
38. Montano, L., Aranguibel, F., Boffill, M., Goodall, A.H., Janossy, G., and Thomas, H.C. 1983. An analysis of the composition of the inflammatory infiltrate in autoimmune and hepatitis B virus-induced chronic liver disease. *Hepatology* 3:292–296.
39. Si, L., Whiteside, T.L., Schade, R.R., Starzl, T.E., and Van Thiel, D.H. 1984. T-lymphocyte subsets in liver tissues of patients with primary biliary cirrhosis (PBC), patients with primary sclerosing cholangitis (PSC), and normal controls. *J. Clin. Immunol.* 4:262–272.
40. Hashimoto, E., Lindor, K.D., Homburger, H.A., Dickson, E.R., Czaja, A.J., Wiesner, R.H., and Ludwig, J. 1993. Immunohistochemical characterization of hepatic lymphocytes in primary biliary cirrhosis in comparison with primary sclerosing cholangitis and autoimmune chronic active hepatitis. *Mayo Clin. Proc.* 68:1049–1055.
41. Snook, J.A., Chapman, R.W., Sachdev, G.K., Heryet, A., Kelly, P.M., Fleming, K.A., and Jewell, D.P. 1989. Peripheral blood and portal tract lymphocyte populations in primary sclerosing cholangitis. *J. Hepatol.* 9:36–41.
42. Trowbridge, I.S., and Thomas, M.L. 1994. CD45: An emerging role as a protein tyrosine phosphatase required for lymphocyte activation and development. *Annu. Rev. Immunol.* 12:85–116.
43. Chang, H.L., Lefrancois, L., Zaroukian, M.H., and Esselman, W.J. 1991. Developmental expression of CD45 alternate exons in murine T cells. Evidence of additional alternate exon use. *J. Immunol.* 147:1687–1693.
44. Ratech, H., Denning, S., and Kaufman, R.E. 1997. An analysis of alternatively spliced CD45 mRNA transcripts during T cell maturation in humans. *Cell. Immunol.* 177:109–118.
45. McCall, M.N., Shotton, D.M., and Barclay, A.N. 1992. Expression of soluble isoforms of rat CD45. Analysis by electron microscopy and use in epitope mapping of anti-CD45R monoclonal antibodies. *Immunology* 76:310–317.
46. Morimoto, C., and Schlossman, S.F. 1993. P. Rambotti Lecture. Human naive and memory T cells revisited: New Markers (CD31 and CD27) that help define CD4+ T cell subsets. *Clin. Exp. Rheumatol.* 11:241–247.
47. Morimoto, C., Letvin, N.L., Boyd, A.W., Hagan, M., Brown, H.M., Kornacki, M.M., and Schlossman, S.F. 1985. The isolation and characterization of the human helper inducer T cell subset. *J. Immunol.* 134:3762–3769.
48. Morimoto, C., Letvin, N.L., Distaso, J.A., Aldrich, W.R., and Schlossman, S.F. 1985. The isolation and characterization of the human suppressor inducer T cell subset. *J. Immunol.* 134:1508–1515.
49. Tedder, T.F., Cooper, M.D., and Clement, L.T. 1985. Human lymphocyte differentiation antigens HB-10 and HB-11, II. Differential production of B cell growth and differentiation factors by distinct helper T cell subpopulations. *J. Immunol.* 134:2989–2994.

50. Sanders, M.E., Makgoba, M.W., Sharrow, S.O., Stephany, D., Springer, T.A., Young, H.A., and Shaw, S. 1988. Human memory T lymphocytes express increased levels of three cell adhesion molecules (LFA-3, CD2, and LFA-1) and three other molecules (UCHL1, CDw29, and Pgp-1) and have enhanced IFN-gamma production. *J. Immunol.* 140:1401–1407.

51. Sanders, M.E., Makgoba, M.W., and Shaw, S. 1988. Human naive and memory T cells: Reinterpretation of helper-inducer and suppressor-inducer subsets. *Immunol. Today* 9:195–199.

52. Morimoto, C., Letvin, N.L., Rudd, C.E., Hagan, M., Takeuchi, T., and Schlossman, S.F. 1986. The role of the 2H4 molecule in the generation of suppressor function in Con A-activated T cells. *J. Immunol.* 137:3247–3253.

53. Rothstein, D.M., Sohen, S., Daley, J.F., Schlossman, S.F., and Morimoto, C. 1990. CD4+CD45RA+ and CD4+CD45RA- T cell subsets in man maintain distinct function and CD45RA expression persists on a subpopulation of CD45RA+ cells after activation with Con A. *Cell. Immunol.* 129:449–467.

54. Hedlund, G., Hansson, J., Ericsson, P.O., Sjogren, H.O., and Dohlsten, M. 1995. Expression of CD11a and CD45R isoforms defines distinct subsets of CD8+ TCR alpha beta and TCR gamma delta CTL in vivo. *Immunol. Rev.* 146:82–94.

55. Leon, M.P., Spickett, G., Jones, D.E., and Bassendine, M.F. 1995. CD4+ T cell subsets defined by isoforms of CD45 in primary biliary cirrhosis. *Clin. Exp. Immunol.* 99:233–239.

56. Volpes, R., van den Oord, J.J., and Desmet, V.J. 1991. Memory T cells represent the predominant lymphocyte subset in acute and chronic liver inflammation. *Hepatology* 13:826–829.

57. Schlaak, J.F, Lohr, H., Gallati, H., Meyer zum Buschenfelde, K.H., and Fleischer, B. 1993. Analysis of the in vitro cytokine production by liver-infiltrating T cells of patients with autoimmune hepatitis. *Clin. Exp. Immunol.* 94:168–173.

58. Lohr, H.F., Schlaak, J.F., Gerken, G., Fleischer, B., Dienes, H.P., and Meyer zum Buschenfelde, K.H. 1994. Phenotypical analysis and cytokine release of liver-infiltrating and peripheral blood T lymphocytes from patients with chronic hepatitis of different etiology. *Liver* 14:161–166.

59. Lohr, H., Manns, M., Kyriatsoulis, A., Lohse, A.W., Trautwein, C., Meyer zum Buschenfelde, K.H., and Fleischer, B. 1991. Clonal analysis of liver-infiltrating T cells in patients with LKM-1 antibody-positive autoimmune chronic active hepatitis. *Clin. Exp. Immunol.* 84:297–302.

60. Lohr, H.F., Schlaak, J.F., Lohse, A.W., Bocher, W.O., Arenz, M., Gerken, G., and Meyer zum Buschenfelde, K.H. 1996. Autoreactive CD4+ LKM-specific and anticlonotypic T-cell responses in LKM-1 antibody-positive autoimmune hepatitis. *Hepatology* 24:1416–1421.

61. Lohr, H., Treichel, U., Poralla, T., Manns, M., and Meyer zum Buschenfelde, K.H. 1992. Liver-infiltrating T helper cells in autoimmune chronic active hepatitis stimulate the production of autoantibodies against the human asialoglycoprotein receptor in vitro. *Clin. Exp. Immunol.* 88:45–49.

62. Hoshino, Y., Enomoto, N., Izumi, N., Kurosaki, M., Marumo, F., and Sato, C. 1995. Limited usage of T-cell receptor beta chains and sequences of the complementarity determining region 3 of lymphocytes infiltrating in the liver of autoimmune hepatitis. *Hepatology* 22:142–147.

63. Tanaka, A., Iwabuchi, S., Takatori, M., Ohno, A., Yamada, H., Hashimoto, N., Ikeda, Y., Kato, T., Nishioka, K., Iino, S., and Yamamoto, K. 1997. Clonotypic analysis of T cells in patients with autoimmune and viral hepatitis. *Hepatology* 25:1070–1076.

64. Hingorani, R., Choi, I.H., Akolkar, P., Gulwani-Akolkar, B., Pergolizzi, R., Silver, J., and Gregersen, P.K. 1993. Clonal predominance of T cell receptors within the CD8+ CD45RO+ subset in normal human subjects. *J. Immunol.* 151:5762–5769.

65. Monteiro, J., Hingorani, R., Choi, I.H., Silver, J., Pergolizzi, R., and Gregersen, P.K. 1995. Oligoclonality in the human CD8+ T cell repertoire in normal subjects and monozygotic twins: Implications for studies of infectious and autoimmune diseases. *Mol. Med.* 1:614–624.

66. Takahashi, F., and Das, K.M. 1985. Isolation and characterization of a colonic autoantigen specifically recognized by colon tissue-bound immunoglobulin G from idiopathic ulcerative colitis. *J. Clin. Invest.* 76:311–318.

67. Nagai, T., and Das, K.M. 1981. Detection of colonic antigen(s) in tissues from ulcerative colitis using purified colitis colon tissue-bound IgG (CCA-IgG). *Gastroenterology* 81:463–470.

68. Das, K.M., Sakamaki, S., Vecchi, M., and Diamond, B. 1987. The production and characterization of monoclonal antibodies to a human colonic antigen associated with ulcerative colitis: Cellular localization of the antigen by using the monoclonal antibody. *J. Immunol.* 139:77–84.

69. Mandal, A., Dasgupta, A., Jeffers, L., Squillante, L., Hyder, S., Reddy, R., Schiff, E., and Das, K.M. 1994. Autoantibodies in sclerosing cholangitis against a shared peptide in biliary and colon epithelium. *Gastroenterology* 106:185–192.

70. Ferran, C., Sheehan, K., Dy, M., Schreiber, R., Merite, S., Landais, P., Noel, L.H., Grau, G., Bluestone, J., and Bach, J.F. 1990. Cytokine-related syndrome following injection of anti-CD3 monoclonal antibody: Further evidence for transient in vivo T cell activation. *Eur. J. Immunol.* 20:509–515.

71. Lehmann, V., Freudenberg, M.A., and Galanos, C. 1987. Lethal toxicity of lipopolysaccharide and tumor necrosis factor in normal and D-galactosamine-treated mice. *J. Exp. Med.* 165:657–663.

72. Tiegs, G., Hentschel, J., and Wendel, A. 1992. A T cell-dependent experimental liver injury in mice inducible by concanavalin A. *J. Clin. Invest.* 90:196–203.

73. Gantner, F., Leist, M., Lohse, A.W., Germann, P.G., and Tiegs, G. 1995. Concanavalin A-induced T-cell-mediated hepatic injury in mice: The role of tumor necrosis factor. *Hepatology* 21:190–189.

74. Mizuhara, H., O'Neill, E., Seki, N., Ogawa, T., Kusunoki, C., Otsuka, K., Satoh, S., Niwa, M., Senoh, H., and Fujiwara, H. 1994. T cell activation-associated hepatic injury: Mediation by tumor necrosis factors and protection by interleukin 6. *J. Exp. Med.* 179:1529–1537.

75. Rincon, M., Anguita, J., Nakamura, T., Fikrig, E., and Flavell, R.A. 1997. Interleukin (IL)-6 directs the differentiation of IL-4-producing CD4+ T cells. *J. Exp. Med.* 185:461–469.

76. Watanabe, Y., Morita, M., and Akaike, T. 1996. Concanavalin A induces perforin-mediated but not Fas-mediated hepatic injury. *Hepatology* 24:702–710.

CHAPTER 12

HOW IS THE LIVER UNIQUE?

I. NICHOLAS CRISPE
Yale University School of Medicine, New Haven, CT

In this volume, contributions from experts in diverse fields of liver-related immunology have reviewed the developmental biology, transplantation immunology, defensive functions, and potential for immunopathology in liver T cells. The aim of this final chapter is to bring together these disparate threads and to weave a tapestry depicting the immunological uniqueness of the liver. At this stage, this is an impressionist exercise and it appears premature to try to lay down a definitive paradigm. Instead, the discussion will proceed through the evaluation of a series of hypotheses concerning the distinctive immunological properties of the liver. At the time of writing, all of these hypotheses appear plausible, and an even-handed evaluation of the evidence for each will be attempted.

"THE LIVER IS A SITE OF THYMUS-INDEPENDENT T CELL DEVELOPMENT"

The liver contains an unusual mixture of lymphocytes, in which conventional $CD4^+$ and $CD8^+$ $TCR\alpha\beta^+$ cells are accompanied by NK cells, $TCR\gamma\delta$ cells and NK-T cells. These other lymphocyte populations have all been proposed to develop independently of the main thymic pathway (1,2). Other tissue sites that display such an unusual complement of lymphoid cells include the bone marrow and the intestinal epithelium, and both of these sites have also been proposed as sites of extrathymic T cell development.

This paradigm has been most fully explored in relation to the intestinal epithelium, where rare cells express the protein RAG-1 (3), which is required for lymphocyte receptor gene rearrangement, has no other known function, and is widely regarded as a marker for sites of lymphocyte development. In addition, chimeric animals in which

T Lymphocytes in the Liver: Immunobiology, Pathology, and Host Defense, Edited by I. Nicholas Crispe
ISBN 0-471-19218-X

the bone marrow has been replaced in thymus-deprived irradiated hosts show repopulation of the intestinal lymphocytes, including both TCRαβ and TCRγδ cells, with bone-marrow-derived cells (4). These data support the idea that the intestine is a site for extrathymic T cell differentiation. However, the experiments involved lethal irradiation, which is known to cause tissue changes that may provoke unphysiological lymphocyte differentiation events. This is well documented in the thymus of RAG-2-deficient mice, where the differentiation block resulting from the inability of precursor T cells to rearrange the TCRβ locus is partially overcome after irradiation (5).

Apparently contradictory results come from congenitally athymic (nude) mice, in which intestinal lymphocytes are very rare. The interpretation of this observation is complicated, since the defect in nude mice which prevents the development of a thymus also creates an abnormality in the skin, resulting in brittle hairs that fracture, leaving the mouse bald (hence: nude). Critics of the nude mouse data therefore argue that the nude mouse could have defects in intestinal epithelium, preventing the normal role of this tissue in supporting T cell development. This criticism is supported in some measure by the observation that neonatal thymectomy prevents the development of intestinal intraepithelial T cells (reviewed in reference 6). These contradictions could be resolved if the thymus were necessary, but not sufficient, for intestinal intraepithelial T cell development. One *ad hoc* hypothesis would be that the thymus releases immature cells with one TCR locus (probably either β, γ, or δ) fully rearranged, but without rearrangement at the other locus requiring an in-frame rearrangement to make a TCR (for example, α). These cells would then rearrange with low frequency in niches around the body where a conducive cytokine environment can induce RAG gene re-expression. Bone marrow transplantation into irradiated hosts could replace this population of partly differentiated precursor cells, accounting for the successful result of these experiments.

These debates about the interpretation of data bearing on the origin of intestinal intraepithelial lymphocytes also apply to the evidence for intrahepatic thymus-independent T cell development. In the liver, as in the intestine, there is RAG-1 gene expression in a subset of lymphocytes (7). In thymectomized, bone-marrow-reconstituted radiation chimeras, donor-derived lymphocytes with the distinctive $TCR\alpha\beta^{intermediate}$ phenotype repopulate the liver (8). Such cells are reduced in absolute number, but increased in frequency, in the livers of nude mice (2). This and other evidence for the intrahepatic development of these cells is reviewed in detail in Chapter 4.

The overwhelming majority of the data suggest that liver lymphocytes with the distinctive $TCR\alpha\beta^{intermediate}$ phenotype, like intestinal intraepithelial lymphocytes with the distinctive $CD8\alpha^{+}\beta^{-}$ phenotype, develop without the same need for a thymic environment as conventional circulating $CD4^{+}$ and $CD8^{+}$ $TCR\alpha\beta^{+}$ T cells. Furthermore, these cells have a distinctive tissue distribution. This could be due to unique patterns of recirculation, based on distinctive adhesion molecules. However there is very little exchange of either intestinal intraepithelial or intrahepatic lymphocytes between parabiosed mice (9), suggesting that instead they are largely sessile and supporting the idea that they develop *in situ*. The alternative hypothesis is that these two T cell populations develop from a common precursor pool, which might undergo an early stage of development in the thymus before seeding the peripheral tissues early in life.

Where might such a common pool of cell reside? Lymphocytes in the NK-T cell/TCR$\alpha\beta^{\text{intermediate}}$ category are abundant in the bone marrow (10), an environment in which B cell receptor (i.e., immunoglobulin) genes are induced to undergo rearrangement by cytokines synthesized by stromal cells. It is therefore possible that the TCR$\alpha\beta^{\text{intermediate}}$ cells of the liver, and the CD8$\alpha^{+}\beta^{-}$ cells of the intestinal epithelium, are local differentiation products of a common pool of incompletely differentiated precursors that are abundant in bone marrow. Such cells may have passed through the thymus early in life, but their further development is not thymus-dependent. However, evidence for such a common pool of extrathymic, partly differentiated T-lineage cells is entirely lacking. We have conducted experiments to identify such cells, using rapid repopulation of the thymic cortex as an assay for cells more differentiated than circulating hematopoietic stem cells (I. N. Crispe, unpublished data). These experiments were uniformly unsuccessful, but it is not difficult to think of technical reasons for the failure. The issue of local intrahepatic versus systemic differentiation of relatively thymus-independent T cells therefore remains open.

"THE LIVER IS A SITE OF IMMUNE PRIVILEGE"

Privileged sites are anatomical locations at which antigenic material, particularly transplanted allogeneic tissue, fails to induce an immune response. The classical privileged sites, namely the hamster cheek pouch and the anterior chamber of the eye, have recently been joined by the testis, in which tolerance appears to prevail because of the local expression of Fas ligand, which engages with the Fas death receptor on incoming T cells and causes them to undergo apoptosis rather than deliver allograft rejection. Testis is also a privileged tissue, which may be readily transplanted to allogenic hosts (11). The liver is a privileged tissue in this sense, since liver allografting leads to a weak rejection response accompanied by the induction of systemic tolerance (reviewed in Chapter 5). But it is not so clear that the liver is a privileged site for the transplantation of other tissues. This question is of interest in the diabetes field, where the transplantation of pancreatic islets of Langerhans offers the prospect of radical cure of the disease. But histocompatible islets are in short supply. Furthermore, current models of insulin-dependent, juvenile-onset diabetes envisage an autoimmune pathogenesis initiated by T cells. To meet the dual therapeutic goals of islet replacement and prevention of autoimmune attack, it would be very helpful to know whether transplantation into the liver would result in immune privilege. The limited data available suggests that this is so (12).

The analysis of the mechanisms of oral tolerance has led to experiments in which antigen-presenting cells are introduced into the portal vein, leading to their passage into the liver (reviewed in Chapter 6). This typically results in systemic transplantation tolerance. One reproducible feature of such portal vein tolerance is that it is dependent on intact Kupffer cell function, since depletion or inactivation of these cells prevents the tolerance (13–15). Another feature of portal vein tolerance is that it is transferable to another animal through the intravenous adoptive transfer of liver lymphocytes, giving rise to the idea that it is due to the induction of regulatory cells (potentially "suppressor T cells") (16,17). Finally, depletion of TCRγδ cells also interferes with portal vein tolerance, suggesting that they may be the regulatory cells involved (17,18). All of these phenomena could be incorporated into an umbrella model in which antigenic cells introduced into the portal vein are trapped in the liver and interact with Kupffer cells, resulting in the activation of TCRγδ cells, which in turn specifically suppress conventional T cells and induce transplantation tolerance. The mechanism of this suppression could be either through specific killing of activated conventional $CD4^+$ and $CD8^+$ T cells, or through the secretion of suppressive cytokines. However, as Dr. Mowat argues in Chapter 6, evidence for this model is circumstantial at best and none of its main tenets have been subjected to a decisive experimental test.

"LIVER TOLERANCE IS DUE TO IMMUNE DEVIATION"

While the initial response against an antigenic challenge appears to result in the mobilization of all the effector mechanisms, long-lasting immune responses frequently polarize into one of two types: inflammatory responses in which the dominant cytokines include the IL-1s, IL-12, TNFα, and IFNγ, and humoral responses in which the dominant cytokines include IL-4 and IL-5. These two types of responses are sustained by $CD4^+$ T cells in distinct states of terminal differentiation, termed Th1 in the case of inflammatory responses and Th2 in the case of humoral responses. $CD8^+$ T cell responses tend to be supported by Th1 $CD4^+$ cells, and suppressed by Th2 $CD4^+$ cells. These two differentiation states tend to be mutually exclusive within any one immunological niche, since Th1 cells secrete IL-12, which inactivates Th2 cell differentiation, while Th2 cells secrete IL-4, which suppresses Th1 cells (19,20). This state of affairs produced two corollaries. One is that an initially undifferentiated immune response can become polarized in response to the local cytokine environment, and once polarized it tends to stay polarized. The other is that an immune response can appear to be inactivated or suppressed, when in fact the polarity of the response has simply switched to the alternative cytokine pattern. This latter process is termed immune deviation.

The anterior chamber of the eye has long been understood as a site of immune privilege, into which allogeneic or xenogeneic tissue may readily be transplanted. Recent experimental work, particularly from Streilein and colleagues, has shown that this is due to immune deviation (termed ACAID, for anterior chamber acquired immune deviation). The introduction of antigen at this site results in a Th2 response, so Th1-dependent phenomena, including graft rejection, are suppressed (21).

Several of the examples of liver tolerance discussed in this book act on inflammatory immune responses driven by Th1 cytokines. This is certainly the case in liver transplantation tolerance, failure to clear hepatitis B virus and chronic malaria, where in each case the major effector cells are $CD8^+$ T cells. If the cytokine environment of the liver were biased towards the generation of Th2 responses, the difficulty in generating an inflammatory immune response would be comprehensible as an example of immune deviation. In liver transplantation, the induction of tolerance is accompanied by hematopoietic chimerism in which liver-derived mononuclear cells recirculate through the host. The biological effect of these cells is not known, but one possible effect could be the polarization of the host immune response towards Th2, and against inflammatory effector functions.

How far is it reasonable to speak of the intrahepatic cytokine environment as biased? One piece of circumstantial evidence comes from the cellular composition of the intrahepatic lymphocytes. In mice, they are enriched for NK-T cells that express an intermediate level of TCR$\alpha\beta$ with very restricted clonal diversity, along with markers typical of NK cells. In humans, the NK cell marker CD56 is coexpressed with the TCR$\alpha\beta$ on many liver lymphocytes. Therefore NK-T cells appear to be a conserved feature of the liver environment. Very little is known about the specificity and function of these strange lymphocytes, which are rare in the major peripheral lymphoid organs but are much more abundant in the liver and the bone marrow. But one of their properties is the secretion of large amounts of IL-4 (22). Even in lymphoid organs where they are rare, these cells have been proposed to influence the polarization of conventional $CD4^+$ T cell responses towards the Th2 pattern. It is therefore plausible that the prevalence of these cells in the liver suppresses inflammatory immune responses by immune deviation.

A newly identified player in this environment is IL-18, also termed interferon-γ inducing factor, or IGIF. This cytokine was recently cloned from a liver cDNA library, and is an IL-1-like cytokine synthesized by Kupffer cells (23). Like IL-1α, it is synthesized as a transmembrane protein and cleaved from the Kupffer cell membrane by the protease ICE (24). IL-18 alone does not directly determine the differentiation pathway of $CD4^+$ cells, but has recently been shown to synergize with IL-12 in promoting Th1 responses by amplifying the effect of IL-12 (25). IL-18 could therefore effect a rapid switch in intrahepatic T cells responses from Th2-dominant to Th1-dominated, and relieve immune deviation, but only when IL-12 is present.

"LIVER TOLERANCE IS DUE TO ACTIVATION-INDUCED CELL DEATH"

The induction of peripheral immune tolerance could act by immune deviation, the induction of functional anergy, or by peripheral deletion. Our own experiments, and those of others, suggest that the liver is a focus of peripheral T cell apoptosis in several TCR transgenic models (reviewed in Chapter 2). The common features of these models are: the coexpression on the majority of T cells of CD8 and an MHC class I–restricted TCR specific for a known antigenic peptide, the induction of rapid peripheral T cell deletion by a series of injections of the specific peptide dissolved in saline, and the transient appearance of large numbers of apoptotic T cells in the liver, coinciding with the disappearance of these cells from the peripheral lymphoid organs (26). We have therefore proposed that the liver is a specific site for the apoptosis of $CD8^+$ cells during peripheral deletion. This could be accounted for by several different mechanisms. Most simply, T cells undergoing peripheral deletion could express membrane markers characteristic of cells at an early stage of apoptosis, leading to their recognition by Kupffer cells or other resident liver cells and the trapping of the

T cells in the liver, where their already activated apoptosis program proceeds to conclusion. Alternatively, the liver could present antigen in such a way that large numbers of T cells are trapped at this site. In this case, the T cell apoptosis could have occurred at any site where the cells were trapped. In a model where T cells undergo expansion prior to deletion, such apoptosis has in fact been seen in other organs including the kidneys and the lungs (27). Finally, the liver could sequester activated T cells and induce their apoptosis, either through the cytotoxic action of resident liver lymphocytes (28), through toxic molecules such as galectin-1 (29,30), or simply through the deprivation of survival signals.

Any of these mechanisms could explain two aspects of liver tolerance, the resistance of allografted livers to T cell–mediated rejection and the systemic tolerance induced by the introduction of allogeneic antigen-presenting cells into the portal vein. In transplantation, we have proposed that incoming host cytotoxic $CD8^+$ cells in a transplanted liver undergo apoptosis before they can induce tissue damage, similar to the situation in the allografted testis (11). In portal vein tolerance, the mechanism would be simply the trapping and apoptosis of any T cells that traverse the liver and encounter their specific antigen presented by Kupffer cells.

The experimental evidence for the accumulation of apoptosing $CD8^+$ T cells in the liver during peripheral T cell deletion is not yet accompanied by any data concerning the mechanism. Questions in need of resolution are: Are the cells really extracted from the circulating T cell pool, or do they accumulate by some other mechanism? If they are extracted, is it from blood delivered via the hepatic artery or the portal vein? What is the molecular basis for their retention, and does it involve adhesion molecules specifically expressed on activated T cells or markers of membrane damage expressed on diverse cell types? Are $CD4^+$ T cells subject to the same process? Do the cells enter the liver already programmed to undergo cell death or is the apoptotic signal delivered *in situ*? And if the latter, what is the lethal effector mechanism?

"CHRONICITY OF LIVER INFECTIONS IS DUE TO LIVER TOLERANCE"

Chronicity is a frequent, but not a universal consequence of infection of the liver by pathogens. One chapter describes the immunology of an infection of the liver, *Listeria monocytogenes*, that is readily cleared in immunocompetent animals. In contrast, two chapters deal with viral hepatitis and with malaria, infections of the liver that commonly become chronic. We will evaluate the potential mechanisms that could explain these very different outcomes.

Probably the best-understood viral disease of the liver is infection with hepatitis B virus (HBV). In Chapter 7 Dr. Chisari discusses the mechanisms of HBV clearance and persistence first in terms of the relationship between the specificity of the response and the prospect of clearance. Broadly, strong responses that result in virus clearance are polyclonal and multispecific cytotoxic T lymphocyte (CTL) responses mediated by classical $CD8^+$ $TCR\alpha\beta^+$ cytotoxic cells, while in weak responses that coexist with chronic infection the $CD8^+$ CTL response is of narrower specificity. This may reflect the high mutation rate in HBV, which is a potential mechanism of immune escape shared with human immunodeficiency virus (HIV). However, other mechanisms may limit the ability of the CTL system to clear HBV. One is the sheer number of hepatocytes potentially infected. Established HBV may infect almost every hepatocyte, which in a human number around 10^{11}. Since there are around 10^{12} T lymphocytes, but the precursor frequency for most antigens is typically around 10^{-4}, specific precursors would therefore number around 10^{8} and could be outnumbered by infected cells by up to 10^{3} to one. Each precursor could potentially give rise to a clone of several thousand cells, and each cytotoxic effector could potentially kill several targets in succession, but the CTL response is clearly stretched to the limit in such a widespread infection. To explain the cases in which HBV is apparently cleared, Dr. Chisari proposes a novel hypothesis, namely that in addition to cytotoxic effector function, CTL-derived inflammatory cytokines can suppress viral replication and even effect virus inactivation in infected hepatocytes without causing hepatocyte death. In support of this hypothesis, the adoptive transfer of CTL into transgenic mice expressing the whole HBV genome resulted in an inflammatory response during which the downregulation of HBV antigen expression could be blocked by antibodies against IFNγ or TNFα.

Both the CTL-based and the cytokine-based mechanisms of HBV elimination would be suppressed by the intrahepatic environment. As in the context of liver allograft rejection, CTL responses are not readily mounted in the liver due to activation-induced cell death affecting primarily $CD8^+$ T cells. In addition, we have already considered the cytokine environment of the liver in terms of immune deviation. The presence of abundant NK-T cells favors the suppression of inflammatory $CD4^+$ and $CD8^+$ T cell responses, and the promotion of responses dominated by IL-4 and IL-5. This bias would tend to suppress the induction of IFNγ and TNFα, either by $CD8^+$ CTL or by $CD4^+$ Th1 cells. Whichever of the two mechanisms of HBV clearance discussed in Chapter 7 is the more important *in vivo*, it is not surprising that the clearance of HBV sometimes fails. Furthermore, the weak immune response observed in chronic HBV could be the cause of the chronicity; alternatively it could be an effect of the widespread expression of HBV antigens in the liver and lead to the induction of apoptosis in HBV-specific CTL and purging of the peripheral repertoire of HBV-reactive cells, an effect parallel to the systemic tolerance generated by a liver allograft (described in Chapter 5).

Hepatitis C virus (HCV) presents a very different picture, in which a low viral load is accompanied by a strong $CD4^+$ Th1 and $CD8^+$ CTL immune response, but the infection is nevertheless chronic. Here, local tolerance and systemic immunity coexist, and there is no evidence for purging of the T cell repertoire. But the local suppression of CTL by deletion or a Th2-dominated cytokine environment may allow the virus to persist.

Malaria parasites in hepatocytes behave immunologically very much like HCV. Only a small minority of hepatocytes are infested, so neither the limits of the specific CTL number nor intrahepatic purging of the specific CTL from the repertoire are plausible mechanisms. Yet the liver stages of *Plasmodium sp.* persist, and there is little specific immunity and no T cell memory. Infection of the hepatocytes by sporozoites probably occurs directly, rather than via infection of Kupffer cells, and there is no obvious pathology and no inflammation. This may be due to the well-adapted invasion mechanisms of the parasite, which avoid tissue injury; alternatively it may be due to the Th2-dominated local environment in which inflammatory immune responses are difficult to start. A protective immune response may be generated by pretreatment of mice with IL-12, suggesting that a proinflammatory cytokine environment is required for immunity. Once this environment is established, parasites could be cleared either by CTL-mediated elimination of infected hepatocytes, or by intracellular killing mediated through nitric oxide. Inducible nitric oxide synthetase is induced by proinflammatory cytokines including IFNγ (31), which in turn is induced by the abundant Kupffer cell product, IL-18.

A common feature of HBV, HCV, and malaria is the need for an immune response dominated by $CD8^+$ CTL and $CD4^+$ Th1 cells. The liver environment appears to induce apoptosis in the former and to suppress the latter by immune deviation. Yet some pathogens of the liver are subject to immune clearance. Effective immune responses must somehow be delivered, despite the tolerogenic local environment.

"DEFENSE AGAINST LIVER PATHOGENS MUST OVERCOME LIVER TOLERANCE"

To understand how immune defense can function in the liver, we must ask: how is the immune response to *Listeria monocytogenes* different to the HBV, HCV, and malaria responses? *L. monocytogenes* is an intracellular bacterium that infects both Kupffer cells and hepatocytes. The bacteria are endocytosed, and in an acidic intracellular compartment elaborate Listeriolysin O, an enzyme which degrades the endosome and allows the organisms to escape into the cytoplasm (reviewed in Chapter 8). There they engage polymerized actin of the host cells and allow themselves to be translocated and spread from cell to cell. Rapid spread of the *Listeria* organisms is followed by an immune response in which their antigenic peptides are processed through the MHC class I pathway and recognized by classical, $CD8^+$ CTL. In immunocompetent mice, the immune response leads to clearance of the *Listeria* organisms. The clearance is compromised in both $CD8^+$ cell-deficient and perforin-deficient mice, suggesting that cytotoxicity is important for the elimination of the pathogen.

One possible explanation of the different outcome in infection by *Listeria sp.* is that the bacteria have not evolved a silent mode of infection; instead, they cause tissue damage leading to inflammation. In particular, they infect Kupffer cells and stress these cells by rupturing their endosomes. As macrophages, Kupffer cells have the potential to make IL-12. They are also able to make IL-18; the two cytokines acting together could reverse immune deviation and allow a protective inflammatory immune response to be delivered. But the local production of IL-12 and IL-18 by infected Kupffer cells in *Listeria* infection has not yet been documented.

This line of argument raises two issues. One is the extent to which Kupffer cell involvement is crucial in generating a protective immune response in the liver. Do all examples of "liver tolerance" specifically disable or bypass Kupffer cells? Another is the relationship between the cytokine environment and the mechanism of $CD8^+$ T cell deletion. Could a Th2-dominated environment be essential for the intrahepatic apoptosis of $CD8^+$ cells?

"AUTOIMMUNE LIVER DISEASE IS NOT REALLY AUTOIMMUNE"

The liver displays several patterns of inflammation associated with lymphocyte infiltrates and liver damage, collectively termed "autoimmune liver disease." These diseases, described in Chapter 10 by Dr. Gershwin and colleagues and in Chapter 11 by Dr. Mehal, are currently classified into three entities: autoimmune hepatitis (AIH), primary biliary cirrhosis (PBC), and primary sclerosing cholangitis (PSC). In each case, a distinctive histology is coupled with characteristic autoantibodies, T cell infiltrate, and a human leukocyte antigen (HLA) association. We will deal with each of these phenomena in turn, evaluate the argument that these observations support an autoimmune pathogenesis, and provide alternative hypotheses.

Classification of a disease as autoimmune implies that specific B or T lymphocytes recognize components of self, make an inappropriate immune response, and thereby cause tissue damage. There are several clear and unequivocal examples driven by antibody: Graves disease, in which agonistic antibodies are made against the thyroid stimulating hormone receptor, and myaesthenia gravis, in which inhibitory antibodies are made against the acetylcholine receptor. A long list of diseases are candidates for T cell–driven autoimmunity (including insulin-dependent diabetes mellitus, multiple sclerosis, rheumatoid arthritis, and ulcerative colitis). In each case candidate antigens come and go, but never has the target auto-antigen been unequivocally identified. Against this background, it is prudent to doubt the validity of the autoimmune paradigm and to consider other interpretations.

A variety of pathogenic mechanisms could masquerade as autoimmunity. The most obvious is an immune response against a covert pathogen. This is quite distinct from "molecular mimicry," the hypothesis that a useful defensive immune response may cross-react on self-molecules and cause tissue damage. Instead, defense against the pathogen could be achieved at the expense of killing enough tissue cells to cause disease. For example, immune responses against intracellular mycobacteria can cause gross tissue damage, yet are not believed to be autoimmune because the pathogen is known.

The three varieties of autoimmune liver disease are associated with distinct but overlapping sets of autoantibodies. In PBC, antibodies include anti-mitochondrial specificities (such as pyruvate dehydrogenase), while in PSC these antibodies are missing, but there are instead antibodies against smooth muscle and against neutrophil granule proteins. In AIH, anti-smooth muscle antibodies are accompanied by those against microsomal antigens (including cytochrome P450) or cytokeratins. Are these autoantibodies evidence of an autoimmune pathogenesis? Possibly—but the alternative interpretation is that they are simply consequences of tissue damage. If this were the case, the distinct patterns of tissue damage would account for the liberation of different sets of self-molecules in an immunogenic form. An example is the antibodies against cardiac muscle synthesized after myocardial infarction (32). Autoantibodies have even been proposed as a homeostatis mechanism to help clear intracellular debris liberated by necrosis (33,34). With these alternative interpretations available, the existence of autoantibodies is not strong evidence for self-reactivity as the primary agent of disease.

The three diseases all feature infiltrates in which T cells are predominant. In AIH and PSC these are mainly of $CD8^+$ cells, while in PBC $CD4^+$ cells are more abundant. This supports the hypothesis that PBC is a distinct disease entity, but does not support an autoimmune pathogenesis. The $CD4^+$ cell infiltrate in PBC could be a response to pathogen-derived antigens presented through the endocytic/MHC class II processing pathway, while the $CD8^+$ cell responses in AIH and PSC could result from the processing and presentation of antigens through the proteasome/MHC class I pathway. In the case of the $CD8^+$ cells, the liver presents a unique alternative mechanism. The trapping of $CD8^+$ cells during a systemic immune response (described in Chapter 2) could result in the local accumulation of cells expressing Fas ligand, thereby causing direct damage to Fas-expressing hepatocytes without a requirement for recognition of any self- or exogenous antigen through the T cell antigen receptor. Similar "collateral damage" appears to be involved in liver injury that results from the injection of the T cell mitogen, concanavalin A (35), although in that case the cytotoxic effect is mediated by TNFα (36).

The three autoimmune liver syndromes are linked to different sets of HLA types. Like many putatively autoimmune diseases, all three are linked to DR4. In addition, PSC is strongly linked to Dw52a, while PBC in Europeans is linked to B8 and DR3. Other HLA alleles influence prognosis within the diagnostic categories (reviewed in Chapter 11). Strong linkage to a set of HLA types is taken as evidence that a disease is influenced by Ir genes, which are allelic variants of MHC molecules that are able to determine whether a response is made to a particular antigen. The nature of Ir gene effects is well understood in molecular terms. MHC molecules, including human HLA-A, -B, -C and -DR, function by holding antigenic peptides in a groove on the apical surface of the molecule. Only in this form are peptides recognized by T cells. The sides and floor of this peptide-binding region are composed of charged and hydrophobic residues, which form a three-dimensional surface that includes deep pockets. These charges, and the shape of the groove, vary between allelic forms of the molecule. Peptides are bound to the MHC molecule through two or three specific residues (termed anchor residues) that fit the pockets. This allows certain peptides, but not others, to bind to any MHC molecule (37). Thus particular HLA alleles can only offer a limited set of peptides for T cell recognition.

In the context of autoimmunity, particular HLA alleles are potentially able to contribute to the disease by acting as Ir genes and presenting self-peptides to T cells. However, if these diseases were consequences of a series of occult infections, Ir gene effects could also predispose to pathology. In this case a disease-promoting allele would be interpreted as a nonresponder gene that fails to bind and present a critical antigenic peptide. This prevents an effective immune response and results in a chronic infection.

The weakness of the direct evidence for autoimmune disease, in the face of extensive investigation, suggests that a paradigm shift may be in order. AIH, PSC, and PBC may not be autoimmune diseases in any sense, but instead covert infections to which the defensive immune response causes collateral tissue damage, similar to the pathology created in many tissues by *Mycobacterium tuberculosis*. Is it really credible that the pathogens causing AIH, PSC, and PBC could have evaded detection until now? To address this point, consider duodenal ulcers. This very common condition was "known" to be due to an imbalance in gastic acid production until *Helicobacter pylori* was identified as the cause (38,39).

"LIVER TOLERANCE IS A CONSEQUENCE OF LIVER ANATOMY"

The unusual immunological properties of the liver may reflect the arrangement of its dual blood supply, sinusoidal structure, slow blood flow, incomplete fenestrated endothelium, and dense resident macrophage (Kupffer cell) bed, as well as its unique populations of lymphocytes. This structure (reviewed in Chapter 1) means that circulating T cells that traverse the intestinal vasculature and the portal vein enter a sinusoidal space in which they are presented with the opportunity to interact with abundant intensely phagocytic, potentially antigen-presenting macrophages without the need for them to traverse endothelial walls. Thus, both L-selectin high naive T cells (which would normally encounter APCs only in lymphoid tissue) and L-selectin low activated cells (which elsewhere traverse tissues) directly encounter the Kupffer cells. There has been little analysis of the antigen-presenting function of Kupffer cells, but the evidence available suggests that they are indifferent APCs (40). A unique aspect of the T cell–Kupffer cell interaction appears to be a circuit in which the Kupffer cell elaborates IL-18, causing the T cell to make IFNγ and IL-6, which in turn causes the Kupffer cell to make inducible Nitric oxide synthetase (iNOS) (31). NO release from the Kupffer cell could then result in immunosuppression.

The sinusoidal endothelium is unusual in its expression of ICAM-1 as well as ICAM-2 (reviewed in Chapter 1). Thus, slowly passing activated T cells that express high-avidity Lymphocyte Function-Associated antigen-1 (LFA-1) molecules on the membrane may be immobilized by direct adhesion to the endothelial cells. Whether this results in apoptosis, facilitated encounter with other cell populations (such as Kupffer cells or resident NK-T cells), or passage through into the space of Disse and thus to the lymphatic system is not known.

The incompleteness of the sinusoidal endothelium means that T cells traversing the sinusoids may make direct contact with hepatocytes. These cells express receptors for the uptake of molecules from the blood, including the asialoglycoprotein receptor (41), which also appears to have a role in the clearance of damaged hepatocytes (42), and these receptors may interact with the distinctive membrane glycosylation patterns of activated T cells, resulting in their immobilization. The antigen-presenting functions of hepatocytes are not fully understood. They express a low level of MHC class I molecules, which could result in the partial activation leading to inactivation of $CD8^+$ T cells due to low ligand density. Intriguingly, the hepatocyte is one of the cell types that constitutively express CD95 (Fas) (43,44) making these cells vulnerable to damage induced by CD95L (FasL) expressed on the membrane of activated T cells. A recent line of discussion in immunobiology is the possible function of CD95L, as well as CD95, as a signaling molecule. The potential for unique signals delivered by CD95-expressing hepatocytes to CD95L-expressing T cells further complicates the two-way signaling between intrahepatic T cells and the sinusoids within which they reside.

EPILOGUE

The contributions in this book make it absolutely clear that the liver is a distinctive immunological environment, in which the strong possibility of extrathymic T cell development coexists with a tolerogenic environment in which T cell suppression, immune deviation, and clonal deletion may all play a part. Antigens that are present in the liver are processed and presented in a poorly understood manner, leading to local and often systemic T cell tolerance. Trying to understand this situation, we are confronted with multiple overlapping mechanisms that may explain these effects.

Unraveling these mechanisms is not purely an academic exercise. The liver is the site of several chronic infections of global importance, including hepatitis B and malaria, in which immune defenses appear to be inadequate. If we understand the cellular and molecular basis of liver tolerance, we may be able to intervene to tip the balance of these pathological relationships in favor of the host. Liver is also a frequent site for the metastasis of many cancers, a phenomenon which may be attributable to adhesion molecules or nutritional requirements, but could also be due to local immunological tolerance towards antigenic tumors. The prevalence of food allergy in the developed world suggests that physiologically useful oral tolerance, which may involve antigen presentation in the liver, can break down with disastrous consequences. Finally, therapeutic efforts to induce specific tolerance to autoantigens, and to histocompatibility antigens in the context of tissue transplantation, would benefit from more precise knowledge of how to make the tolerogenic environment of the liver work for us.

REFERENCES

1. Ohteki, T., Okuyama, R., Seki, S., Abo, T., Sugiura, K., Kusumi, A., Ohmori, T., Watanabe, H., and Kumagai, K. 1992. Age-dependent increase of extrathymic T cells in the liver and their appearance in the periphery of older mice. *J. Immunol.* 149:1562–1570.
2. Hai, T. Watanabe, H., Seki, S., Sigura, K., Hirokawa, K., Utsuyama, M., Takahashi-Iwanaga, H., Iwanaga, T., Ohteki, T., and Abo, T. 1992. Ontogeny and development of extrathymic T cells in mouse liver. *Immunology* 77:556–563.
3. Guy-grand, D., Vanden Broecke, C., Briottet, C., Malassis-Seris, M., Selz, F., and Vassalli, P. 1992. Differential expression of the recombination activity gene RAG-1 in various populations of thymocytes, peripheral T cells and gut thymus-independent intraepithelial lymphocytes suggests two pathways of T cell receptor gene rearrangement. *Eur. J. Immunol.* 22:505–510.

4. Poussier, P., Edouard, P., Lee, C., Binnie, M., and Julius, M. 1992. Thymus-independent development and negative selection of T cells expressing T cell receptor alpha/beta in the intestinal epithelium: Evidence for distinct circulation patterns of gut- and thymus-derived T lymphocytes. *J. Exp. Med.* 176:187–199.
5. Guidos, C.J., Williams, C., Wu, G.E., Paige, C.J., and Danska, J.S. 1995. Development of CD4+CD8+ thymocytes in RAG-deficient mice through a T cell receptor beta chain-independent pathway. *J. Exp. Med.* 181:1187–1195.
6. Lefrancois, L., and Puddington, L. 1995. Extrathymic intestinal T-cell development: Virtual reality? *Immunol. Today* 16:16–21.
7. Collins, C., Norris, S., McEntee, G., Traynor, O., Bruno, L., von Boehmer, H., Hegarty, J., and O'Farrell, C. 1996. RAG1, RAG2 and pre T cell receptor alpha chain expression by adult hepatic T cells: Evidence for extrathymic T cell maturation. *Eur. J. Immunol.* 26:3114–3118.
8. Sato, K., Ohtsuka, K., Hasegawa, K., Yamagiwa, S., Watanabe, H., Asakura, H., and Abo, T. 1995. Evidence for extrathymic generation of intermediate T cell receptor cells in the liver revealed in thymectomized, irradiated mice subjected to bone marrow transplantation. *J. Exp. Med.* 182:759–767.
9. Poussier, P., Edouard, P., Lee, C., Binnie, M., and Julius, M. 1992. Thymus-independent development and negative selection of T cells expressing T cell receptor alpha-beta in the intestinal epithelium: Evidence for distinct circulation patterns of gut and thymus-derived T lymphocytes. *J. Exp. Med.* 176:187–199.
10. Sykes, M. 1990. Unusual T cell populations in adult murine bone marrow. Prevalence of CD3+CD4-CD8- and alpha beta TCR+NK1.1+ cells. *J. Immunol.* 145:3209–3215.
11. Bellgrau, D., Gold, D., Selawry, H., Moore, J., Franzusoft, A., and Duke, R.C. 1995. A role for CD95 ligand in preventing graft rejection. *Nature* 377:630–632.
12. Goss, J.A., Flye, M.W., and Lacy, P.E. 1996. Induction of allogeneic islet survival by intrahepatic islet pre-immunization and transient immunosuppression. *Diabetes* 45:144–147.
13. Callery, M., Kamei, T., and Flye, M. 1989. Kupffer cell blockade inhibits induction of tolerance by the portal vein route. *Transplantation* 47:1092–1094.
14. Squiers, E., Salomon, D., Pickard, L., Howard, R., and Pfaff, W. 1990. Abrogation of the induction of portal venous tolerance in cardiac transplant model resulting from Kupffer cell inhibition by gadolinium. *Transplantation* 50:171–173.
15. Sato, K., Yabuki, K., Haba, T., and Maekawa, T. 1996. Role of Kupffer cells in the induction of tolerance after liver transplantation. *J. Surg. Res.* 63:433–438.
16. Koyamada, N., Ohteki, T., Abo, T., Fukimori, T., Ohkouchi, N., Satomi, S., Taguchi, Y., Kusumi, A., Mori, S., and Kumagai, K. 1993. Induction of specific tolerance by hepatic double negative CD4-8- alpha-beta T cells of mice immunized with allogeneic cells via the portal vein. *Cell. Immunol.* 149:107–116.
17. Gorczynski, R.M. 1994. Adoptive transfer of unresponsiveness to allogeneic skin grafts with hepatic gamma delta T cells. *Immunology* 81:27–35.
18. Gorczynski, R.M., Cohen, Z., Leung, Y., and Chen, Z. 1996. Gamma-delta TcR+ hybridomas derived from mice preimmunized via the portal vein adoptively transfer increased skin allograft survival in vivo. *J. Immunol.* 157:574–581.
19. Mosmann, T., and Coffman, R.L. 1989. Th1 and Th2 cells: Different patterns of lymphokine secretion lead to different functional properties. *Annu. Rev. Immunol.* 7:145–173.
20. Abbas, A.K., Murphy, K.M., and Sher, A. 1996. Functional diversity of helper T lymphocytes. *Nature* 383:787–793.

21. Streilein, J.W., Takeuchi, M., and Taylor, A.W. 1997. Immune privilege, T cell tolerance and tissue-restricted autoimmunity. *Hum. Immunol.* 52:138–143.

22. MacDonald, H.R. 1995. NK1.1+ T cell receptor alpha-beta cells: New clues to their origin, specificity and function. *J. Exp. Med.* 182:633–638.

23. Tsutsui, H., Nakanishi, K., Matsui, K., Higashino, K., Okamura, H., Miyazawa, Y., and Kaneda, K. 1996. IFN-gamma-inducing factor up-regulates Fas ligand-mediated cytotoxic activity of murine natural killer cell clones. *J. Immunol.* 157:3967–3973.

24. Gu, Y., Kuida, K., Tsutsui, H., Ku, G., Hsiao, K., Fleming, M.A., Hayashi, N., Higashino K., Okamura, H., Nakanishi, K., Kurimoto, M., Tanumoto, T., Flavell, R.A., Sato, V., Harding, M.W., Livingston, D.J., and Su, M.S. 1997. Activation of interferon gamma inducing factor mediated by interleukin-1 beta converting enzyme. *Science* 275:206–209.

25. Robinson, D., Shibuya, K., Mui, A., Zonin, F., Menon, S., Sava, T., Hartley, S.B., Kastelein, R., Bazan, F., and O'Garra, A. 1997. IGIF does not drive Th1 development but synergizes with IL-12 for interferon-gamma production and activates IRAK and NF-kappaB. *Immunity* 7:571–581.

26. Huang, L., Soldevila, G., Leeker, M., Flavell, R.A., and Crispe, I.N. 1994. Liver is the site of T cell destruction during peripheral deletion. *Immunity* 1:741–749.

27. Wack, A., Dellaporta, P., Crispe, I.N., and Kioussis, D. 1997. Multiple sites of post-activation CD8+ T cell disposal. *Eur. J. Immunol.* 27:577–583.

28. Winnock, M., Garcia Barcina, M., Lukomska, B., Huet, S., Saric, J., Balabaud, C., and Bioulac-Sage, P. 1995. Human liver-associated lymphocytes: An overview. *J. Gastroenterol. Hepatol.* 10:S43–S46.

29. Perillo, N.L., Pace, K.E., Seilhamer, J.J., and Baum, L.G. 1996. Apoptosis of T cells mediated by galectin-1. *Nature* 378:736–739.

30. Lotan, R., Belloni, P.N., Tressler, R.J., Lotan, D., Xu, X.C., and Nicholson, G.L. 1994. Expression of galectins on microvessel endothelial cells and their involvement in tumour cell adhesion. *Glycoconj. J.* 11:462–468.

31. Roland, C.R., Walp, L., Stack, R.M., and Flye, M.W. 1994. Outcome of Kupffer cell antigen presentation to a cloned murine Th1 lymphocyte depends on the inducibility of nitric oxide synthase by IFN-gamma. *J. Immunol.* 153:5453–5464.

32. Golan, D.T., and Kursbaum, A. 1976. Anti-heart autoantibodies in ischemic heart disease patients. *Clin. Exp. Immunol.* 26:86–90.

33. Kay, M.M., Sorenson, K., Wong, P., and Bolton, P. 1982. Antigenicity, storage and ageing: Physiologic autoantibodies to cell membranes and serum proteins and the senescent cell antigen. *Mol. Cell. Biochem.* 49:65–85.

34. Avrameas, S. 1991. Natural antibodies: From "horror autotoxicus" to "gnothi seauton." *Immunol. Today* 12:154–159.

35. Tiegs, G., Hentschel, J., and Wendel, A. 1992. A T cell-dependent experimental liver injury in mice inducible by concanavalin A. *J. Clin. Invest.* 90:196–203.

36. Gantner, F., Leist, M., Lohse, A.W., Germann, P.G., and Tiegs, G. 1995. Concanavalin-A induced T cell mediated hepatic injury in mice: The role of tumor necrosis factor. *Hepatology* 21:190–198.

37. Matsumura, M., Fremont, D.H., Peterson, P.A., and Wilson, I.A. 1992. Emerging principles for the recognition of peptide antigens by MHC class I molecules. *Science* 257:927–934.

38. Peterson, W.L. 1991. Helicobacter pylori and peptic ulcer disease. *N. Engl. J. Med.* 324:1043–1048.

39. Cover, T.L., and Blaser, M.J. 1992. Heliobacter pylori and gastroduodenal disease. *Annu. Rev. Med.* 43:145–153.

40. Rubenstein, D., Roska, A.K., and Lipsky, P.E. 1986. Liver lining sinusoidal cells express class II major histocompatibility antigens but a poor stimulators of fresh allogeneic T lymphocytes. *J. Immunol.* 137:1803–1810.

41. Huseby, N.E., Mortensen, B., and Smedsrod, B. 1993. Clearance of circulating gamma-glutamyltransferase by the hepatic galactose receptor. Variability in clearance rate due to carbohydrate heterogeneity of the enzyme. *Biochem. Biophys. Acta* 1156:283–287.

42. Dini, L., Autuori, F., Lentini, A., Oliverio, S., and Piacentini, M. 1992. The clearance of apoptopic cells in the liver is mediated by the asialoglycoprotein receptor. *FEBS Lett.* 292:174–178.

43. Ogasawara, J., Watanabe-Fukunaga, R., Adachi, M., Matsuzawa, A., Kasugai, T., Kitamura, Y., Itoh, N., Suda, T., and Nagata, S. 1993. Lethal effects of the anti-Fas antibody in mice. *Nature* 346:806–809.

44. Ni, R., Tomita, Y., Matsuda, K., Ichihara, A., Ishimura, K., Ogasawara, J., and Nagata, S. 1994. Fas-mediated apoptosis in primary cultured mouse hepatocytes. *Exp. Cell. Res.* 215:332–337.

INDEX